Stuttering and Related Disorders of Fluency

Other Volumes in the Series

General Principles of Therapy

Dysarthria and Apraxia

Language Handicaps in Adults

Voice Disorders

Phonologic-Articulatory Disorders

Hearing Disorders

Language Handicaps in Children

Stuttering Disorders

Aphasia and Related Neurogenic Language Disorders

CURRENT THERAPY OF COMMUNICATION DISORDERS

Series Editor
William H. Perkins, Ph.D.

Stuttering and Related Disorders of Fluency

Richard F. Curlee, Ph.D.

Professor
Department of Speech and Hearing Sciences
The University of Arizona
Tucson, Arizona

1993
THIEME MEDICAL PUBLISHERS, INC.   **New York**
GEORG THIEME VERLAG   **Stuttgart · New York**

Thieme Medical Publishers, Inc.
381 Park Avenue South
New York, New York 10016

STUTTERING AND RELATED DISORDERS OF FLUENCY
Richard F. Curlee

Library of Congress Cataloging-in-Publication Data

Stuttering and related disorders of fluency / [edited by] Richard F.
  Curlee.
       p.   cm.—(Current therapy of communication disorders)
    Includes bibliographical references and index.
    ISBN 0-86577-442-0 (Thieme Medical Publishers).—ISBN
  3-13-783401-5 (G. Thieme Verlag)
    1. Stuttering.   I. Curlee, Richard F. (Richard Frederick, 1935–
  II. Series.
    [DNLM: 1. Stuttering—therapy.   WM 475 S9372]
  RC424.S768   1993
  616.85'54—dc20
  DNLM/DLC
  for Library of Congress   92-49795
                                                              CIP

Important note: Medicine is an ever-changing science. Research and clinical experience are continually broadening our knowledge, in particular our knowledge of proper treatment and drug therapy. Insofar as this book mentions any dosage or applications, readers may rest assured that the authors, editors, and publishers have made every effort to ensure that such references are strictly in accordance with the state of knowledge at the time of production of the book. Nevertheless, every user is requested to carefully examine the manufacturers' leaflets accompanying each drug to check on his own responsibility whether the dosage schedules recommended therein or the contraindications stated by the manufacturers differ from the statements made in the present book. Such examination is particularly important with drugs that are either rarely used or have been newly released on the market.

Some of the product names, patents, and registered designs referred to in this book are in fact registered trademarks or proprietary names even though specific reference to this fact is not always made in the text. Therefore, the appearance of a name without designation as proprietary is not to be construed as a representation by the publisher that it is in the public domain.

Printed in the United States of America.

5   4   3   2   1

TMP ISBN 0-86577-442-0
GTV ISBN 3-13-783401-5

Contents

Contributors vii

Foreword *William H. Perkins, Ph.D.* ix

Preface xi

1. Identification and Management of Beginning Stuttering   1
    Richard F. Curlee, Ph.D.

2. Differential Evaluation–Differential Therapy for Stuttering
    Children 23
    Hugo H. Gregory, Ph.D., and Diane Hill, M.A.

3. Treating School-Age Stutterers 45
    Carl W. Dell, Jr., Ph.D.

4. Behavioral Treatment of Stuttering Children 68
    Janis Costello Ingham, Ph.D.

5. Therapy for School-Age Stutterers: An Update on the Fluency
    Rules Program 101
    Charles M. Runyan, Ph.D., and Sara Elizabeth Runyan, M.A.

6. Management of Stuttering: Treatment of Adolescents and
    Adults 115
    David Prins, Ph.D.

7. Intensive Fluency Training of Chronic Stutterers 139
    Megan Neilson, Ph.D., and Gavin Andrews, M.D.

8. Transfer and Maintenance of Treatment Gains of Chronic
    Stutterers 166
    Roger J. Ingham, Ph.D.

9. **Cluttering: Another Fluency Syndrome** 179
    David A. Daly, Ed.D.

10. **Stuttering Associated with Acquired Neurological Disorders** 205
     Nancy Helm-Estabrooks, Sc.D.

     Index 220

Contributors

Gavin Andrews, M.D.
Clinical Research Center for Anxiety
  Disorders
University of New South Wales at St.
  Vincent's Hospital
Darlinghurst, New South Wales
Australia

Richard F. Curlee, Ph.D.
Department of Speech and Hearing
  Sciences
The University of Arizona
Tucson, Arizona

David A. Daly, Ed.D.
School of Education
University of Michigan
Ann Arbor, Michigan

Carl W. Dell, Jr., Ph.D.
Department of Speech Pathology and
  Audiology
Eastern Illinois University
Charleston, Illinois

Hugo H. Gregory, Ph.D.
Stuttering Programs
Department of Communication
  Sciences and Disorders
Northwestern University
Evanston, Illinois

Nancy Helm-Estabrooks, Sc.D.
Aphasia Research Center
Boston V.A. Medical Center
Boston, Massachusetts

Diane Hill, M.A.
Department of Communication
  Sciences and Disorders
Northwestern University
Evanston, Illinois

Janis Costello Ingham, Ph.D.
Department of Speech and Hearing
  Sciences
University of California, Santa
  Barbara
Santa Barbara, California

Roger J. Ingham, Ph.D.
Department of Speech and Hearing
  Sciences
University of California, Santa
  Barbara
Santa Barbara, California

Megan Neilson, Ph.D.
Clinical Research Center for Anxiety
  Disorders
University of New South Wales at St.
  Vincent's Hospital
Darlinghurst, New South Wales
Australia

William H. Perkins, Ph.D.
Department of Communications and
  Arts and Sciences
University of Southern California
Los Angeles, California

David Prins, Ph.D.
Department of Speech and Hearing
    Sciences
University of Washington
Seattle, Washington

Charles M. Runyan, Ph.D.
Department of Speech Pathology and
    Audiology
James Madison University
Harrisonburg, Virginia

Sara Elizabeth Runyan, M.A.
Department of Speech Pathology and
    Audiology
James Madison University
Harrisonburg, Virginia

Foreword

This second volume on stuttering in the *Current Therapy* series is a splendid account of the mainstream treatment ideas and procedures in the waning years of the 20th century. All of these therapies have merit, yet none are offered as a panacea. Bear in mind, too, that this volume presents stuttering as seen primarily through the eyes of American speech pathologists, who have done more with this problem than any other professional group. The views elsewhere in the world are sometimes different.

Moreover, psychiatrists and clinical psychologists have vested interests in stuttering as well, and have therapies which differ from those presented here. Then, of course, those who do the stuttering have their views, too, as to the nature of the problem and what can best be done about it. Those views, as expressed through their self-help group literature, are also different.

Stuttering is, indeed, a perplexing problem. One of its peculiarities is that no procedure seems to benefit everyone, yet most procedures seem to help someone. In fact, some evidence suggests that fluency improvement, avoidance reduction, and self-help groups are approximately equal in client satisfaction. Perhaps this is because people seek the program with the most potential satisfaction for them, and steer clear of those they do not like.

As you will see from these chapters, stuttering is almost as much an enigma now as it ever was. Why this is so is in itself a puzzle. Is stuttering so complex that it defies scientific solution? Or have we not yet found the right direction and asked the right questions? Certainly, some fundamental issues concerning therapy remain unanswered. For instance, the recovery prospect of up to 80% of children who start to stutter is intriguing when compared to the therapy success with 8 out of 10 children. One must wonder how much of this success would have occurred without therapy. Yet, lacking clear criteria for determining who will recover and who will not, wisdom dictates initiating therapy as soon after onset as possible.

It is similar with adults for whom stuttering has become a way of life. Why are they so resistant to recovery while children are so prone to it? Many who undertake therapy for chronic stuttering will eventually relapse for unknown reasons. Equally obscure is why therapy sometimes, perhaps often, results in relatively permanent improvement. Even more troubling is the prospect that achievement of fluency by therapeutic intervention can be used as a clinically sanctioned avoidance device. We have no evidence that this does happen, but more important, we have no evidence that it does not.

Therapy of stuttering is a challenging business. It is fraught with pitfalls, glorious opportunities, and great satisfactions. Some excellent tools for meeting this challenge are offered in this volume. If used with care, concern, and sensitivity, they can unlock doors for clients and also intellectually curious clinicians.

William H. Perkins, Ph.D.

Preface

The Egyptian hieroglyphic symbol (Fig. 1) below is said to represent stuttering. If so, it is one of the earliest references to an impairment of human communication and indicates that stuttering has been disrupting the communication efforts of speakers for as long as the histories of human civilization have been recorded, and most likely longer. The earliest references to the treatment of stuttering are attributed to the Greek historian, Herodotus, writing some 2400 years ago. Since that time an extraordinary variety of medical, surgical, psychological, and behavioral treatment practices have been employed. This volume selectively samples from the variety of contemporary clinical management procedures used with children and adults who stutter or have a related fluency disorder.

Of the ten chapters that follow, five focus on the evaluation and treatment of children who stutter. This emphasis reflects my belief that treating children who stutter is the most effective way to manage this problem. Such treatment typically results in better, longer-lasting results than those achieved with adults, and

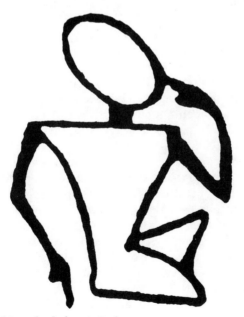

Figure 1. Egyptian hieroglyph for stuttering.

complete remissions of stuttering, or "cures", are not uncommon among children who stutter. In contrast, complete, permanent remissions of the chronic stuttering problems of adults are so sufficiently infrequent that their occurrence may legitimately be viewed as bordering on the miraculous. Nevertheless, most adults who stutter can be helped so that routine everyday communication is not a significant problem for them much of the time. Therefore, three chapters address the challenges of effecting clinically significant, durable changes in the persistent stuttering problems of adolescents and adults. The remaining two chapters in this volume describe the evaluation and management of clients who present a number of the same signs and symptoms that characterize idiopathic, or developmental, stuttering but whose problems differ sufficiently to warrant coverage in separate chapters.

In the initial chapter, I have described the procedures that I use when evaluating young children who may be beginning to stutter. The symptoms and signs that are elicited during case history interviews and observed during clinical evaluations are discussed, and guidelines for choosing among several clinical management alternatives are suggested. Finally, I describe several parent intervention strategies that are intended to modify the child's environment, thereby preventing the development of a chronic stuttering problem.

Chapter 2, by Hugo Gregory and Diane Hill, details a differential evaluation process that results in the selection of one of three treatment strategies for stuttering children and their parents. The approach described can be employed with both preschool and school-age children and involves a skillful blend of both counseling and therapy techniques. Some focus on parents' and children's reactions to disfluent speech; others, on specific techniques that are intended to assist a young child learn how to speak more fluently. Together, they comprise an eclectic integration of both fluency and stuttering management treatment strategies.

In Chapter 3, Carl Dell presents a philosophy of managing stuttering and describes how this philosophy guides his therapy with children who stutter during their early elementary school years. It is a clinical management philosophy for stuttering that has stood the test of time since its beginnings a number of years ago in the work and writings of Charles Van Riper. This chapter focuses on how clinicians can go about "removing the mystery of stuttering" for both stuttering children and their parents and contains a wealth of ideas and suggestions for working with a child this age.

The philosophy that guides the treatment program described by Janis Ingham in Chapter 4 rests on the premise that diagnostic and treatment decisions should rely primarily on observations of stuttering children's speaking behavior. The therapy techniques she recommends were derived from principles of behavioral management that have been supported by laboratory and field experiments. An appendix details the procedures she uses to systematically increase the length and complexity of a stuttering child's utterances from highly structured, short responses to self-generated, spontaneous conversations in naturalistic contexts.

Chapter 5, by Chuck and Sara Runyan, concludes this initial section of chapters on managing childhood stuttering with an update of their fluency rules program for school-age children who stutter. These rules, which employ meaningful vocabulary for school-age children, can be conceptualized as descriptions of speaking behaviors that are incompatible with stuttering. The Runyans describe how school-age children can learn to use such speaking behaviors on a treatment schedule that is compatible with the caseload and time constraints of most elementary school systems.

The treatment procedures advocated by David Prins in Chapter 6 are derived, in part, from social learning and self-efficacy theories. From this perspective, many of the problems of adolescents and adults who stutter stem from their reactions to their own speech disruptions that have become, over the years, an integral part of their speech production process. He believes that these reactions of chronic stutterers must be modified if therapy is to be successful and describes a thoughtful strategy that focuses therapy procedures on the management of stuttering.

Chapter 7 details the intensive fluency training procedures employed by Meg Neilson and Gavin Andrews in Sydney, Australia. These procedures are aimed at modifying the speech production process in ways that are believed to be incompatible with the act of stuttering, and then generalizing this newly acquired way of speaking to everyday communication activities on a permanent basis. This 3-week program is responsible for gathering much of the empirical information that has been published on the effectiveness of intensive fluency-training treatment programs, and the data collected provide impressive support of its efficacy.

Most adolescents and adults who stutter, as well as some children, have considerable difficulty transferring treatment gains they achieve in the clinic to many everyday speaking situations. Moreover, some relapse of treatment gains over time is also commonly reported. In Chapter 8, Roger Ingham critically examines some of the thorny methodological problems involved and describes a performance-contingent transfer and maintenance procedure that he has employed successfully with a wide age-range of clients who stutter. He also shares some misgivings about a number of other procedures that he has found to be relatively ineffective. As with most complex human problems, there do not appear to be any simple or easy answers.

In recent years, cluttering has begun receiving much greater attention from scientists and clinicians in this country. Until then, most of what was known and published about this syndrome came from the work of European physicians and speech specialists. Chapter 9, by David Daly, reviews the information available on cluttering, its nature, and possible causes. He concludes that cluttering is an independent fluency syndrome that frequently co-occurs with stuttering and relates some of his clinical experiences with children and adults who present this complex pattern of signs and symptoms. I suspect that many clinicians may begin seeing some of their stuttering clients from a new perspective after reading this chapter.

Like cluttering, the stutter-like disruptions of speech that occasionally accompany neurological lesions also have received substantially increased coverage in professional journals during the past decade or so. In Chapter 10, Nancy Helm-Estabrooks carefully examines the evidence that a variety of neurological disorders can produce speech disruptions that patients and clinicians alike view as "stuttering." She argues convincingly that such problems do not reflect a unitary disorder and describes a battery of observations and tests for evaluating such patients.

Finally, she reviews the variety of treatment procedures that have been employed with them and concludes that successful treatment outcomes depend largely on the skill with which clinicians implement a therapy plan that effectively addresses the strengths and deficits that uniquely characterize each specific patient.

Contributors were selected so that a broad range of current clinical management perspectives would be presented by clinicians whose research and clinical experience permit them to write with both understanding and authority on the topic that each was assigned. Each was asked to describe the procedures that he or she uses when evaluating and treating a child or an adult with the assigned fluency disorder and to do so in sufficient detail that these procedures could be adopted by clinicians interested in such problems. Each was also asked to summarize the likely treatment outcome of using these procedures. The result is a remarkable collection of the strategies and techniques currently employed with clients who stutter or present one of the other fluency disorders covered. In short, it is a storehouse of the clinical wisdom now available for managing such problems effectively.

Richard F. Curlee, Ph.D.

Identification and Management of Beginning Stuttering

Richard F. Curlee, Ph.D.

Introduction

Stuttering most often begins insidiously during the course of a child's otherwise normal speech and language development. It affects about 5% of the population, and incidence is highest during the preschool years.[1] For at least 20% of these children, stuttering will persist, often worsening, and if it continues past puberty, it is likely to become a life-long disability.[2] Significant educational, vocational and/or personal adjustment problems are common among those who continue to stutter as adults.[1] It is widely believed that identification and appropriate clinical intervention with young incipient stutterers comprise the most effective management strategy for preventing stuttering from becoming a chronic, long-term disability.[3–6]

If stuttering is severe or has been a chronic problem for some period of time, accurate diagnosis is seldom a problem. Most such children can be readily distinguished from nonstuttering children, even those who are also highly disfluent.[7,8] Nevertheless, the speech of many preschool-age children who are just beginning to stutter often sounds very much like that of other children their age much of the time.[9] Their stuttering is episodic and varies substantially in frequency and severity from day to day, or one situation to another. Few, if any, signs of stuttering may be observed during a clinical evaluation. Thus, identifying stuttering among these children can pose a significant diagnostic challenge for even experienced, expert clinicians.

In spite of such difficulties, there seems to be a consensus among many clinicians who have focused their clinical work and research on children who stutter that most young, incipient stutters can be reliably identified and effectively treated. In the last decade, a number of diagnostic approaches have been recommended for differentiating these children from their nonstuttering peers, some of whom may also be highly disfluent.[3,5,6,10] While there is substantial agreement across these diagnostic protocols, there is also considerable disagreement on some of the specific diagnostic signs that have been proposed. Moreover, even if clinicians agree that a child has begun to stutter, they may disagree on whether or not treatment should begin immediately, and if so, what kind of treatment would be most appropriate.

Such disagreement is not surprising. A variety of different treatments have apparently resulted in successful outcomes for many young children who stutter.[2,11] Nevertheless, many also stop stuttering without receiving any professional help.[1,2,12] It is my belief that clinical management of these children should rely heavily on the empirical information that is available on stuttering and its onset and remission. This kind of information is used to support the procedures that will be described for eliciting signs and symptoms of incipient stuttering during a case history interview and a subsequent clinical examination. Guidelines will also be proposed for making appropriate clinical management decisions for those children whose stuttering seems likely to persist unless effective professional intervention is initiated.

Clinical Evaluation

Diagnosis of beginning stuttering relies on observing patterns of signs and symptoms that distinguish those children who are at risk for becoming chronic stutters from their nonstuttering peers. Such patterns include both qualitative and quantitative differences in speech disruptions as well as a child's reactions to these disruptions. Unfortunately, there is no sign or symptom that unequivocally confirms or excludes this diagnosis, and the patterns of signs and symptoms that are observed are varied and can be inconclusive. Fortunately, all problems are repetitive by nature; therefore, ongoing follow-up observations of a child suspected of stuttering will be rewarded in time by the emergence of a pattern of signs and symptoms that either supports a diagnosis of beginning stuttering or permits the clinician to conclude that a child's nonfluencies do not signal the onset of such problems.

Most young, incipient stutterers are accurately identified by parents during the case history interview. Subsequent clinical observations of the child merely confirm what has already been learned from the parents. Nevertheless, it is not unusual for some children to evidence none of the speech disruptions, or struggle, or frustration that the parents have described. Even more important, the child may also evidence lags in speech-language acquisition that have been overlooked by the parents. In these instances, further observation and testing are needed before appropriate plans for clinical intervention can be made.

Medical diagnoses rely on the symptoms reported by patients, clinical signs observed by physicians, and a variety of objective test findings to identify the etiology of an abnormal medical condition or disorder. A diagnosis of incipient stuttering involves a differentiation of children who are beginning to stutter from their nonstuttering peers and a determination of the kind of clinical intervention, if any, that may be needed. Thus, this task requires clinicians to gather the information that is needed to arrive at one of the following diagnostic conclusions:

1. The child is evidencing few, if any, signs of beginning stuttering, and it is unlikely that he or she is developing such problems.

2. The child is evidencing inconsistent signs of beginning stuttering, and further observation and testing are needed.

3. The child is evidencing consistent signs of beginning stuttering, and an appropriate clinical management plan should be developed and initiated.

4. The child is already evidencing a number of signs of chronic stuttering, and remission is unlikely in the absence of direct professional intervention.

The evaluation procedures to be described should provide clinicians with the information needed to support one of these conclusions. First, a detailed case history is obtained from the parent(s). Next, the child is observed and tested. Finally, the results of the evaluation are summarized and interpreted for the parent(s) and appropriate clinical management options are discussed. It is my preference to obtain this information during a series of diagnostic sessions across several days so that there is sufficient time to analyze the information that has been obtained and prepare for subsequent meetings.

Case History Interview

Interviews with parents who suspect that their child may be beginning to stutter need to include a review of the child's overall development and acquisition of speech and language as well as a careful exploration of the parents' fluency concerns. Many children who stutter also evidence other speech or language-learning difficulties,[11,13] and in some cases, these difficulties will constitute a much more significant problem than does stuttering. Any concerns that arise during the interview about the child's development can be explored further by using one of several standardized questionnaire/interview instruments that screen a child's acquisition of communication skills.

The importance of information obtained from case history interviews can not be overemphasized. Parents have opportunities to observe their children at times and under circumstances that are not available to clinicians. Such observations of real-life situations also enjoy a validity that clinic observations do not. Thus, these interviews provide clinicians an opportunity to elicit recollections of key events and descriptions of symptoms that may be critical in making a diagnosis of incipient stuttering. The clinician can also learn what kinds of information or help the parents may need. Finally, if clinical management is needed, this interview initiates the beginning of a relationship between the clinician and parents that is likely to be highly significant to the child's ultimate clinical outcome.

It is my experience that descriptions of specific speech behaviors are seldom elicited during explorations of parents' concerns about their child's speech disruptions. It is unusual for parents to be able to describe their child's fluency difficulties in diagnostically useful terms (e.g., part-word repetitions or sound prolongations or tense pauses) initially. Most simply express concern about "his stuttering" and may seem somewhat perplexed or frustrated if asked to describe the child's "stuttering" in greater detail. Nevertheless, most can readily identify the kinds of disfluencies that are bothering them when simulated by a clinician. Some may even recall specific examples they have observed, which strengthens the credibility of their reports. Simulations of specific stuttering signs can be useful also in helping parents' recall how many units of repetition they commonly observe, their tempo, and whether or not increases in pitch or loudness accompany the child's speech disruptions. With patience, a clinician should be able to obtain descriptions of a child's speech from the parents which clearly suggest that the child is either beginning to stutter or that the parents are reacting to essentially normal, age-appropriate nonfluencies. It is my experience that parental misdiagnoses of stuttering seldom occur. I can recall only a handful of such cases after over 20 years of clinical practice.

The signs and symptoms that I have found useful for identifying beginning stuttering and for determining when to initiate treatment are organized below as two groups of questions. Answers to the first group of questions help distinguish beginning stuttering from the nonfluencies of nonstuttering children. The second group of questions help differentiate beginning stutterers from confirmed, chronic stutterers. Even though a child may have begun to stutter, direct professional intervention may not be necessary, but once chronic stuttering patterns are established, remission is unlikely, and direct professional intervention should begin as soon as possible. A brief discussion of the rationale and selected supporting references accompany each question.

INDICATORS OF BEGINNING STUTTERING

1. What kinds of speech disruptions are eliciting parental concern?   There is extensive overlap in the types of speech disruptions that have been observed in groups of both stuttering and nonstuttering children.[11,14,15] Among those who are beginning to stutter, however, within-word (sound/syllable) repetitions and occasional sound prolongations, especially those that are longer than 1 second, occur much more frequently than among nonstuttering peers.[3,15–18] Within-word repetitions can be evenly paced and stressed, but if more than two units of repeats per repetition are frequently observed, the child is likely stuttering.[15] In contrast, if the parents are concerned primarily about revisions, interjections, or repetitions of multisyllable words and phrases, the types of speech disruptions that appear to reflect linguistic encoding processes,[19] it is unlikely that the child is beginning to stutter.

2. Have the child's speech disruptions changed since the parents first became concerned? Beginning stuttering is episodic, with the frequency and severity of a child's speech disruptions varying from one day to another, and situation to situation, and several days may pass on occasion with no problems being observed by the parents.[2,11,20] It is important to inquire if stuttering seems to be limited to only a few situations, such as display talking at home or talking to the teacher at preschool, or if it has been observed during many of the child's conversational interactions.[3,5,10] As stuttering persists, within-word speech disruptions typically occur less episodically and more consistently from one situation to another, and extended periods of fluent speech occur less often. A child whose stuttering initially consisted only of effortless repetitions may now be prolonging sounds much of the time.[4] In general, as within-word speech disruptions become more frequent and consistent and occur in clusters more often, a child is increasingly evidencing the signs of chronic stuttering.[21]

3. How long have the parents been concerned about the child's fluency?   Remission of stuttering can occur at any age,[18,22] but around half of these remissions occur within the first year of the onset of stuttering.[1] In addition, remissions seem to occur more often among mild than among severe stutterers.[12,22] Thus, if stuttering persists beyond a year and if increases in the frequency or severity of stuttering have occurred, the likelihood of remission probably has decreased, and the need to initiate some form of clinical intervention should be carefully re-evaluated.

4. How valid do the parents' concerns about stuttering appear to be?   When parents are able to describe their child's speech disruptions in detail and to document its patterns of occurrence with specific examples that are commonly reported when children are beginning to stutter, it is highly unlikely that their fears are ill-founded. Such details ordinarily reflect careful, purposeful observations and lend credibility to their concerns that the child may be beginning to stutter. In addition, many parents also report that the child's fluency difficulties have been noticed and commented on by friends or relatives. Such adverse reactions to a child's speech by different observers usually indicate that the child's speech is deviant and that a speech problem exists.

INDICATORS OF CHRONIC STUTTERING

1. Do the child's speech disruptions consist predominantly of sound prolongations, tense pauses, and within-word repetitions that are accompanied by noticeable tension?   Most often stuttering begins insidiously so that the disfluencies of young beginning stutterers can be quite similar to those of their nonstuttering peers much of the time[14]; however, some children evidence many of the characteristics of chronic stutterers from the beginning.[10,20,23] Indeed, systematic observations of a group of preschool stutterers soon after onset found all of the types of speech disruptions noted above,[15] and in a subsequent study, Yairi and Ambrose[23] classified more than a third of their large group of preschoolers as having abrupt onsets of stuttering. Regardless, if a child's disfluencies persist and become increasingly characterized by noticeable effort and tension and by interruptions or cessation of articulator movement, airflow, and phonation, the risk that chronic stuttering problems will continue, perhaps for life, has increased.[2,3,5] As was noted earlier, eliciting this kind of descriptive information about the child's speech disruptions from parents can be facilitated if the clinician simulates such difficulties for them.

2. Has the child evidenced negative emotional reactions or expressed concern about speech disruptions or about speaking in general?   It is not unusual for parents of young beginning stutterers to comment that their child seems to be unaware of his or her speech disruptions and that they have observed no signs of the child's concern. As stuttering persists and the child becomes older and encounters the reactions of other children to the stuttering, a number of emotional and cognitive reactions are likely to emerge.[3,11] Early reactions of young children to stuttering include frequent blinking and breaking of eye contact during speech disruptions.[4,24] Some beginning stutterers may evidence occasional frustration, especially on those occasions when their speech disruptions are especially frequent or severe.[10] Such emotional reactions ordinarily precede any admissions by a child that he or she is having difficulty with speech (e.g., "Mommy, I can't talk right" or "Daddy, I can't say that word") or indications that he or she is attempting to avoid talking or saying specific words, all of which are commonly observed among adult stutterers. If observed in a child, these are clearly signs of chronic stuttering.[10]

A thorough case history interview with the parents should provide clinicians with a clear impression of the kinds of fluency difficulties that are likely to be observed when the child is evaluated. At the conclusion of the case history interview, the clinician should summarize these impressions for the parents and address any questions or concerns that they may have. It is not unusual for parents to feel that something they did, or did not do, may have caused the problem or made it worse. I like to assure parents that we will never know why their child began having fluency difficulties and that their guilty feelings are understandable but are likely the result of an overactive sense of parental responsibility. I then note that rather than worrying about what might have initiated the child's stuttering, we need to focus on what can be done to promote its remission.

This is also a good time to review with the parents the plans for observing and testing the child and to provide them with information on stuttering that has been prepared specifically for parents[25,26] and which they can read at home. In addition, if the child's speech disruptions have been characterized as highly episodic, it may be a good idea to see if the parents can bring a recording from home of the kinds of speech disruptions that are causing them concern. Finally, if there is reason to suspect that other speech-language difficulties may be present, there is ample time to develop a diagnostic plan that will screen other speech-language skills as well as permit observations of the child's fluency difficulties across a variety of speaking tasks of varying complexity and difficulty.

Clinical Observations and Tests

An evaluation of a child who is suspected of stuttering should include observations of the child conversing with both parents and clinician while performing speaking tasks that vary in structure, complexity, and communicative stress. Recordings of the evaluation, videotape if possible, are needed for subsequent fluency and language analyses. Videotapes may also be helpful later when discussing some of the child's specific problem behaviors with the parents and for helping them to become more aware of communication interaction patterns that need to be changed. A "typical" diagnostic plan might include the following:

- The child and parents are observed and recorded while interacting with one another in unstructured play. This provides a sample of the child's speech with familiar people under unstressful circumstances and permits observation of parent-child interaction patterns.

- The clinician joins the child and parents, and after a few minutes, asks the parents to wait in another room while the evaluation proceeds. Subsequent discussions of diagnostic findings with the parents can be significantly facilitated if they are able to observe the remainder of the evaluation from the adjoining room.

- Formal speech-language screening tests are usually administered early in a diagnostic session. Administration may be modified to accommodate a child's stuttering. For example, those language tests that use repetitions of words, phrases, or sentences can be used to see if changes in stuttering occur with changes in the length and complexity of responses if utterances are modeled at slower rates. Such test findings can also supplement observations of the child's language development obtained from analyses of a language sample. Similarly, tasks for obtaining speech samples for phonological or articulatory analyses can use auditory models to elicit responses if stuttering frequently occurs when pictures are used for elicitation.

- Observations of the child's fluency while talking during unstructured play can be compared with those recorded earlier with the parents and can also be used for any language analyses that may be indicated. If the child is stuttering frequently, clinicians can attempt to determine if modifying the speaking task or the child's manner of speaking reduces its frequency. For example, those tasks that require short, descriptive, concrete responses often elicit less stuttering than longer, less-representative, informational narratives. Similarly, speaking in unison with the clinician, rhythmic recitations, whispering, or speaking slowly or with exaggerated inflections often results in reduced stuttering. If a child seldom stutters or has yet to stutter during the evaluation, the clinician can also see if stuttering increases when the child is asked to describe some past activity or future plan or how to find his or her house, by bombarding the child with rapidly spoken questions, by interrupting or challenging or disagreeing with him or her, or by using any other tactic that increases the difficulty or communicative stress of the task.

- The clinical examination should also include routine screening examinations of hearing and of the peripheral speech mechanism, including performance on diadochokinetic tasks.

A major goal of this portion of the diagnostic evaluation is observation of the kinds of speech disruptions that have been reported by the parents. Occasionally, a clinician may be uncertain that a child is evidencing the kinds of fluency difficulties that have been reported. At such times it can be helpful to review a video recording of the session with the parents to see if the child's speech has been atypically fluent or dysfluent during the evaluation. In contrast, if the concerns of the parents are confirmed through observations of the child's speech, the focus of the evaluation shifts from that of problem identification to assessment of the variability of the problem and its severity. Consequently, it is important to obtain samples of the child talking with different partners and while engaged in different speaking tasks. Five- and 10-minute speech samples are commonly recommended for such purposes.[27] At a minimum, I try to obtain recordings that contain at least 3 minutes of the child talking, for quantifying each of the speaking tasks and situations sampled. To evaluate the consistency of a child's disfluencies across different settings, recordings with different conversation partners, both outside and within the clinic, are needed.[27] I count each word or syllable as either stuttered or not stuttered, counting each only once regardless of how long or how many types of disruptions are involved. Then I count the number of words or syllables in the sample. Each count is repeated, and if they agree, that number is used to calculate the percent words or syllables stuttered (i.e., %WS/%SS). If the counts do not agree, a third count is needed, and the modal or median count is used to calculate the child's rate of stuttering. Repeating these samples at 2- to 4-month intervals and comparing measures of stuttering frequency and severity provide the information needed in deciding whether or not to initiate direct intervention with the child.

As was noted earlier, a substantial number of children who begin to stutter stop without receiving any professional treatment. Unfortunately, there is no way of distinguishing, with any certainty, between those children whose stuttering is transient and who do not require therapy and those whose stuttering seems unlikely to remit in the absence of direct clinical intervention. One way of attempting to make this distinction is to evaluate those children whom you have decided are stuttering in terms of indicators that characterize beginning stuttering versus those that are indicative of a chronic stuttering syndrome. As long as a child is evidencing the signs of beginning stuttering predominantly, a clinician may choose to monitor the child's speech every few months to see if stuttering decreases, or stops, without any treatment being provided. In contrast, if chronic stuttering signs predominate, there is reason to believe that remission is unlikely unless some form of direct professional intervention occurs.[10] As before, two groups of indicators, expressed as questions, will be presented. Each question should be answered on the basis of observations of the child's speech during the diagnostic evaluation and subsequent analyses of video recordings of the session. These answers will serve as guidelines for deciding when and how to intervene with a specific child.

INDICATORS OF BEGINNING STUTTERING

1. Does the frequency of the child's speech disruptions indicate beginning stuttering problems?   The frequency of all disfluencies and of stuttered (or within-word) speech disruptions should be determined. If the child's disfluencies (all types) exceed 10% of the words or syllables uttered, the child may be having fluency problems.[5,6,15] If stutterings (or within-word disfluencies) exceed 2 to 3% of the words or syllables uttered, stuttering should be suspected.[3,4,6,15] If these frequency guidelines are exceeded substantially, and with some consistency, the greater the likelihood that a child is stuttering. Even if only a few speech disruptions are perceived as unequivocal instances of stuttering by an experienced clinician, that is sufficient evidence to conclude that the child has begun to stutter.

2. Do the type, duration, and prosodic characteristics of the speech disruptions indicate that the child is stuttering?   If a child's speech disruptions consist predominantly of frequent revisions, interjections, or multisyllable word and phrase repetitions, and if the frequency of within-word speech disruptions is relatively low, and if the child's speech disruptions ordinarily sound smooth, evenly paced, effortless, then he or she is probably not beginning to stutter. In contrast, if within-word repetitions often sound unevenly paced and stressed, faster in tempo, louder or increased in pitch, are marked by interrupted airflow or voicing or by replacement of the vowel by /ʌ/ in the repeated syllable, the child is probably stuttering.[3,10,20]

Stuttering children's within-word repetitions often exceed two units per instance,[3,15,17] and if multiple types of dysfluencies characterize many speech disruptions and, more often than not, form clusters of disfluencies on adjacent words or syllables, stuttering is clearly indicated.[21] If it is apparent that a child's speech disruptions are becoming more conspicuous and occurring more frequently and consistently across settings, it is possible that the child's stuttering may be evolving into a chronic problem that will require direct treatment.

3. *Do observations of the child and parents in conversational interactions suggest that modifications in their patterns of interaction may lead to improvements in the child's fluency?*   Findings from empirical studies of parent-child conversational interactions and stuttering are inconsistent.[28–32] Nevertheless, there are a number of clinicians who rely, at least partially, on manipulating parents' conversational behavior as a means of managing the fluency problems of beginning stutterers.[33–36] Uncontrolled clinical trials and a number of case studies have reported promising clinical outcomes. Parent behaviors that are believed to be of importance include: speaking rate, length and complexity of utterances, interruptions, turn-switching pauses, correcting/directing child's speech, and other behaviors. Review of the video recording of the parents and child conversing during the evaluation may identify interaction patterns that warrant further study or modification. Such video recordings can also be used to initiate parent training if this intervention option is selected.[35]

As many as half of all stuttering remissions occur within the first year of their onset.[1] Consequently, if stuttering persists beyond a year, some form of clinical intervention should be considered, even if a child's stuttering is largely free of tension and effort and there is no apparent concern, because his or her chances of remission would appear to be decreasing. If stuttering persists and speech disruptions become longer, more complex, and effortful, it is increasingly likely that the child will begin to voice concern about them and to evidence frustration, apprehension, and avoidance reactions about stuttering and speaking.[11,20] If such signs are consistently present for several months without sign of amelioration, it is my view that direct clinical intervention has to be initiated for that child to have a reasonable chance of stopping stuttering. Consequently, the indicators of chronic stuttering that follow focus on those signs which suggest that a child is using muscle tension and physical effort to initiate speech or to terminate speech disruptions and that negative cognitive and emotional reactions to these disruptions are apparent and commonplace.

INDICATORS OF CHRONIC STUTTERING

1. *Are the child's speech disruptions frequently accompanied by signs of tension or struggle?*   If prolongations constitute a fourth or more of all a child's stutterings (or within-word dysfluencies), are 1 second or longer, or involve fluctuations in loudness or pitch or abrupt terminations, the signs of chronic stuttering are clearly present.[3,6,10,15,17,20] Tense pauses between words that precede the effortful initiation of words are also frequently observed among chronic stutterers.[3,10,20] Other commonly observed signs include: extraneous articulatory postures and a variety

of nonspeech facial or body movements such as blinks, winks, turning of the head, or curling of the upper lip during speech disruptions.[3,10,20,24] Somewhat different, but related, signs include substituting words, whispering, or using other unusual techniques or "tricks" to assist in speaking, tapping a finger rhythmically to "get started" or slowing down portions of utterances.[11,20] All such signs are commonly viewed as accessory behaviors that are acquired as a consequence of stutterers' efforts to cope with involuntary disruptions of their speech.[18]

2. Does the child express concern or negative emotional reactions about his or her speech disruptions? As children get older and stuttering persists, it is not uncommon for them to seem embarrassed or frustrated about their fluency disruptions and to leave an impression, perhaps admit directly, that they often feel apprehensive or fearful about talking.[11,20] Some children cry or stop talking or ask with evident emotion, "What's wrong with me?" as their stuttering begins to disrupt their efforts to communicate. In contrast, other young stutterers, when asked, may calmly state that they stutter or comment that talking is difficult or that words get "stuck." A communication attitude test[37] appropriate for school-age children is currently under development and may be useful in quantifying young stutterers' beliefs about their speech. Wingate[18] views such cognitive/emotional reactions as symptoms that are commonly associated with chronic stuttering but not obligatory symptoms of the syndrome. In contrast, some clinicians, such as Sheehan,[38] believe that seeing oneself as being disabled by dysfluent speech and reacting with negative emotions to speaking and stuttering are obligatory components in the cluster of symptoms that are always present to some extent in chronic stuttering syndromes. This view is consistent with my own clinical experience.

3. Do repeated evaluations of the child's speech indicate that treatment should be initiated or changed? If systematic evaluations of the frequency and severity of stuttering find similar or increased rates of stuttering in speech samples within and outside the clinic across several follow-up evaluations, it is unlikely that significant or lasting improvements in stuttering will occur unless a change in the child's clinical management is initiated. If the child's speech is only being monitored, then some form of intervention should begin. If intervention with only the parents has been used, then some change in those tactics is indicated, which could include direct therapy with the child. If direct therapy does not result in clear-cut improvements in the child's stuttering within about 6 weeks,[39] then treatment should be terminated, at least for a while, and referral to another clinic or clinician considered.

Oftentimes diagnostic evaluations of suspected young stutterers find that a child's speech-language skills test substantially below age expectation.[13,40,41] In my experience, such problems most often involve difficulties in the use of age-appropriate language forms (i.e., phonology, morphology, syntax) among preschool stutterers or of language-learning disabilities among older, school-age stuttering children. If treatment of these "other" speech-language problems is initiated, then some attention to the child's fluency problems is often needed to ensure that stuttering does not worsen. Moreover, it is also possible that deficits in these "other" speech-language capacities may contribute to a child's fluency problem or hamper its remission.[42,43] Thus, treatment of such "other" problems also may be viewed as a form of indirect treatment of a child's stuttering.

Case Selection Criteria

Following initial observations and testing of the child, clinicians need to integrate the information that was obtained from their examination of the child with that obtained from the parents. Most often information from these two sources is complementary and provides a sound basis for drawing a diagnostic conclusion. Occasionally, there are substantial discrepancies, and these discrepancies need to be resolved through further interviews, observations, or testing. In my experience, substantial differences in the problem behaviors described by parents and those observed during clinical examinations usually reflect inconsistent occurrence of the behavior rather than inaccurate parent descriptions. Thus, I ordinarily assume that parents' descriptions are accurate and will be confirmed, ultimately, by direct or taped observations.

As noted earlier, evaluations of children suspected of stuttering result in one of four diagnostic conclusions. These conclusions will be listed below, followed by brief sketches of the patterns of signs and symptoms that frequently characterize each conclusion.

1. The child is evidencing few, if any, signs of beginning stuttering, and it is unlikely that he or she is developing such problems. These children are often highly nonfluent with speech disfluencies (all types) exceeding 10% of the syllables or words uttered. High frequencies of interjections and word and phrase repetitions often seem to reflect the child's efforts to maintain his or her speaking turn while engaged in linguistic encoding processes. The frequency of stuttering (or within-word dysfluencies) ordinarily falls below 2 to 3% of the words or syllables uttered and such dysfluencies are perceived to be effortless and free of excessive muscle tension.

2. The child is evidencing inconsistent signs of beginning stuttering, and further observation and testing is needed. Some of these children may be described by parents as having a severe stuttering problem but show few, if any, such signs while being tested and observed by the clinician. This suggests that stuttering is not a consistent problem for the child, which some clinicians believe is a positive prognostic sign, but there has to be some concern that even infrequent episodes of severe stuttering may be a forerunner of significant fluency problems in the future. Other children may have spoken little during an evaluation, answering questions with short utterances or a shrug of the shoulders. The result, of course, is that little stuttering is likely to have been observed. In such cases, video recordings from home or follow-up evaluations at the clinic will ultimately determine whether or not the child is beginning to stutter and, if so, what clinical management approaches should be tried. It has been my experience that many of these children stop stuttering without my intervening with either the parents or the child.

    There are still other children who show some of the early signs of stuttering but who do not comply with standardized speech-language testing instructions and for whom there is reason to suspect that other speech-language skills may not be age-appropriate. Treatment decisions, of course, should largely be determined by the results of these tests. If management of a syntactic or phonological impairment is needed, treatment procedures will often need to incorporate fluency-enhancing manners of speaking (e.g., speaking slowly, rhythmically, whispering) to ensure that the child's stuttering does not worsen as a result of therapy. Again, follow-up clinical evaluations will provide clinicians with the information needed to make such decisions.

3. The child is evidencing consistent signs of beginning stuttering, and an appropriate clinical management plan should be developed and initiated. These children usually evidence more than 5% stutterings (or within-word dysfluencies), and their speech is seldom completely free of such speech disruptions for any extended period of time. They commonly avert their eyes and show signs of muscle tension during speech disruptions (e.g., increases in pitch, loudness, or tempo). If asked why he or she came to the clinic, many may answer, "Because of my stuttering." Some may also evidence irritation or frustration if they are having unusual difficulty speaking but otherwise are likely to show little concern. Although this cluster of signs may also be present at the onset of stuttering, it occurs more frequently, in my experience, among preschool-age children who have been stuttering a year or more. If these signs are observed across the multiple speech sample environments that are systematically monitored in follow-up evaluations, some type of clinical intervention is clearly indicated in my opinion.

4. The child is already evidencing a number of signs of chronic stuttering, and remission is unlikely in the absence of direct professional intervention. Speech is often hard work for these children. Stutterings (or within-word dysfluencies) are frequent, sometimes in excess of 15% syllables stuttered, usually sound effortful, and often are accompanied by a variety of blinks, facial twitches, lip tremors, or posturings of the articulators. Signs of frustration and avoidance are not uncommon, even among preschoolers, and usually increase with age. The signs of chronic stuttering syndrome may be present in some children soon after stuttering onset but are seldom observed consistently until a child has been stuttering for several years. There are several reasons why these children should receive direct treatment for their stuttering without delay. First, stuttering this severe constitutes a significant communication handicap for most children. Second, remissions occur less frequently among severe stutterers.[12,22] Finally, there is reason to believe that successful treatment outcomes, with no recurrences, occur more frequently among young children who stutter than among older teens and adults.[44]

It would, of course, be convenient if every child's signs and symptoms clustered in only one of these diagnostic categories. In actuality many of them evidence signs in more than one. If there is substantial uncertainty about which diagnostic conclusion is appropriate for a specific child, further observation and testing are needed. Ordinarily, the most problematic decisions involve the selection of an appropriate clinical management plan. The reason, of course, is the lack of empirical findings on which to base such clinical decisons.

A strong case for active clinical intervention with every beginning stutterer can be made. There are a variety of direct[45] and indirect[46] treatment approaches that have been tried with young stutterers and that have resulted in reports of substantial improvements in stuttering. Furthermore, improvements in young stutterers' fluency often generalize to other speaking situations without special training. Indeed, some of these young stutterers stop stuttering completely, which seldom occurs among older teens and adults.[2] And most important, there is no credible evidence that intervening with these young stutterers will be harmful. So, why might some clinicians hesitate in recommending therapy for a beginning stutterer?

First, there is substantial evidence that most beginning stutterers are likely to stop stuttering whether they receive professional intervention or not.[1,12,22,44,47,48] Some of these remissions may reflect a natural growth or maturation process. Others might result from common sense, folk remedies employed by the parents, or an effective behavioral compensation adopted by the child while trying to cope with stuttering. Regardless, a significant proportion of these young children do not require professional treatment in order to stop stuttering. So, it is clearly appropriate for a clinician to question whether treatment is necessary for a specific child and when it should be recommended, with all of the accompanying fees and time commitments involved. Such questions arise because of the lack of published treatment trials that have used untreated comparison groups to control for the high remission rate among this age group of young stutterers. Even single-subject studies which demonstrate that decreases in a child's stuttering are clearly related to the treatment employed can not determine whether some of these children would have stopped stuttering at some later time without treatment. So, there is good reason for clinicians to feel uncertain when trying to decide what to recommend for a specific child.

My preference in dealing with such uncertainty is to let the parents decide. This places the decision for what are clearly elective procedures in the appropriate hands, the parents'. It also provides them an initial experience with the type of clinical partnership that needs to be established for effective management of the child's fluency difficulties. Consequently, once initial observations and testing of the child are completed, a meeting should be scheduled and both parents encouraged to attend. This meeting, which may need to be scheduled so that working parents can attend, provides parents an opportunity to raise questions that may have arisen since the case history interview or as a result of reading informational material they have been provided.

I like to begin this session by chatting briefly with the parents and attempt to set them at ease as we begin the task ahead. Then, I might ask how the child's speech has been at home or inquire about questions or concerns that may have arisen since we last met. This would be followed by a careful summary of the signs that have been reported and observed during the diagnostic evaluation and an exploration of the parents' reactions to this information. It is important to verify that these signs have also been observed by the parents and, therefore, are likely to be accepted by them as common or typical for their child. Then, if it appears that the child is stuttering, it is crucial to try to relate these clinical findings to the information that is available about the remission of stuttering in young children and to the treatment outcomes of children this age who have been treated recently at the clinic. Once this has been accomplished, the parents are prepared for the clinician to review the clinical management alternatives that seem most appropriate for their child. If more than one alternative may be appropriate, which is often the case, it is my view that the parents should decide what to do, even if an alternative that is less preferred by the clinician is selected.

A few parents may need to be told that their child does not appear to be evidencing abnormal dysfluencies, that there is no reason for further concern on their part. In more than 20 years of clinical practice, I have evaluated only a few children whom parents suspected were stuttering but whose fluency was unequivocally normal. Moreover, their parents seemed relieved and satisfied when they were told that their child was not stuttering. Nevertheless, some clinicians report that some parents do not appear to accept that nothing is wrong with their child's speech in spite of the clinician's findings. If such should occur, follow-up monitoring evaluations are one way to assure parents that any developing speech problems that warrant professional attention will not be overlooked.

For some parents, the preferred clinical management alternative is to systematically monitor their child's speech for awhile to see if stuttering is transient and decreases substantially with the passage of time. Others may wish to try managing the problem indirectly by modifying some of the ways they interact with their child, especially in conversation. Many parents choose this alternative, in my experience. Perhaps they feel less apprehensive or concerned when they are actively involved in trying to resolve their child's problem. In any event, when parents choose this alternative, there is usually no problem in obtaining their cooperation in changing some of their behaviors.

Another clinical management alternative is initiating therapy directly with the child. This alternative may or may not include using indirect management procedures concurrently with the parents. Again, that is their decision. If parents are highly concerned about their child's dysfluencies, perhaps unnecessarily so, they may choose to initiate direct therapy sooner than clinicians who prefer to begin by monitoring the child's speech for a while or by working with the parents. In contrast, a few parents may wish to avoid placing their child in therapy even though he or she is already showing consistent signs of chronic stuttering and will agree only to monitoring the speech initially. It has been my experience that parents ordinarily want to do the best they can to help their child, and under such circumstances it is important to try to understand their reluctance to begin therapy. Perhaps they need additional time in order to accept the possibility that their child's "problem" is unlikely to be a transient phase of speech development and that it warrants professional intervention. Perhaps there are financial or transportation difficulties. Regardless, if parents feel supported and understood at such times, it will usually not be long before they decide to try therapy if the child continues to evidence significant fluency difficulties. And while this alternative may only delay the inevitable, there is no evidence that even several months' delay in beginning treatment will be harmful to such children in the long run.

Thus, the concluding interview of a diagnostic evaluation is most often an initial clinical management session. It should educate the parents about stuttering and enlist them as full partners in the clinical management of their child. They need to know that there are no guarantees, that some children continue to stutter as adults even with professional intervention, but that the odds strongly favor their child stopping stuttering regardless of what they decide to do initially. These sessions can be filled with questions, long pauses, and much uncertainty. But if the parents have confidence in the clinician, they will likely leave the session feeling that they have made the right decision for their child and family and that there is every reason to believe that their child's fluency difficulties will not be a severe, lifelong handicap. Thus, a successful session results in the parents feeling empowered, through the support and assistance of the clinician, to manage their child's stuttering successfully.

Clinical Management

As has been noted in several previous sections, a variety of treatment strategies have been used with apparent success with young children who are beginning to stutter. Indirect strategies are those that try to improve the child's speech by targeting the environment or some other aspect of the child's behavior for change. Traditionally, indirect strategies have relied on play therapy, parent counseling, general parenting instruction, modification of parent-child interactions, and a number of other intervention procedures to accomplish the goals. In contrast, direct strategies have largely relied on response-contingent conditioning programs, fluency training, and/or stuttering modification procedures to decrease stuttering. Many clinicians, of course, use several different procedures that often combine elements of both direct and indirect strategies in their clinical work with stutterers.[49] Several subsequent chapters in this volume describe the direct clinical management of young stutterers. The remainder of this chapter, therefore, will be devoted to indirect management.

Indirect management strategies are used most often with children of preschool age who are stuttering but who have not yet begun to evidence consistent signs of tension or struggle in association with their stuttering and who seldom seem to notice or evidence concern about it. Although descriptions of play therapy with young stutterers[50,51] have been absent from the professional literature in recent years, it would not be surprising if these procedures continue to be used by clinicians whose training and experience have been based on psychodynamic perspectives of behavior. Play therapy has been used traditionally to attack the problems of children that are believed to be symptomatic of family and environmental conflicts. It is thought that children are best able to express such conflicts through play and, with the help of the clinician, ultimately master them. It should also be noted that various aspects of play therapy can be combined with speech therapy to promote a child's self-expression and to facilitate the establishment of an effective therapeutic relationship with a child.[52] Parent counseling is frequently used as an adjunct to other treatment procedures employed with a child, such as stuttering therapy[4,34,52] and play therapy.[51] A diverse range of procedures and goals has been included in clinicians' descriptions of parent counseling activities in the literature. Some focus on the emotional reactions of parents to their child and his or her stuttering and try to promote helping the child feel accepted, more secure; on decreasing stress and family conflicts; and on the expression and acceptance of feelings within the family.[33,34] Other clinicians describe counseling procedures that are intended to improve parents' skills in listening, disciplining, and managing a child's behavior.[53] This type of parenting skills training appears to be applicable and of possible benefit to all children, not just those who stutter. It is usually carried out in an instructional format rather than in self-exploratory discussions that ordinarily characterize many counseling sessions. Still other clinicians focus on having parents modify their communicative interactions with the stuttering child, such as having them ignore stuttered utterances but react positively to fluent utterances.[54] Some believe that the content and style of parents' interactions should be modified,[32] while others emphasize changing parents' speaking rate, utterance length and complexity, turn-switching pauses and interruptions, and other conversational patterns.[34,39,55] This strategy targets for change those parent behaviors that elicit and reinforce fluency, those that model desirable speaking behaviors for the child, and those that are suspected of disrupting the child's fluency. The following indirect clinical management procedures reflect this strategy.

Treatment Goals

The overall goal of these procedures for managing beginning stuttering is to decrease the likelihood that stuttering will persist and become a chronic problem for the child as an adult. This strategy seems most appropriate when used for the initial clinical management of those young stuttering children who do not evidence consistent accessory behaviors or associated features of stuttering or to supplement the direct treatment of children who are chronic stutterers. It can also be used with parents of children manifesting only ambiguous clinical signs of stuttering (whose speech is being systematically monitored) who are anxious to be actively involved in their child's management. Finally, it may also be tried for a 4- to 6-week period of trial therapy for children evidencing the signs of chronic stuttering syndrome if the parents are reluctant to initiate direct treatment. However, it should not be continued as the only management approach with such children unless substantial improvements in the child's speech are promptly achieved and maintained.

It has been proposed elsewhere[10] that as tense postures and movements of the speech production mechanism come to characterize an incipient stutterer's dysfluencies and embarrassment, apprehension, frustration, and avoidance of his or her reactions to speaking and stuttering, the less likely that child is to stop stuttering. This view hypothesizes that these motor, emotional, and cognitive signs, which are characteristic of chronic stutterers, are largely self-reinforcing responses that prevent the production of speech that is free of stuttering. In time, this likely results in the establishment of neurophysiological patterns that can be modified only partially in most adults. Thus, the frequent, consistent occurrence of such motor, emotional, and cognitive responses ultimately produces the relatively irreversible condition of chronic stuttering syndrome.

The specific objectives of the clinical management procedures that will be described include:

1. Monitoring the child's speech in order to document improvement and determine if changes in procedures or strategy are warranted.
2. Modifying situations, activities, and/or behaviors that disrupt the child's speech.

3. Modifying parental communication behaviors during interactions with the child.

Treatment Procedures

Indirect management of incipient stuttering begins when the parents decide that this is the best treatment alternative for them and their child. If the parents have been given *Stuttering and Your Child: Questions and Answers*[25] following the case history interview, the clinician can use the information provided in that publication to begin considering some of the things that parents can do to help a child who stutters. This is an initial step in helping parents begin to identify those activities and behaviors that appear to disrupt the child's speech and increase his or her stuttering as well as those that facilitate more fluent speech. The parents will also need to be enlisted as active participants in the ongoing monitoring of the child's stuttering. There are many ways in which these objectives can be accomplished satisfactorily. What follows is one such way.

MONITORING STUTTERING

Systematic monitoring of a child's stuttering, both at home and in the clinic, is necessary to determine whether satisfactory improvement is occurring or whether changes in treatment strategy or procedures are needed. Weekly recordings of the child's speech during unstructured play with the parents should be reviewed and analyzed every 2 weeks. If appropriate, recordings of the child interacting with a sibling should be included, especially if parents report that stuttering is worse when talking with that brother or sister. Monitoring at the clinic should ordinarily occur at 3-month intervals. However, for those children whose stuttering is steadily decreasing on at-home recordings, and elsewhere by parent report, follow-up visits may be delayed until 6 months has passed. In contrast, children whose stuttering worsens substantially between scheduled follow-up visits should be seen, if possible, during the period of heightened stuttering. During each clinic visit, 5- to 10-minute samples of the child conversing with a parent and with the clinician during play should be obtained. Other samples should include recordings of a narrative task or the retelling of a story and of the child engaged in conversation with someone who speaks rapidly and frequently interrupts and bombards the child with questions.

From these recordings percentages of total disfluencies, of words or syllables stuttered, and of within-word dysfluencies that are sound prolongations should be calculated. If accessory behaviors are present, the percentage of stutterings that are accompanied by such behaviors should be determined. For some children, measures of the duration of "typical" instances of stuttering and of three of the longest instances of stuttering may assess an aspect of stuttering severity that is missed by frequency measures.[27] Some clinicians also measure a child's overall speaking rate (e.g., syllables or words per minute), but there is insufficient normative information on the speaking rates of preschool-age children to permit useful interpretation of such information in my opinion. Consequently, it is my practice to measure speaking rates of young children only if treatment plans involve the manipulation of their speech rates.

All of the frequency and duration measures of stuttering gradually decrease when indirect management strategies are successful. It should be noted, however, that consistent, continuous decreases across samples and time are rarely observed. In my experience, frequency of stuttering usually continues to wax and wane somewhat from one day to another and situation to situation but becomes more intermittent and less noticeable across monthly intervals. Finally, if these management strategies are successful, the at-home and in-clinic recordings will be free of stuttering and the parents' daily logs, which will be discussed in the following section, will report that no stuttering has been observed elsewhere.

MODIFYING SITUATIONS

One way to help parents begin to identify specific situations that influence the child's stuttering is to have them maintain a daily log that lists the activities, circumstances, and persons involved when the child's stuttering is observed to be substantially increased or decreased. The log should also provide the parents' overall assessment of the child's stuttering that day. In my experience, parents often do not complete this task reliably unless they are provided a form that needs to be completed daily until the next visit. Charts recommended by Gregory and Hill[5] and Zwitman[53] can be easily adapted to obtain the observations most appropriate for a specific child. Information from this log and from conversations with the parents is used to identify those speaking situations and tasks that are associated with increased stuttering. This log, which records parents' overall assessment of the child's fluency day by day, supplements the systematic measures of stuttering that are obtained from at-home and in-clinic recordings, and is useful in evaluating how widespread the changes in the child's stuttering are.

After a list of situations that are identified with increased stuttering has been developed, the parents should select the one they wish to work on first. Such lists commonly include: talking while excited, competing for listeners' attention, speaking under time pressure, reciting or performance talking for others, etc. The clinician needs to help the parents determine how best to accomplish the task selected. Some situations, such as performance talking, can be easily handled by eliminating requests that the child "tell Grandma what you did in school yesterday." Others, such as competing with siblings for the floor during dinnertime conversations, likely will require changes in everyone's conversational behavior. In any event, once a plan of attack is agreed upon by the parents, the results of its implementation should be charted on the daily log. As each situation is modified successfully, another is selected until all of the activities and behaviors that appear to disrupt the child's fluency have been addressed appropriately.

MODIFYING COMMUNICATION BEHAVIORS

Soon after the parents decide to participate in an indirect treatment program, I like to have them record a 5- to 10-minute interaction with the child, similar in nature to that described by Mallard.[35] The parent and child need to be alone in the room. They can not be watching television or listening to the radio or recordings. The child is to choose the toy, game, or activity he or she plays with, and the parent cannot be reading or engaged in any other activity. If possible, a video camera should be used for the recording. At a subsequent clinical appointment, the parents and clinician view the recorded interactions together, and each parent is asked to evaluate his or her interaction with the child, what does the parent like, what should be changed. Often, the clinician may wish to direct a parent's attention to speaking rate, turn-switching pauses, interruptions, the number and type of questions asked, or corrections of the child's speech. During such sessions, the parent needs to select a behavior that he or she wishes to change during recorded interactions with the child over the following 2 weeks. These interactions are reviewed with the clinician at the next session and a decision is made as to whether further changes in that behavior are needed or whether some other communication behavior should be worked on for the next 2 weeks.

These videotaped interactions are intended to get parents to spend some time each day talking to the child in a relaxed, unhurried manner and to become more sensitive to how they communicate with each other. Often, they may be encouraged to pause a second or so before responding to the child, to speak slower, to use shorter, less complex utterances, or to ask fewer questions. If warranted, they should be urged to avoid interrupting the child, finishing his or her sentences, rushing the child, or correcting his or her speech. Such changes in parents' communication behavior are intended to decrease the child's stuttering during these interactions and encourage them to adopt these changes during other conversational exchanges with the child. If this strategy is successful, of course, the child's stuttering should decrease and ultimately result in the remission of stuttering.

Expected Outcomes

Clinical records are subject to a number of biases. The data from these records apply only to those families who chose to obtain assistance for a child's stuttering at a specific clinic; in this case, university speech-language training clinics. The data are incomplete because clients stop treatment for a variety of reasons: The child begins school; the family moves or is disrupted by loss of employment, divorce, or illness; or the family decides to terminate therapy, apparently satisfied, even though the child still stutters occasionally. Even those whose treatment ends only after there is no evidence of stuttering for several months may not return to the clinic if stuttering recurs. For these and other reasons, clinical records are basically anecdotal reports. Their validity is always open to question. The expected outcomes summarized below are based on such records and should be interpreted accordingly.

About half of the children whose intervention consists only of monitoring stuttering through parent reports and recorded speaking samples in the clinic at 3- to 6-month intervals can be expected to stop stuttering. As a group, these children probably evidence less frequent and less consistent stuttering at the time of their initial evaluation than do those whose parents decide to participate in an indirect management program. Those who do not improve substantially or stop stuttering during follow-up monitoring evaluations should be seen in indirect, direct, or a combined treatment program.

Of those children seen in indirect treatment only, or who did not show appropriate improvements while being monitored, again about half are likely to stop stuttering within 6 months to a year of directed parent intervention. Some may have stopped, of course, without any intervention. About a fourth of the children who stutter only are ultimately seen in direct treatment, and most have been stuttering a year or longer and are usually evidencing more severe symptoms. In addition, of course, all of those stuttering children having concomitant speech-language problems would also be seen in direct therapy. Of all those stuttering children seen in direct therapy, a few will show no progress and need to be dismissed or referred elsewhere. Of those remaining, about half can be expected to be dismissed with little if any continuing stuttering problems remaining. For the other half, referral for their continuing problems to another clinic or school program needs to be considered, even though some improvement may have occurred. Overall, the indirect treatment strategy that has been summarized can be expected to result in the remission of stuttering in about three-fourths of the preschool children whose clinical management begins within a year of stuttering onset.

Conclusion

Diagnostic evaluation procedures and guidelines for identifying incipient stuttering and for deciding which children may be evidencing transient difficulties and which seem likely to continue to stutter unless professional intervention is initiated have been described. Such decisions, at present, rely heavily on the experience and judgment of individual clinicians since data from adequately controlled clinical studies are not available. Based on the data that are available, and some 25 years of clinical experience, it has been argued that while most children who begin to stutter do not require direct clinical management, they should be monitored systematically for at least a year after onset. Monitoring only, or accompanied by indirect treatment procedures, should continue until there is no improvement or there is remission of stuttering. Direct treatment should begin once a child evidences persistent signs of chronic stuttering.

Suggested Readings

Conture EG, Fraser J (eds): *Stuttering and Your Child: Questions and Answers*. Memphis, Speech Foundation of America, 1989.
    This short publication provides information and advice about stuttering for parents in a question-and-answer format by a panel of clinicians with substantial experience working with children who stutter.
Egolf D, Shames G, Johnson P, Kasprisin-Burelli A: The use of parent-child interaction patterns in therapy for young stutterers. *J Speech Hear Disord* 1972; 37:222–232.
    This early article describes the changes in stuttering observed when the contents and style of parents' conversational interactions are modified.
Starkweather CW: Talking with the Parents of Young Stutterers, in Gruss JF (ed): *Counseling Stutterers*. Memphis, Speech Foundation of America, 1981.
    This short chapter focuses on how parents can facilitate the development of a child's self-esteem and model appropriate communication behaviors.
Zwitman DH: *The Disfluent Child*. Baltimore, University Park Press, 1978.
    This brief text describes a clinical management program that instructs parents on how to react to disfluent speech, improve the child's self-concept and feelings of security, and respond to misbehavior.

References

1. Andrews G: The Epidemiology of Stuttering, in Curlee RF, Perkins WH (eds): *Nature and Treatment of Stuttering: New Directions*. San Diego, College-Hill Press, 1984.
2. Curlee RF: Stuttering Disorders: An Overview, in Costello JM (ed): *Speech Disorders in Children*. San Diego, College-Hill Press, 1984.
3. Adams MR: The Young Stutterer: Diagnosis, Treatment, and Assessment of Progress, in Perkins WH (ed): *Stuttering Disorders*. New York, Thieme-Stratton, 1984.
4. Conture EG: *Stuttering*, ed 2. Englewood Cliffs, NJ, Prentice-Hall, 1990.
5. Gregory HH, Hill D: Stuttering Therapy for Children, in Perkins WH (ed): *Stuttering Disorders*. New York, Thieme-Stratton, 1984.
6. Pindzola RH, White DT: A protocol for differentiating the incipient stutterer. *Lang Speech Hear Serv Schools* 1986; 17:2–15.
7. Westby CE: Language performance of stuttering and nonstuttering children. *J Commun Disord* 1979; 12:133–145.
8. St. Louis KO, Hinzman AR, Hull FM: Studies of cluttering: Disfluency and language measures in young possible clutterers and stutterers. *J Fluency Disord* 1985; 10:151–172.
9. Yairi E: Disfluencies of normally speaking two-year-old children. *J Speech Hear Res* 1981; 24:490–495.
10. Curlee RF: A Case Selection Strategy for Young Disfluent Children, in Perkins WH (ed): *Stuttering Disorders*. New York, Thieme-Stratton, 1984.
11. Bloodstein O: *A Handbook on Stuttering*, ed 4. Chicago, National Easter Seal Society, 1987.
12. Glasner PJ, Rosenthal D: Parental diagnosis of stuttering in young children. *J Speech Hear Disord* 1957; 22:288–295.
13. Blood GW, Seider R: The concomitant problems of young stutterers. *J Speech Hear Disord* 1981; 46:31–33.
14. Johnson W, Associates: *The Onset of Stuttering*. Minneapolis, University of Minnesota Press, 1959.
15. Yairi E, Lewis B: Disfluencies at the onset of stuttering. *J Speech Hear Res* 1984; 27:154–159.
16. McDearmon JR: Primary stuttering at the onset of stuttering: A reexamination of data. *J Speech Hear Res* 1968; 11:631–637.
17. Zebrowski PM: Duration of the speech disfluencies of beginning stutterers. *J Speech Hear Res* 1991; 34:483–491.
18. Wingate ME: *Stuttering Theory and Treatment*, New York, Irvington Publishers, 1976.
19. Wexler K, Mysak E: Disfluency characteristics of 2-, 4-, and 6-year-old males. *J Fluency Disord* 1982; 7:37–46.
20. Van Riper C: *The Nature of Stuttering*, ed 2. Englewood Cliffs, NJ, Prentice-Hall, 1982.
21. Hubbard C, Yairi E: Clustering in the speech of stuttering and nonstuttering preschool children. *J Speech Hear Res* 1988; 31:228–233.
22. Sheehan JG, Martyn MM: Stuttering and its disappearance. *J Speech Hear Res* 1970; 13:279–289.
23. Yairi E, Ambrose NG: Onset of stuttering: Age, sex, onset type, and other factors. *Asha* 1990; 32:144.
24. Conture EG, Kelly EM: Young stutterers' nonspeech behavior during stuttering. *J Speech Hear Res* 1991; 34:1041–1056.
25. Conture EG, Fraser J (eds): *Stuttering and Your Child: Questions and Answers*. Memphis, Speech Foundation of America, 1989.
26. Cooper EB: *Understanding Stuttering*. Chicago, National Easter Seal Society, 1990.
27. Costello JM, Inghan RJ: Assessment Strategies for Stuttering, in Curlee RF, Perkins WH (eds): *Nature and Treatment of Stuttering: New Directions*. San Diego, College-Hill Press, 1984.
28. Wall M, Starkweather CW, Cairns H: Syntactic influences on stuttering in young child stutterers. *J Fluency Disord* 1981; 6:283–298.
29. Meyers SC, Freeman FJ: Mother and child speech rates as a variable in stuttering and disfluency. *J Speech Hear Res* 1985; 28:436–444.
30. Meyers SC, Freeman FJ: Interruptions as a variable in stuttering and disfluency. *J Speech Hear Res* 1985; 28:428–435.
31. Meyers SC: Verbal behaviors of preschool stutterers and conversational partners: Observing reciprocal relationships. *J Speech Hear Disord* 1990; 55:706–712.
32. Egolf D, Shames G, Johnson P, Kasprisin-Burelli A: The use of parent-child interaction patterns in therapy for young stutterers. *J Speech Hear Disord* 1972; 37:222–232.
33. Bailey AA, Bailey WR: Managing the environment of the stutterer. *J Child Commun Disord* 1982; 6:26–39.
34. Rustin L: *Assessment and Therapy Programme for Dysfluent Children*. Tucson, Communication Skill Builders, 1987.
35. Mallard AR: Family intervention in stuttering therapy. *Semin Speech Lang* 1991; 12:265–278.
36. Kelly EM, Conture EG: Intervention with school-age stutterers: A parent-child fluency group approach. *Semin Speech Lang* 1991; 12:309–321.

37. Brutten GJ, Dunham SL: The Communication Attitude Test. *J Fluency Disord* 1989; 14:371–377.
38. Sheehan J: Conflict Theory of Stuttering, in Eisenson J (ed): *Stuttering: A Symposium*. New York, Harper & Row, 1958.
39. Gregory H: Therapy for school-age children. *Semin Speech Lang* 1991; 12:323–334.
40. St. Louis KO, Hinzman A, Mason N: A descriptive study of speech, language and hearing characteristics of school-age stutterers. *J Fluency Disord* 1988; 13:331–356.
41. Louko LJ, Edwards ML, Conture EG: Phonological characteristics of young stutterers and their normally fluent peers. *J Fluency Disord* 1990; 15:191–210.
42. Adams MR: The demands and capacities model I: Theoretical elaborations. *J Fluency Disord* 1990; 15:135–142.
43. Starkweather CW, Gottwald SR: The demands and capacities model II: Clinical applications. *J Fluency Disord* 1990; 15:143–158.
44. Shearer WM, Williams JD: Self-recovery from stuttering. *J Speech Hear Disord* 1965; 30:288–290.
45. Adams MR: The Differential Assessment and Direct Treatment of Stuttering, in Costello JM (ed): *Speech Disorders in Children*. San Diego, College-Hill Press, 1984.
46. Guitar B: The Indirect Treatment of Stuttering, in Costello JM (ed): *Speech Disorders in Children*. San Diego, College-Hill Press, 1984.
47. Wingate ME: Recovery from stuttering. *J Speech Hear Disord* 1964; 29:312–321.
48. Dickson S: Incipient stuttering symptoms and spontaneous remission of stuttered speech. *J Commun Disord* 1971; 4:99–110.
49. Peters TJ, Guitar B: *Stuttering: An Integrated Approach to its Nature and Treatment*, Baltimore, Williams & Wilkins, 1991.
50. Murphy A, FitzSimmions R: *Stuttering and Personality Dynamics*. New York, Ronald Press, 1960.
51. Wyatt G, Herzan H: Therapy with stuttering children and their mothers. *Am J Orthopsychiatry* 1962; 23:645–659.
52. Van Riper C: *The Treatment of Stuttering*. Englewood Cliffs, NJ, Prentice-Hall, 1973.
53. Zwitman DH: *The Disfluent Child*. Baltimore, University Park Press, 1978.
54. Johnson L: Facilitating Parental Involvement in Therapy of the Preschool Disfluent Child, in Perkins WH (ed): *Stuttering Disorders*. New York, Thieme-Stratton, 1984.
55. Starkweather CW: Talking with the Parents of Young Stutterers, in Gruss JF (ed): *Counseling Stutterers*. Memphis, Speech Foundation of America, 1981.

2

Differential Evaluation–Differential Therapy for Stuttering Children

Hugo H. Gregory, Ph.D.
Diane Hill, M.A.

Our frame of reference for the evaluation and treatment of stuttering children takes into consideration characteristics of the child, environmental conditions, and the way in which these factors interact. Support for this approach is derived from research and clinical experience indicating that individuals who stutter are a heterogeneous group and that differing patterns of factors appear important in the clinical management of each child or adult.[1-7]

We will show how a differential evaluation procedure is used to determine (1) the existence of a problem; and (2) if there is a problem, what variables are related to it. Treatment strategies will be discussed, indicating how each takes into account a child's specific needs. The major emphasis will be on developmental intervention with preschool children, followed by a brief consideration of elementary school-age children who display varying degrees of stuttering behavior and awareness that speech is difficult. The latter discussion will show how the decision-making process with children whose stuttering behavior and awareness are more obvious compares to that with children in the earlier stages of stuttering.

Prevention and Management of Stuttering in the Early Stages of Development

Overview of Differential Evaluation Process

The diagram in Table 2-1 illustrates the differential evaluation procedure used at Northwestern University and shows, in general, how a clinician chooses appropriate evaluation and treatment strategies. The level of initial evaluation is determined by information obtained from the parents.

INITIAL CONTACT BY PARENTS

The evaluation process begins with the parents' first contact, usually a telephone call expressing concern. Ample time (20 to 30 minutes) is needed for a telephone

Table 2-1.   Overview of Differential Evaluation in Therapy*

Parents Identify a Disfluency Problem

|

Telephone Interview

|

Screening Evaluation

Typically disfluent	Borderline atypically disfluent without complicating speech, language, or behavioral factors	Borderline atypically disfluent with complicating speech, language, or behavioral factors	Atypically disfluent stuttering with or without complicating speech, language, or behavioral factors
Strategy I. Preventive parent counseling	Strategy II. Prescriptive parent counseling and limited involvement of the child	In-depth speech and language evaluation	
		Strategy III. Comprehensive therapy program involvement of both parents and child	

*From Gregory, HH, Hill D: Stuttering therapy for children, in Perkins W (ed.) *Stuttering Disorders*. New York: Thieme-Stratton, Inc., 1984.

interview. It is important to listen carefully to the parents' description of what they have noticed about the child's speech, their responses to the child's disfluency/stuttering, and their observations about factors that may have precipitated stuttering or are maintaining it.

Open-ended questions are posed to elicit the best parental insights: "Tell me what your child's stuttering is like." "When did you first become concerned?" "Does it seem to be more noticeable at some times than at others?" "Have you noticed situations in which your child has more trouble?" Follow-up questions are asked to clarify statements by the parent. If a mother says that the child "gets stuck" at the beginning of a sentence, the clinician may give examples of a one-syllable word repetition, a prolongation, or a block to help the parent explain. Once there is some clarification of the fluency pattern, additional questions are asked about the early development of speech and the current status of speech and language skills. It is also important to obtain information about motor development, social development, and health problems. Finally, the parent is asked about advice, evaluation, or treatment that has been received elsewhere. As the telephone interview ends, a decision is made concerning the need for evaluation and how comprehensive it should be.

FLUENCY SCREENING EVALUATION

As can be seen in Table 2-1, a fluency screening evaluation, consisting of 1 hour of observation and testing of the child and 1 hour of feedback to the parents, is scheduled if the parents describe a pattern of speech disruption that is typical of children at the child's age or if stuttering has been observed for 6 months or less and there are no concerns about other aspects of speech and language development. The fluency screening evaluation consists of four parts: (1) a brief case history of speech, language, and fluency development and other factors, such as illness, that may be important; (2) an analysis of fluency in monologue, play, play with pressure, and parent-child interaction; (3) an analysis of parent-child interactive behaviors, such as interrupting, fast-paced turn taking, or asking many questions; and (4) an assessment of speech, language, and hearing.

Decisions following this evaluation may result in utilizing treatment strategy I (preventive parent counseling) or strategy II (prescriptive parent counseling and limited involvement of the child) or in scheduling an in-depth speech and language evaluation (see Table 2-1).*

IN-DEPTH SPEECH AND LANGUAGE EVALUATION

This includes more extensive assessment in each of the four areas mentioned above, with attention given to a more thorough case history; a comprehensive evaluation of speech, language, oral-motor, auditory, and visual-motor skills; and observation of the child's response to the clinician's modeling of an easy, relaxed speech pattern. Ordinarily, an in-depth evaluation leads to the child and parents' involvement in treatment strategy III (comprehensive therapy program with involvement of both parents and child; Table 2-1). However, findings occasionally reveal a recent improvement in fluency, and if there are no other complicating concerns, a less intensive strategy II may be followed.

Evaluation Procedures

Since what we do is similar to widely used diagnostic procedures, they will not be described in detail. Those features that are of particular importance in making decisions about therapy will be highlighted, and brief case illustrations will be provided.

ANALYSIS OF FLUENCY

Information about the quantitative and qualitative characteristics of disfluency in the speech of nonstuttering and stuttering children has helped us be more precise in our evaluations of a child's speech fluency.[2,3,8] Breaks in fluency at the word level (sound and syllable repetitions and prolongations of sounds) usually occur less frequently than nonrepetitive disfluencies and one-syllable word disfluencies in the speech of most children. Therefore, in general, clinicians are more concerned about increases in these within-word disfluencies in a child's speech. In addition, we are more concerned about one-syllable word repetitions

---

*Treatment strategies are described later in this chapter.

and part-word repetitions if there is a higher frequency of units of repetition (two or more), and even more so if increased tension manifests itself in an irregular tempo. Thus, both frequency of specific types of disfluencies and their qualitative features are considered in determining whether a problem exists or the nature of the problem.

In clinical evaluations and parental guidance, we have found it useful to refer to a continuum of disfluent speech behaviors from "More Usual" at one end to "More Unusual" at the other (Table 2-2). Note that in keeping with our research knowl-

Table 2-2. Continuum of Disfluent Speech Behaviors

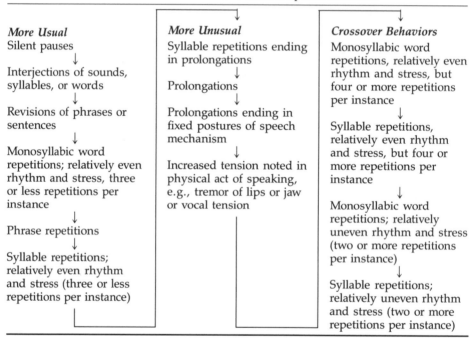

More Usual	More Unusual	Crossover Behaviors
Silent pauses ↓ Interjections of sounds, syllables, or words ↓ Revisions of phrases or sentences ↓ Monosyllabic word repetitions; relatively even rhythm and stress, three or less repetitions per instance ↓ Phrase repetitions ↓ Syllable repetitions; relatively even rhythm and stress (three or less repetitions per instance)	Syllable repetitions ending in prolongations ↓ Prolongations ↓ Prolongations ending in fixed postures of speech mechanism ↓ Increased tension noted in physical act of speaking, e.g., tremor of lips or jaw or vocal tension	Monosyllabic word repetitions, relatively even rhythm and stress, but four or more repetitions per instance ↓ Syllable repetitions, relatively even rhythm and stress, but four or more repetitions per instance ↓ Monosyllabic word repetitions; relatively uneven rhythm and stress (two or more repetitions per instance) ↓ Syllable repetitions; relatively uneven rhythm and stress (two or more repetitions per instance)

More Usual: Typical disfluencies in preschool children's speech listed in the order of expected frequency (hesitations the most frequent). These disfluencies are relatively relaxed, as, for example, noted by repetitions being even in rhythm and stress; however, if any are noticeably tense, then they are considered atypical. *More Unusual*: Atypical disfluencies that are very infrequent in the speech of children. More characteristic of what listeners perceive as stuttering. If in a speech sample of 200 syllables or more, there is more than 2% atypical disfluency (stuttering), this should be a basis for concern, especially if airflow or phonation is disrupted between repetitions (one-syllable word or part-word syllable) or if a schwa sounding vowel is substituted in the repetition of a syllable (for example, muhmuhmuhmama). Blocks and other signs of increased tension and fragmentation of the flow of speech should be a basis for immediate attention. *Crossover Behaviors*: On the continuum, such qualitative features as the number of repetitions per instance, the stress pattern involved, and the presence of tension distinguish typical and atypical disfluencies. *Total Disfluency*: More than 10% total disfluency (nonrepetitious and repetitious) should signal a reason for concern. These children are very disfluent. Research indicates that highly disfluent children are also likely to show a higher frequency of atypical disfluency which is more likely to be noticed by a listener. *Summary Statement*: Although most typical disfluencies are characterized by the fragmentation of a sentence or a phrase unit, most children show some part-word syllable repetition. Crossover behaviors include more fragmentation of the word, and finally, atypical disfluencies include more fragmentation of the syllable (the core unit of speech) and increased tension. Experience indicates that increased tension is the principal factor leading to more serious disruption of speech.

edge and clinical experience,[9-13] we have labeled the latter two types of disfluencies in column 1 and the first two in column 2 as "crossover behaviors" from "typical" to "atypical." Often the stress pattern and number of repetitions per instance of these disfluencies will mark an evolution into stuttering. Thus, noting the occurrence of such crossover behaviors helps in identifying early indications of stuttering. This continuum is also useful in helping clinicians and parents compare a child's disfluencies with what is usual in children's speech and with what types of disfluencies are more unusual or characteristic of stuttering. The more frequently the more unusual or atypical disfluencies occur, the greater the concern about the development of a stuttering problem.

The speaking situations in the screening evaluation include: (1) a monologue based on picture descriptions (action-picture story sequences), (2) play dialogue (comfortable conversational interaction with a clinician while playing with a toy village or other objects, (3) play with pressure in which the clinician's responsiveness systematically varies (loss of eye contact, verbal interruption, challenging or disagreeing, competition in play, hurrying the child), and (4) parent-child interaction (parents and child interact while exploring a standard set of play materials and games). Story telling (guided telling of a familiar story with pictured material, e.g., "The Three Bears") is added in the in-depth evaluation to assess the relationship between language formulation and fluency.

Samples are videotaped and analyzed utilizing the Systematic Disfluency Analysis (SDA) procedure.[14] Verbatim transcriptions of 200 syllables from each speaking situation are studied. In addition to the identification of disfluency types (such as those listed in the continuum), audible and visible qualitative features and the combining of several disfluency types in one instance of disfluency are also noted. Percentages of typical and atypical (stuttering) disfluency are determined. It has been our clinical experience that if a child has 2% or more of atypical disfluencies (stuttering) on any one of the 200-syllable samples, then there is reason to give careful consideration to beginning therapy. Several clinicians have pointed out that the child's total disfluency should also enter into the decision-making process, and we consider 10% total disfluency another reason for considerable concern. Even though a child may be below criterion (less than 2%) on atypical fluency disruptions (stuttering), 10% or greater frequency of total disfluency warrants further evaluation to determine the factors (e.g., some verbal expressive deficit) that may be contributing to such a high occurrence.

We emphasize the importance of scoring verbatim transcriptions, documenting the types of disfluencies, including audible and visible features, before commenting on the pattern of disfluency. It is difficult for clinicians to focus on eliciting a high-quality sample while noting qualitative features at the same time. In keeping with the continuum concept and data from the SDA, we classify patterns into the following diagnostic categories:

Typically Disfluent: Less than 10% typical disfluency and less than 2% atypical disfluency (stuttering);

Borderline Atypically Disfluent: 10% or more typical disfluency and/or 2 to 3% atypical disfluency;

Atypically Disfluent/Stuttering: 3% or more atypical disfluency and/or 10% or more total disfluency.

The following example presents a summary of information from the SDA.

Danny, age 3 years, 11 months

	MONOLOGUE	PLAY	PRESSURE PLAY	STORY RETELLING
% Typical disfluency	3.0	5.0	7.5	1.5
% Atypical disfluency	1.5	5.0	11.0	1.5
% Total disfluency	4.5	10.0	18.5	6.7

Danny was considered to be typically fluent in the monologue and story-telling situations, but he emitted significantly elevated amounts of stuttering, as well as a sizable increase of more typical disfluency, in the play with pressure situation and particularly in the parent-child interaction. The demands placed on him by the clinician and the parent appeared to be cues for speech disruption. An initial hypothesis was that psychosocial factors were of significance in this case and that speech-language developmental factors were not significant.

The following pattern of increased stuttering and typical disfluency is very different.

Christy, age 3 years, 9 months

	MONOLOGUE	PLAY	PRESSURE PLAY	STORY RETELLING
% Typical disfluency	15.5	5.5	6.0	11.5
% Atypical disfluency	1.0	.5	0.0	5.5
% Total disfluency	16.5	6.0	6.0	17.0

Here, it appears that the demands for increased language formulation had a disrupting effect on the flow of communication, particularly in retelling "The Three Bears" story. Christy was normally fluent when she was free to choose what to talk about in the play situation. The high amounts of more typical disfluency were of as much concern as the indication of beginning stuttering in terms of her further evaluation and treatment. In future evaluations, we would want to carefully assess her receptive and expressive language skills with a specific focus on vocabulary and word finding.

These two examples illustrate the importance of sampling fluency across several speaking situations. Parents sometimes report that their child did not stutter during previous evaluations. If a clinician spoke to the child in a relaxed, accepting manner, and made few demands, it is not surprising that stuttering was not elicited. We use the pressure play situation to assess the effect of this kind of demand.

CASE HISTORY

The history should include information such as the informant's statement of the problem, any family history of stuttering, general development and medical factors, speech and language development, and environmental conditions. This background helps to focus the clinical examination on factors that may be contributing to a problem and, in turn, have a direct bearing on treatment. For example, we need to know how an informant's perception of a child's speech compares to that of the clinician or even with the child's own evaluation. It may be that the parents are hypersensitive about speech fluency. Knowledge of family history may be important in terms of what it implies about the likelihood of parental sensitivity about disfluency or the possibility of a genetic link. Today's parents have read about stuttering being inherited, and they want information about it (see the chapter by Kidd,[15]). If there is a history of language delay, the present status of language should be evaluated more extensively and carefully.

As an adjunct to the case history, we have also used such scales as the Holmes Social Readjustment Scale for Children,[16] which provides information from the parents about life situations that the child is asked to manage. Examples of such life events include moving to a new home, starting a new activity, having a mother who goes to work, staying with a baby-sitter, or being enrolled in a day care center. One can readily see how this information may help the clinician and parents understand how the child's need to cope with a situation may be influencing the development of speech and language skills.

PARENT-CHILD INTERACTION ANALYSIS

First explored by Kasprisin-Burelli and colleagues[17] and by Mordecai,[18] these analyses supplement case history reports and begin the process of directly observing the parents and the child and mapping out suggestions for communicative and interpersonal change. When counseling parents, it is important not to confuse the information gained from observing parents interacting with their children with the idea that parents are causing the stuttering. Rather, styles of interacting may be contributing to the growth or maintenance of stuttering.

The analysis of a 10- to 15-minute interaction is based on a verbatim transcription of a parent's and child's utterances and can be used as a baseline to assess change. The following examples of interactive behaviors, if identified, are targeted for intervention: verbal interruptions, asking many questions, asking a second question before an initial one has been answered, filling in words, guessing what the child is about to say, constant corrections of the child's verbal and nonverbal behavior, verbal or nonverbal reactions to disfluency in the child's speech, and rapidly paced conversation involving poor turn taking.

The clinician should look at the ratios of a parent's questions versus comments, questions and statements of demand versus instances of praise and support (recall Sheehan's demand-support ratio[19]), and parent utterances versus those of the child. The parent's speech rate and adequacy of pauses for providing time for the child to initiate an utterance should be observed also. Finally, such negative interpersonal patterns as annoyance, bribery, and threats to elicit behavior in contrast to more positive patterns such as offering choices, rewarding, encouraging, and sharing should be noted as well.

It is even more significant to document the occurrence of stuttering as it relates to certain parental behaviors. One 3-year-old whom we saw recently reacted with increased stuttering when he was verbally interrupted in the parent-child interaction situation. These interruptions were characteristic of the mother and became one of the principal targets of change for the parent. A final comment is that we should make sure that we know how both parents, mother and father, may be interacting in ways that increase stuttering.

EVALUATION OF SPEECH, LANGUAGE, AND OTHER BEHAVIOR

Our clinical experience is in agreement with that in other reports[20–22] that there is a higher prevalence of articulation and language disorders in stuttering children. We have observed that the potential impact of these delays, or deficits, varies not only in terms of the severity of the problem but also in relation to the child's awareness level, frustration tolerance, and reactions from individuals in the environment.

Here is an illustration of what we mean:

> Joey, by his parents' report, had been noticeably disfluent since he began to speak. His speech and language development was delayed and he was difficult to understand. At age 3, while he was enrolled in therapy for a phonological disorder, the parents observed that he was stuttering and became very anxious about it. They were confused because he had made great progress, and his speech was much more intelligible, for which they were thankful, but now he was stuttering. The parents observed that Joey was more fluent in structured utterances, but that there were frequent disruptions in the flow of speech during more spontaneous, connected speech. During stutterings, he seemed to increase speech loudness, "widen" his mouth, and show more pitch variability. Observation of parent-child-sibling interactions revealed a pattern of rapidly paced conversation and poor turn taking. Frequently, more than one person spoke at the same time. Joey had to talk louder and louder and faster and faster to be heard. His older brother also spoke rapidly and often interrupted Joey.

In this case, it is clear that both child factors (delay in speech and language development and an existing stuttering problem) and environmental factors (communicative stress in the family) should receive attention. Thus, both Joey and his family were involved in therapy.

Children who have attention problems, who are passive and withdrawn, or who are fearful or perfectionistic may also need therapy directed to these problems as we give attention to speech. Also, either before therapy or during treatment, we may solicit the consultation of a clinical psychologist about problems such as these.

Differential Therapy

In keeping with the thesis of this chapter, differential therapy, what we stress in treatment, is based on the findings of a differential evaluation.[4,6,23,24] Commonalities exist in intervention, but procedures are modified, to some extent, for each child. In general, most clinicians intervene first to modify communicative stress in the environment. More in-depth evaluation and intervention may or may not be necessary.

TREATMENT STRATEGY I. PREVENTIVE PARENT COUNSELING: CHILD TYPICALLY DISFLUENT

1. Parent Feedback.   We describe how speech develops and include information about the occurrence of disfluency, perhaps by using the continuum depicted in Table 2-2. Using the results of the SDA, we help parents to understand the basis for our present judgment that their child's disfluency is typical for his or her age. We encourage them to agree or disagree that the samples we have gathered are representative of the speech pattern about which they are concerned. If they say, "He usually repeats words five or six times and sometimes covers his mouth," and if only a screening evaluation has been done, a more extensive evaluation should be conducted, or strategy II (prescriptive parent counseling) may be undertaken.

2. Discuss Interactive Styles.   Some communicative and interpersonal situations that are frequently related to increased disfluency and stuttering, such as those covered in the previous section on parent-child interaction analysis, are described for the parents. We reinforce the appropriate and positive behaviors they report and discuss possible parent-child interactions that may require further monitoring. For example, it is usually helpful for all parents if we mention the value of commenting more and questioning less to encourage more conversation and to impose fewer verbal demands at this critical period of the child's speech and language development. It is also useful to describe Sheehan's demand-support ratio in this regard.[19] In general, we encourage the parents to give attention and time to their children, to express appreciation for what they do in the way of childhood tasks, and to be reasonable in their demands, based on the child's age and readiness.

3. Increase Understanding of Communicative Stress.   The concept of time pressure in communication is discussed. We give such concrete examples as an adult beginning to talk just before or immediately after a child speaks, or asking a second question before a child has finished answering the first. We emphasize how children during their preschool years, when speech and language are developing and important emotional and social development is taking place, may show increased disfluency as they attempt to compete.

4. Increase Understanding of Speech and Language Development.   Findings of the speech and language evaluation are discussed and suggestions are provided for monitoring and supporting development in any area that is only marginally within normal limits on formal testing. Normative guidelines are provided.

5. Provide Information through Reading.   Parents read section on speech interactions and nonverbal communication in such books as *If Your Child Stutters: A Guide for Parents*[25] and *Stuttering and Your Child: Questions and Answers*.[26] These publications reinforce the information given in counseling sessions and serve as future references for the parents.

One counseling session, or possibly two, are usually sufficient to complete these tasks. A schedule of monthly phone contacts is planned to confirm continued normal fluency development. The parents are also encouraged to call whenever they are concerned. Normally, follow-up contacts continue for 3 to 6 months, with a fluency recheck at the end to formally assess the child's disfluency across speaking situations.

TREATMENT STRATEGY II. PRESCRIPTIVE PARENT COUNSELING, BRIEF THERAPY WITH THE CHILD: CHILD BORDERLINE ATYPICALLY DISFLUENT WITHOUT COMPLICATING SPEECH OR LANGUAGE FACTORS

1. Parent Feedback.   Based on observations and information obtained during the screening evaluation, feedback is given to the parents regarding the clinician's judgment that their child is showing some borderline stuttering behaviors. The parents and the child are then scheduled to attend four biweekly sessions that are 1 hour in length. At these sessions, the child is involved in fluency-enhancing activities, and parents participate in discussions, observations of their child and possibly other children, and activities with the child and clinician, and finally with the child.

2. Charting Disfluent Episodes.   The parents are instructed in how to identify disfluencies and in charting episodes of unusual disfluency using the form shown in Table 2-3. These charts are used to discuss patterns of child factors and environmental factors that the parents observe to be related to increases in the child's disfluency. Parents are asked to choose one at a time to solve. For example, one mother discovered that her daughter stuttered more in the morning while dressing. As she analyzed the reasons why, she realized that the two of them were "battling" about the choice of what to wear. The solution that the mother chose was to lay out two clothing choices and leave it up to her 3½-year-old to decide which to wear. The result was a decrease in conflict and in the child's disfluency, and a mom who was pleased with her successful management of the situation.

3. Modeling Positive Communicative Styles Conducive to Increased Fluency.   During each session, the child is involved in games that promote fluency. While the child is with the clinician, the parents and another clinician watch from an observation room, as the clinician with the child models communication behaviors that are

Table 2-3.   Chart of Disfluent Episodes

Person	*Message*	*Type of Disfluency*	*Child Awareness*	*Listener Reaction*	*Fluency Disruptors*
Mother talking on the phone	Child interrupted his mother and wanted her attention	Irregular rhythm on syllable repetitions in the first word of the sentence	Overall tense, but not aware of disfluencies	Mother said she would talk as soon as she finished	Getting listener attention, not tolerant of delay

supportive to fluency development. Such behaviors include speaking in a more easy, relaxed manner; giving the child time to respond to comments, questions, or instructions; reduced direct questioning and increased commenting; allowing a short pause before replying to the child's statement; and reinforcing the child when appropriate. While the parents are watching, the clinician observing with them comments about the conversational interaction between the child and the other clinician and highlights these fluency-enhancing behaviors. In this way, parents learn vicariously before they enter the situation and participate with the child. Then, as they begin to participate, they have an opportunity to practice the behaviors they saw modeled. Gradually, in successive sessions, parents assume more and more of the clinician's role. The clinician who is observing provides written feedback commenting on the parents' behavior, saying, for example, "Good commenting today. Did you notice how much more conversation you had with Julie? You were also successful in increasing the time you allowed for her to answer your questions. Great!"

4. *Re-assessment of Child and Parent-Child Interaction.*   At the conclusion of four sessions, follow-up fluency analyses and parent-child interaction analyses are used to evaluate progress. If the child's fluency is within normal limits, plans are made for monthly telephone contacts for 3 to 6 months. In some cases, additional prescriptive parent-child sessions are recommended. In a few cases, more intensive and more direct treatment of a child is carried out as parent counseling continues. If, at any time after dismissal, parents have concerns about increases in the child's disfluency, the clinician can advise by telephone or see the family as soon as possible.

TREATMENT STRATEGY III. COMPREHENSIVE THERAPY PROGRAM: CHILD BORDERLINE ATYPICALLY DISFLUENT WITH COMPLICATING SPEECH OR LANGUAGE FACTORS OR ATYPICALLY DISFLUENT (DEMONSTRATING MORE DEFINITE STUTTERING BEHAVIORS) WITH OR WITHOUT COMPLICATING SPEECH, LANGUAGE, OR BEHAVIORAL FACTORS

Children are enrolled in the comprehensive program when they are judged to be demonstrating atypical patterns of disfluency. Generally, these patterns have persisted for 6 months or longer. Oftentimes, parents report that there has been a decrease in their cyclic variation. We assume that greater cyclic variation means a less well-established problem. In addition, the observed differences in speech fluency have not resolved with maturation, the parents' attempts to utilize the information they have been provided on communication interaction, or the family's involvement in a program such as prescriptive parent counseling. The majority of children in this program are 3 or 4 years old.

The child is seen for at least two 30- to 50-minute sessions each week, and the parents participate in a parent group session and a portion of their child's therapy session once a week. Depending on the severity of the problem, more frequent sessions may be necessary. Typically, the child and parents take part in this format for two 10-week sessions and, if needed, children continue to receive individual therapy with parent participation until treatment goals are met. Clinicians should organize their programs as they think best, but less than two individual sessions for a child each week is not likely to succeed.

The following procedures are more specific to strategy III.

1. *Facilitating the Child's Fluency.*   For more than 20 years, we have based our approach to fluency development in children on the principles of modeling (observational learning), counterconditioning, and modified programmed instruction. Children develop more fluent speech by observing first the clinician, and then the mother, speak in a pattern that we call "slower, more easy, relaxed speech." This speech pattern counters the tension that may exist, and it is taught, beginning with shorter utterances and progressing to those of gradually increasing length and complexity. An analysis of the literature on early intervention indicates a trend toward the use of such fluency-enhancing procedures[23,24,27–29] with preschool children with fluency problems.

The desired result is for a young preschool child to speak in a slower, easy, relaxed manner with adequate loudness and appropriate inflection. Because children 2 to 5 years old are still developing perceptual, speech-motor, and vocal skills, the clinician's model must be quite obvious at first. Speech rate is slow and smooth, which enables the child to perceive the model's easy approach, followed by smooth movement. Rate of speech is normalized as instruction in easy relaxed speech moves from words to phrases and longer utterances, and as these modifications become more stable in the child's speech. Thus, slow speech is not the goal. More relaxed speech with easy approaches to its initiation, smooth movements, normal rate, and natural inflection is the desired outcome.

Initially, instructions to the child should be general and encourage close attention to the clinician's models through listening and watching. The clinician might say: "We're going to play a game, and I'm going to show you how to play. Watch me and listen. I want you to name this just like I do." While engaging the child's interest, the clinician not only verbally models slower and more easy relaxed speech, but also moves in a relaxed manner and provides visual, rhythmic cues such as moving cards or pieces of a game smoothly and slowly across a table or rolling a ball gently. Listening to and watching the model is also reinforced—"I like the way you listened and waited for your turn."

When the child learns to attend and evidences some understanding, the child is asked to imitate a word or phrase "doing it just like I did." Whenever possible, we begin at the phrase level, because these are more meaningful speech units and more natural inflection is possible. However, many children must begin at the word level in order to produce good-quality, easy, relaxed speech responses. At first, reinforcement is more general, for example, "Good listening, you remembered to tell me the name and the color—blue ball. You said that like I did." As the child is more successful, reinforcement becomes more specific. "You said that smoothly; good!" or "That was smooth and easy." As target responses become longer and include several sentences, models will emphasize an easy approach more often and a normalizing of transitions through phrases. Again, reinforcement becomes more specific. "I like the way you said that. You had an easy beginning." Later, "I like the way you said that. You had an easy beginning, and you said it smoothly."

Slower, easy, relaxed speech is learned and stabilized through response imitation and repetition, moving through several hierarchies. These hierarchies involve:

(1) length of response, i.e., single words, phrases, etc.; (2) type of model, i.e., direct model (clinician says, "Sun,"; Child says, "Sun"), delayed model (clinician says, "Sun, Now you tell me,"; child says, "Sun"), intervening model (clinician names a picture, child names another picture), no model (child names picture), and question model (clinician says, "What is this?"; child says what it is, e.g., "ball"); (3) propositionality of response (imitation, recall, stereotyped response, etc.); (4) communication situation (at table, on floor, standing, walking, etc.).

The criterion for response stability is set at 90% for 15 to 20 trials in two consecutive treatment sessions with 100% reinforcement and is followed by two sessions with 50% reinforcement. As speech change is more successful, variables are introduced that create more real-life situations; for example, walking around a building and asking for objects needed for a project. We manipulate generalization and transfer variables related to topic, location, physical activity, people present, etc., depending on how these factors are judged to contribute to increased disfluency and stuttering in a particular child.

2. Increasing Tolerance to Fluency Disrupting Influences.   As the clinician continues to make observations about those factors that tend to disrupt a child's fluency, and the parents share their observations, a hierarchy of factors is developed. A child's hierarchy may include such stimulus conditions as verbal interruption, excitement, competition during a game, noisy environment, asking questions, walking and talking, etc. Before work ends at a given length of utterance (e.g., four-word sentences), desensitization procedures are introduced.[30] Once there is a basal fluency level, a stressor, such as increased excitement, is introduced in a mild manner. The next time, excitement is increased. When fluency begins to break down, the clinician reduces the stress. Later in the same session, after fluency is re-established, the stress is applied again. This procedure is used only by the clinician, not the parents. Children's environments cannot be made optimal; therefore, this process is important in preparing them to maintain increased fluency in real-life communication situations.

3. Developing Competence in Skills with the Potential to Interfere with Fluency.   Our experience is in agreement with reports in the literature[2,20–22] that there is a higher incidence of articulation and language disorders in children who stutter. The children we see often need therapy that focuses on articulation and expressive language, including word retrieval. In most cases, we work on fluency first, stabilizing fluency at the four-word length of utterance, before introducing work on other areas of communication. Syntactic structures can be worked on as we go from shorter, less complex utterances to longer, more complex ones in modifying fluency.

Our approach to helping children with word-finding difficulty is twofold: (1) We help them to learn to cope more appropriately with the time pressure related to word lapses, and (2) we improve skills that facilitate word finding. In helping them feel more comfortable with delays and pauses in the flow of speech, we model delays in our responses to naming objects, commenting "I couldn't remember the name for that. Sometimes it's hard to think of words. Everyone has some trouble thinking of words." We reward increased pause time and desensitize feelings of needing to respond rapidly in such activities as throwing a ball back and forth more slowly with the child. Following this, we may play a game in which a child takes a turn throwing the ball back after thinking of an animal or a fruit. The child is prompted to take time thinking. Parents are encouraged to give ample time for the child to converse and not to fill in words or to interrupt. Rather, parents are advised to provide word choices, perhaps saying, "Were you thinking of a banana, an apple, or an orange?"

In building strategies to facilitate improved word recall, we use activities that accomplish the following: develop word association, categorization, and descriptive skills; build flexibility in word recall, by saying, for example "Think of four things that fly" or "Think of three fruits"or "Think of five green things"; expand vocabulary and word knowledge; and develop specific cues that facilitate the process, for example, saying "Describe the object" or "Think of the first sound," or "Think of what group it belongs in."

In this two-part process, children become more confident in their ability to convey messages. They are able to cope more effectively with the demands of conversational interchange, and word-finding difficulties are less of a fluency-disrupting influence.

The second goal is to develop strategies that facilitate word finding. One way we have done this is by practicing associations between objects and their attributes, stressing semantic associations such as color, size, shape, and function. We then practice describing objects using the various words dealt with in the association exercises.

Generalization and Transfer

We have observed success in generalization and transfer if parents, and sometimes siblings (depending on our judgment of the probable success of doing so), become part of the therapy process. At first, they observe the clinician and the child and follow the clinician's model. In the usual progression, parents are assigned to do at home what they have done in the clinic. In this way, both parents and children are experiencing generalization and transfer. Also, in this manner, the process seems very natural and is usually quite successful.

Summary of Parent Counseling

In describing our three intervention strategies, a variety of parent counseling procedures have been described: such as giving parents information about speech fluency, disfluency, and stuttering; teaching them to chart and discuss episodes of stuttering; helping them to modify communicative and interpersonal stress; and training them to model the behavior we wish their children to acquire. It is important to remember that verbal counseling should always be accompanied by the clinician modeling any changes suggested for the parents.

Parent groups often identify issues that can be particularly troublesome such as appropriate expectations for child behavior, parent-child separation difficulty, and sibling rivalry. Clinicians should be able to handle this type of discussion and remain alert to the possible need for family counseling by another specialist.

It is our belief that the success of therapy is, to a great extent, dependent on the relationship that we establish with parents and on their ability to enter into the problem-solving process with us. We say to them, "We are joining with you in a process that we are hopeful will lead to your child developing normal speech."

Therapy for School-Age Children with More of a Confirmed Problem

Differential Evaluation

Whether the referral is from a parent of teacher or, as in some few cases, results from an expression of concern by a child, we attempt to find what the informant views as a possible problem. The child's speech is screened during conversation and, as appropriate, by having the child read. The need for further evaluation is determined, and the parents and/or teachers are given feedback about our initial impressions. If it appears that treatment will be needed, a more in-depth evaluation is done.

As illustrated in Figure 2-1, evaluation of these children is considered to be a differential process, just as it was in working with preschool children. It includes a

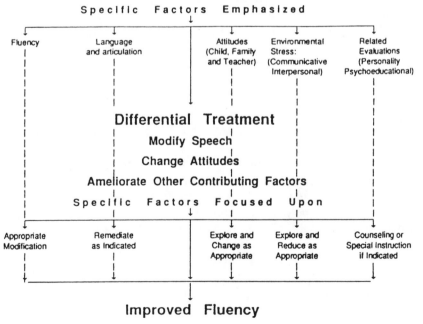

Figure 2-1.   School-age children who stutter—differential evaluation and treatment. Adapted with permission from Gregory and Campbell.[40]

case history, a complete speech analysis, other more formal tests and observations, and in some cases, related examinations by another specialist, such as a psychologist.

Gregory[3,31] provides a detailed description of these procedures, and the reader is referred to chapters on evaluation by Riley and Riley[4] and Williams[32] and books on stuttering therapy (by Conture,[5] Cooper,[27] Gregory,[3] Ham,[33] and Peters and Guitar[34] for additional information about evaluations that can be applied to this system.

Differential Therapy

A differential evaluation results in initial decisions about therapy, but evaluation continues throughout therapy. The latter point will be illustrated clearly as we describe approaches to speech modification.

The following examples indicate how information gained in evaluation determines the direction of therapy:

1. Understanding how a child's perception of his or her problem compares with that of the parents, teachers, and the speech-language pathologist tells us something about a child's sensitivity and motivation and the sensitivity of the child's parents and teachers. If a child shows little concern or interest in therapy, therapy should begin on a trial basis only, or be postponed until motivation is greater. A discrepancy between the way the parents and teachers perceive the child's speech may tell us either about sensitivity on their part or about differences in the stimulus conditions that are associated with stuttering at home and at school. Directions of counseling are determined by this kind of information.

2. From knowledge about how communicative stress (the way people talk with the child) and interpersonal stress (the way people interact with the child and with each other in the child's environment) influence the child's speech, we begin to consider how such factors as time pressure or rapid family pace may need to be modified. Such information, of course, may also have implications for the school environment.

3. Information about speech and language helps to determine if a deficit in receptive or expressive language is associated with the child's stuttering problem and should be taken into consideration in planning therapy.

4. Having knowledge of a child's adjustment has implications for how he or she may respond to therapy or may indicate the need for referral to a clinical psychologist. The more we know about a child's personality, the better we can judge how we should relate to him or her.

SPEECH MODIFICATION

From 6 or 7 to around 11 or 12 years of age, it is difficult to be certain about a child's awareness of his or her problems, the consistency of avoidance behaviors and inhibitory tendencies, and the child's self-image as a person with a speech problem. There is essential agreement among a number of clinical contributors, such as Adams,[35] Bloodstein,[36] Cooper,[27] Costello,[37] Gregory,[3] Shine,[29] Van

Riper,[30] and Williams,[38,39] that procedures should be used to enhance elementary school-age children's confidence in their ability to speak easily and to enjoy communication. As is true of therapy for a preschool child, analysis of stuttering behavior is, in general, viewed as counterproductive, at least until otherwise indicated, as we will explain later.

Less Specific and More Specific Approaches. Historically, the terms "direct" and "indirect" have been used to characterize two general approaches to stuttering therapy for children. "Direct" usually refers to modifying a child's speech, and "indirect" means working with the parents. With elementary school-age children, we work directly with the child's speech, but we consider it more appropriate to think of what we do as "less specific" or "more specific."[3,40] A differential evaluation of how to best modify an elementary school-age child's speech is made during the therapy process. In our view, it is best to begin with a *less specific approach* that emphasizes the development of fluency skills. A *more specific approach* that focuses on residual stuttering can be used to the extent necessary. The latter assumes that certain cues associated with speech and stuttering are stronger and specifically associated with sounds, words, and situations.

In the *less specific approach*, the clinician models an easier, more relaxed approach with smooth movements beginning with words, then phrases, and working up to longer, more complex utterances. There is no analysis of stuttering. For example, in practicing words, initial consonant-vowel (CV) or vowel-consonant (VC) combinations are produced with more relaxed, smooth movements that are slightly slower than usual. The remainder of the word, beyond the initial CV or VC, is produced at a normal rate and with normal prosody. Children who stutter often show a tendency to assume anticipatory articulatory positions for sounds (e.g., at the beginning of a word) such as closing the lips for "p," rather than thinking of the "p" *and* the following vowel as a single *smooth movement*.

With phrases, an easier, more relaxed approach with smooth movements is emphasized on the first CV or VC combination of the first word. The remainder of the word and all subsequent words in the phrase are blended together. In connected speech, the child is instructed to focus on monitoring the beginning of each phrase. We say, "Make an easy relaxed approach, and then let it go, making a smooth movement through the phrase." Rate and prosody should be kept as natural and normal sounding as possible.

Pausing, resisting time pressure, and general relaxation are part of the therapy program. We point out to the child that stuttering involves tension that breaks up the smooth flow of speech and that relaxation should be carried over into the coordinated movements involved in talking.

If the cues associated with stuttering on particular sounds and words are of sufficient strength that stuttering is persistent, then a *more specific approach* is employed *as needed*. For example, (1) child A may need the more specific approach on only a few words, (2) child B may need this attention on several sound transitions, (3) child C may need rather extensive work on several aspects of speech production (sounds, words), and (4) child D may be unable to modify speech fluency to any significant degree without using the more specific approach. The last example is very rare.

The following steps illustrate the more specific approach.

1. The clinician feigns the introduction of tension in her or his speech to produce syllable repetitions, sound prolongations, vocal tension, bilabial blocks, etc. The child imitates some of the "clinician's blocks."

2. The clinician models the modification of this feigned stuttering by, for example, slowing a repetition, shortening a prolongation, or easing the tension in the initiation of a word. The child does the same, imitating the feigned behaviors and modifications modeled by the clinician.

3. Following the clinician's model, the child imitates the actual difficulty he or she is having (e.g., prolonging the /s/ sound at the beginning of words) and then experiments with making the prolongation longer, then shorter, more tense, less tense, etc.

4. Modifying speech is finally evolved into an easier, more relaxed approach with smooth movements.

5. Voluntary disfluency may be modeled and taught if the child is unduly sensitive about disfluency. Children need to understand that some disfluency (e.g., word repetition, phrase repetition, interjections, and revisions) is a normal aspect of speech. Cancellations are used following stutterings that are persistent. Also, time-out contingencies may be employed by the clinician to help children be more effective in carrying out a speech change procedure.

Speech clinicians will recognize that in actual practice elements of the more specific approach can be integrated with the less specific approach. For example, if a child shows particular difficulty being successful with the easier, more relaxed approach with smooth movement on words beginning with /s/, the clinician may include some of the more specific approach by first modeling tension and poor transitions at the beginning of words, and then having the child copy these models and see how approaches to words can vary in tension, length of the /s/ sound, repetition of /s/, repetition of first syllables of words, etc. Then, these productions are contrasted with the easier, more relaxed approach with smooth movements in words and phrases.

Elementary children are very concrete,[41,42] and require considerable repetition to learn well. Repetition is acceptable if the clinician frequently reinforces the child and makes clear what is being learned. Children this age usually generalize more slowly; therefore, transfer activities must be carefully planned and practiced. The school is an excellent environment for planning and practicing carry over to situations of real life. In addition, the child's prognosis will be improved by bringing the parents in at regular intervals to show them what the youngster is learning. In this way, they will be better able to reinforce the child appropriately.

ATTITUDE CHANGE

Some clinicians use a direct approach to attitude change, bringing up topics for discussion, much like they might do with secondary school-age and adult clients. On the other hand, some feel hesitant to focus on a child's thoughts and feelings. We believe that clinicians should keep discussions of speech on a concrete level, making specific comments about speech being more easy and relaxed or making smooth movements in contrast to tense beginnings or broken movements. It can also be helpful to use pictures or models of the speech mechanism. We encourage the children to describe in their words what they think is occurring when they talk, such as: "Words get trapped in my throat," as the child points to the larynx; "I feel tense here," pointing to the chest, or "I repeat and can't stop it." These descriptions can be discussed with reference to a picture of the speech mechanism and how speech is produced.

Analogies between changing a speech skill and the way in which a person learns to modify swinging a baseball bat or tennis racket have been found useful by many clinicians as one way of making activities meaningful to a child who needs concrete explanations.

In terms of feelings, most children feel better when they realize that speech is a more flexible process that can be changed. Our first approach, and one that requires patience and restraint, is to be a good listener. In most cases we should wait until a child brings up situations such as teasing from peers, advice from parents, or how a teacher makes him or her feel about participating in class. As therapy progresses, questions may be asked, such as "How do you feel about talking?," "Where do you like to talk the most?," etc. Once feelings are expressed and acknowledged, the clinician can suggest some possibilities for handling them. For example, teasing can be discussed as a need of the teaser. Acknowledging a problem and saying that you are in therapy to improve will often stop it.

Almost always a child will resist change to some degree. The clinician should recognize this and be understanding about it. We might say, "It feels and sounds funny because it is different." As children get used to more relaxed speech, for example, and as the speech-language pathologist, teachers, parents, and others reinforce it, attitudes change. We also think that reinforcement is key in motivation. We must be sincere about it, but we should be very proud of progress made by a child. Videotaping is a good approach to attitude change about modifying speech. As youngsters watch themselves on television and as people approve (i.e., give positive reinforcement), change becomes more realistic.

PARENT AND TEACHER COUNSELING

It is crucial to the success of therapy that parents understand and participate in the therapy process. One of our most successful procedures, as was discussed in early intervention, is for the parents to learn to modify their speech in the same ways that the child is learning to do. The parents need to learn how stresses, such as time pressure in a communication situation, increase stuttering and make it difficult to change. Therefore, training in proper turn taking in the family can be very important. We have found that most parents can modify this behavior; they simply have not understood the importance of reducing such pressures. One father, who had very high levels of expectation for his 8-year-old son and who talked in a fast, animated way with his son, with little pause time, said, "I thought that was the way to make it interesting." Teachers can also be crucial in helping speech-language pathologists understand how the child responds to classroom activities. Of even more importance, the teacher can support what the clinician is working on with the child in the classroom.

Treatment Results

Most contributors about early intervention[5,6,24,28] have been saying in their formal presentations at professional meetings and through the media that we are highly successful at normalizing speech development and preventing stuttering when proper intervention takes place within 6 months of the observed onset of the problem. In prescriptive parent counseling, which we view as preventive, we are nearly 100% successful after four to six biweekly sessions with parents and children. Only a few of these children show a recurrence that concerns parents or that requires further intervention. As noted before, if parents are concerned, they are urged to telephone immediately, and we give the appropriate counseling or re-evaluation. In the comprehensive therapy program, successful intervention may take 8 to 12 months, but approximately 5% of children have persisting problems that may require referral for family counseling or psychoeducational evaluation and longer-term follow-up. Unfortunately, some parents do not accept recommendations for referral and the needed follow-up. One additional note: Comparing results now with those of 10 years ago,[24] we are seeing children who are younger and sooner after onset, both of which may be contributing to a better outcome.

Comments on the results of therapy for elementary school-age children are based on a philosophy of either succeeding; finding out why we are not succeeding, then taking new steps aimed toward better progress; or deciding that success cannot be expected at the time and discontinuing treatment.[31] One of us (H.H.G.) has been alarmed by the number of teenagers and adults who report that they went to therapy year after year as children and do not feel that they were helped. He now emphasizes that therapy for elementary school-age children that is not producing results that are obvious and rewarding to a child in a period of 3 to 4 months should probably be discontinued. Therapy is successful for about eight out of ten of these youngsters who gain confidence sufficient to be comfortable about communication and are able to speak easily in most situations. About one in ten does not reach this level and will need therapy later, perhaps when there is a greater concern about speaking better. Progress is slow and problematic in another one in ten, due to personal or family problems of adjustment, which leads in many cases to recommending referrals for psychological counseling and guidance.

Suggested Readings

Conture E, Fraser J (eds): *Stuttering and Your Child: Questions and Answers*, Publication no. 22. Memphis, Stuttering Foundation of America, 1989.
   Provides answers to questions most often asked by parents who are concerned about stuttering and their child. Represents careful thought by seven authorities who met together to discuss this topic.
Gregory H (ed): *Stuttering Therapy: Prevention and Intervention with Children*. Publication no. 20 Memphis, Stuttering Foundation of America, 1984
   Focuses on the development of speech fluency in children, determining when a problem exists, and if so, what factors (including emotional and environmental, language, and speech motor) may be contributing to the problem. Discusses prevention and early intervention.
Rustin L (ed): *Parents, Families, and the Stuttering Child*. San Diego, Singular Publishing Group, 1991.
   Concerns the role of parents and families in the management of stuttering, an area that deserves more attention. Brings together information from Great Britain and the United States.

Perkins W (ed): *Stuttering: Challenges of therapy. Semin Speech Lang*, 1991; 12(4).
   Provides information about school-age children who stutter and treatment approaches as practiced by leading authorities in the United States.

References

1. Andrews G, Craig A, Feyer A, Hoddinott S, Howie P, Neilson M: Stuttering: Review of research findings and theories, circa 1982. *J Speech Hear Disord* 1982; 48:226–246.
2. Bloodstein O: *A Handbook on Stuttering*. Chicago, National Easter Seal Society, 1987.
3. Gregory H: *Stuttering: Differential Evaluation and Therapy*. Austin, TX, Pro-Ed, 1986.
4. Riley G, Riley J: Evaluation as a Basis for Intervention, in Prins D, Ingham R (eds): *Treatment of Stuttering in Early Childhood*. San Diego, College-Hill Press, 1983.
5. Conture E: *Stuttering*. Englewood Cliffs, NJ, Prentice-Hall, 1990.
6. Starkweather C, Gottwald S, Halfond M: *Stuttering Prevention: A Clinical Method*. Englewood Cliffs, NJ, Prentice-Hall, 1990.
7. Van Riper C: *The Nature of Stuttering*. Englewood Cliffs, NJ, Prentice-Hall, 1982.
8. Starkweather C: *Fluency and Stuttering*. Englewood Cliffs, NJ, Prentice-Hall, 1987.
9. DeJoy D, Gregory H: The relationship between age and frequency of disfluency in preschool children. *J Fluency Disord* 1985; 10:107–122.
10. Wexler K, Mysak E: Disfluency characteristics of 2-, 4-, and six year old males. *J Fluency Disord* 1982; 7:37–46.
11. Yairi E: Disfluencies of normally speaking two-year old children. *J Speech Hear Res* 1981; 24:490–495.
12. Yairi E: Longitudinal studies of disfluencies in two-year old children. *J Speech Hear Res* 1982; 25: 155–160.
13. Yairi E, Lewis B: Disfluencies in the onset of stuttering. *J Speech Hear Res* 1984; 27:154–159.
14. Campbell J, Hill D: *Systematic Disfluency Analysis*. Unpublished, Evanston, Northwestern University Dept. of Communicative Disorders, 1987.
15. Kidd K: Recent Progress on the Genetics of Stuttering, in Ludlow Cooper J (ed): *Genetic Aspects of Speech and Language*. New York, Academic Press, 1983.
16. Holmes T, Masuda M: Life Change and Illness Susceptibility, in Dohrenwend B, Dohrenwend BS (eds): *Stressful Life Events*. New York, John Wiley & Sons, 1974.
17. Kasprisin-Burrelli A, Egolf D, Shames G: A comparison of parental verbal behavior with stuttering and nonstuttering children. *J Commun Disord* 1972; 5:335–346.
18. Mordecai D: *An Investigation of the Communicative Styles of Mothers and Fathers of Stuttering Versus Nonstuttering Preschool Children during a Triadic Interaction*. PhD dissertation. Chicago, Northwestern University, 1980.
19. Sheehan J: Role-conflict Theory, in Sheehan J (ed): *Stuttering: Research and Therapy*. New York, Harper & Row, 1970.
20. Andrews G, Harris M: *The Syndrome of Stuttering*. London, The Spastic Society Medical Education and Information Unit, Levenham, 1964.
21. Blood G, Seider R: The concomitant problems of young stutterers. *J Speech Hear Res* 1981; 46:31–33.
22. Wall M, Meyers F: *Clinical Management of Childhood Stuttering*. Baltimore, University Park Press, 1984.
23. Gregory H: *Stuttering: Differential Evaluation and Therapy*. Indianapolis, Bobbs-Merrill, 1973.
24. Gregory H, Hill D: Stuttering Therapy for Children, in Perkins W (ed): *Strategies in Stuttering Therapy*. New York, Thieme-Stratton, 1980.
25. Ainsworth S, Gruss J: *If Your Child Stutters: A Guide for Parents*. Memphis, Stuttering Foundation of America, 1981.
26. Conture E, Fraser J: *Stuttering and Your Child: Questions and Answers*. Publication no. 22. Memphis, Stuttering Foundation of America, 1989.
27. Cooper E: Intervention Procedures for the Young Stutterer, in Gregory H (ed): *Controversies about Stuttering Therapy*. Baltimore, University Park Press, 1979.
28. Meyers S, Woodford L: *The Fluency Development System for Young Children*. Buffalo, United Educational Services, 1992.
29. Shine R: Direct Management of the Beginning Stutterer, in Perkins W (ed): *Strategies in Stuttering Therapy*. New York, Thieme-Stratton, 1980.
30. Van Riper C: *The Treatment of Stuttering*. Englewood Cliffs, NJ, Prentice-Hall, 1973.
31. Gregory H: Therapy for elementary school age children. *Semin Speech Language* 1991; 12:323–334.
32. Williams D: The Problem of Stuttering, in Darley F, Spriestersbach D (eds): *Diagnostic Methods in Speech Pathology*. New York, Harper & Row, 1978.

33. Ham R: *Therapy for Stuttering: Preschool through Adolescence.* Englewood Cliffs, NJ, Prentice-Hall, 1990.
34. Peters T, Guitar B: *Stuttering: An Integrated Approach to Its Nature and Treatment.* Baltimore, Williams & Wilkins, 1991.
35. Adams M: The Young Stutterer: Diagnosis, Treatment and Assessment of Progress, in Perkins W (ed): *Stuttering Disorders: Current Therapy of Communication Disorders.* New York, Thieme-Stratton, 1984.
36. Bloodstein O: Stuttering as Tension and Fragmentation, in Eisenson J (ed): *Stuttering: A Second Symposium.* New York, Harper & Row, 1975.
37. Costello J: Treatment of the Young Chronic Stutterer: Managing Fluency, in Curlee R, Perkins W (eds): *The Nature and Treatment of Stuttering: New Directions.* San Diego, College-Hill Press, 1984.
38. Williams D: Stuttering Therapy for Children, in Travis L (ed): *Handbook of Speech Pathology.* New York, Appleton-Century-Crofts, 1971.
39. Williams D: A Perspective on Approaches to Stuttering Therapy, in Gregory H (ed): *Controversies about Stuttering Therapy.* Baltimore, University Park Press, 1979.
40. Gregory H, Campbell J: Stuttering in the School Age Child, in Yoder D, Kent R (eds): *Decision Making in Speech-Language Pathology.* Toronto, BC Decker, 1988.
41. Piaget J, Inhelder B: *The Growth of Logical Thinking from Childhood to Adolescence.* New York, Basic Books, 1958.
42. Flavell J: *The Developmental Psychology of Jean Piaget.* Princeton, NJ, Van Nostrand, 1963.

3

Treating School-Age Stutterers

CARL W. DELL, JR., PH.D.

Introduction

It has been 8 years since I left Van Riper's vineyard of speech pathology. Teaching and supervising in a university department just isn't the same. Although I am an active supervisor, it is a far cry from the full day of therapy with stuttering children that was part of my past. It is interesting that we are promoted only after leaving the battlefield, which makes me feel rather fraudulent. How valid are my ideas now that I have become, for the most part, only a supervisor of the process? It is a topsy-turvy system that allows a spectator to advise clinicians who are working and gaining knowledge about stuttering children.

There are three main points that you will find repeated throughout this chapter. My redundancy is partially due to my current professional role; many of us feel the need to be redundant in classes so that students will retain information. . . . They don't! Secondly, these three points were of fundamental importance to my success in helping stuttering children.

The first main point is that stuttering is intermittent, variable, and largely unpredictable. Although there has been a plethora of words written about stuttering, there is still much to learn. It is the quicksilver speech disorder because of its refusal to follow rules. In fact, one of the few things we can offer with assurance is to beware of those claiming to grasp and understand the many aspects of stuttering.

The second main point involves removing the mystery of stuttering for your clients. Although the subject of stuttering remains shrouded in mystery, the disfluent child needs to experience stuttering in an accepting environment you must create. Words cannot demystify. The only way children discover the reality of stuttering is to stutter without the accompaning emotion. We must lead them to this new awareness.

Finally, the third main point is that we must find methods of informing stuttering children that they have choices when speaking. They may not always be able to speak fluently, but they can learn, with our help, to stutter in less abnormal ways.

Clinical Evaluations: Diagnosing the Young Stuttering Child

Certainly, a great amount of time and effort in recent years have been spent on improving our evaluation techniques for children at risk for stuttering. Our profession has been influenced by the research of Sheehan and Martyn,[1] which indicated that 80% of all children who begin stuttering at an early age outgrow or become fluent with or without professional intervention. The importance of this evidence is at once obvious. With public school caseloads being what they are, the importance of identifying those 80% (incipient stutterers) is necessary if we are to economize our clinical efforts.

Sheehan and Martyn's research report was one of those landmark articles that appears in the literature and forever alters the thinking of all of us working with children who stutter. The 80% figure has been universally accepted and repeated so often that we view it as a fundamental truth about stuttering. It is a concept that many of us have adopted without question. Recently, however, some of us have begun to question the methods and findings of the Sheehan and Martyn report. Hallelujah!

My purpose here is not to quibble over research findings, but rather to point out that not all we hear and read about stuttering is necessarily true.

In my early work in the schools and now at our university clinic, I have not shared the concern of some about the importance of differentiating incipient from chronic stuttering. The reason for this attitude is my distrust of diagnostic tools or sets of procedures that propose to weed out the incipient from the chronic stuttering child. I contend that if there is a universal truth about stuttering, it is that the disorder is intermittent and variable and often eludes our attempts at categorization. I am not comfortable seeing a child for a single diagnostic evaluation and then making confident decisions about treatment based on that one interaction. Indeed, my reluctance intensifies when forced to determine a child's candidacy for therapy based on the diagnostic tools currently available.

There have been many examples over the course of my work with stuttering clients that dramatically point out why I am so cautious when making decisions about a child's qualifications for treatment. Soon after beginning my professional career, I was asked to see a sixth-grade boy whose mother had called the school after hearing that a new speech-language pathologist (SLP) (me) had been hired in the district. I saw her child for nearly an hour. Although he talked reluctantly, he never stuttered during reading or conversational speech. His mother responded angrily when I called to inform her that her son was not a candidate for my regular therapy schedule. "You're the third speech teacher now that has told me that, and I'm getting damn sick of it"! she snapped. I felt hesitant at the time to inform her of my proper professional title. She intimidated me, so I acquiesced, agreeing to see her son on a weekly basis for the rest of the semester. I have always been a pushover for domineering women.

In the following weeks, I talked with the child's principal and teachers at school. None of them could remember hearing the boy stutter. Another local SLP remembered him as a quiet but fluent child who had a demanding, overperfectionistic mother. "The boy's fine. It's his mother who needs the therapy," she told me one day. It was during the fifth week when we were on the playground talking that I heard him stutter for the first time. We were pitching pennies against the wall (I probably could have gotten fired for that) when he started stuttering severely. These were not gentle repetitions and prolongations. Rather, his face was flushed and he was gasping for breath as he tried to speak. I am ashamed to admit that I stood there staring in disbelief at this young boy as he contorted his mouth and face trying to squeak out a sound.

This early experience has always highlighted the implicit dangers of making a confident diagnosis on the basis of a single meeting. Although it is not my intention to diminish the importance of collecting objective data during the initial interview, we must always be careful not to overlook the intermittency and variability of stuttering, particularly when assigning students to our crowded caseload.

Unfortunately most of us do not have the luxury of being able to spend the necessary time required for a thorough diagnosis. We make decisions regarding a child's candidacy for therapy on the basis of a meager amount of data, knowing full well that because of the intermittency and variability of stuttering, our decisions will be tenuous. This is a cause of insecurity for us but it is much better to be tentative than to make bold statements about a child's stuttering disorder when we cannot know all the facts.

Case History

Before seeing the child for a diagnostic examination, I phone the parents or make an appointment with them alone prior to seeing the child. I want to find out when the child began stuttering and to get some idea of how the disorder has progressed since its onset. If possible, I attempt to get them to imitate some of the child's more severe stuttering behaviors. Some parents are either unwilling or unable to demonstrate their child's stuttering. In these cases I demonstrate some typical core behaviors (repetitions, prolongations, and airflow blockages) in a joint effort to help them describe their child's stuttering behaviors. Once the core behaviors have been determined, I imitate differing levels of severity in an attempt to assess the child's current level of stuttering. After I have some idea of core behaviors and severity, I inquire in the same manner about secondary characteristics, that is, the avoidances and physical concomitants of the disorder, and quiz the parents on the physical gesturing the child uses to escape stuttered words. As with the core stuttering, I may need to demonstrate these behaviors. Next, I ask about covert behaviors. That is, what are the negative feelings the child displays that are a result of the broken speech. Broadening the scope of the investigation, I ask if neighbors, friends, or relatives have mentioned their child's speech problem.

Certainly time constraints necessitate a short interview. At this point I am just gathering information needed to make a diagnosis and do not attempt to provide counseling, which will come after I have identified the specific problem. However, I may at this point provide the family with some stuttering literature they can read prior to our next meeting, which will follow the diagnostic evaluation of the child. Speech Foundation of America has three booklets that I have found valuable for this purpose: *Do You Stutter: A Guide for Teens,*[2] *Stuttering and Your Child: Questions and Answers,*[3] and *If Your Child Stutters: A Guide for Parents.*[4] The National Stuttering

Project, a self-help group for people who stutter, also has a good brochure for parents.[5]

After this initial parental interview, I contact the child's teacher prior to the initial diagnostic meeting. From the teacher, I get some idea of core behaviors, severity, secondary characteristics, and covert behaviors the teacher has noticed. As I noted above, these reports may differ. This does not imply that one of the respondents is untruthful or in error. Almost always there is some intermittency and variability in stuttering. After all, a child's performance is often dependent on his or her comfort level in the environment.

Observations and Testing

I regard the stuttering diagnostic as both the easiest and most difficult of all speech diagnostic evaluations. My goal is to obtain a good speech sample or, in the case of an older child, both a speech and reading sample. Superficially that appears to be a relatively easy task, and often it is. Many new clients talk willingly, which makes gathering a speech sample an easy task. However, others, because of their embarrassment over stuttering, are reluctant speakers. Getting a child to speak who is dead set against it is truly difficult. Every SLP who has been in this business for any length of time is an expert at getting hesitant children to speak. Children who stutter are not much different. We need to remove their fears and create an atmosphere that is warm, friendly, and accepting. Most SLPs have more skill at this than they realize. However, if you are having trouble getting a speech sample from a stuttering child, you might try asking fewer questions. Adults are forever talking and questioning youngsters who are reluctant to speak. If you find yourself being unsuccessful, back off and begin some silent play, preferably down on the floor. The floor is the child's world. He or she is comfortable there and, perhaps if we play quietly or introduce some parallel talk, we may find the child beginning to engage in conversation.

Another technique that has helped me get speech from a reluctant child is to stutter voluntarily during our conversation. These are not long, severe stutters but rather mild interruptions in my speech. You do not need to be a stutterer to do this. All of my practicum students routinely stutter while in therapy, and children usually do not react to this atypical behavior. It does, however, seem to reduce some children's anxiety and make them feel comfortable. With a particularly shy child, I have even pretended to stutter on a word, then stopped and explained what just happened: "Oops, I had a little trouble on that word. Let me try it again." This occasional stuttering and a calm attitude regarding it often effectively reduce a child's apprehension about stuttering. It creates an environment in which the child feels safe.

Another difficult aspect of the stuttering diagnostic is the varied number of behaviors that the clinician must catalog. In a short time we need to note core behaviors, secondary characteristics, and covert feelings the child may be experiencing. Many of us do not have the luxury of a video recorder so we must perform this data gathering on-line.

Tests are also available for classifying stuttering severity. Riley's Stuttering Severity Instrument[6] and the Iowa Scale of Stuttering Severity[7] are two examples of objective diagnostic scales that can be used to score a client's responses. I prefer the Riley scale.

Let me at this time issue a word of caution about the validity of formalized testing for stuttering clients because of the intermittency and variability of disfluent children. Formalized test scores may vary dramatically from week to week or even day to day! Another factor affecting test scores is the testing environment. A child's test results may vary depending on the perceived affect of the examining clinician. That is, the mood you set during the diagnostic will often influence how the child responds to testing.

I have found in our clinic that three different practicum students will often gather conflicting data on the same child on the same day. This is due to the child's perception of the examiner and the clinical environment created by a given clinician. I have also gathered diagnostic data at the student union, which yielded yet another conflicting data base.

I have witnessed and heard reports from adult stutterers who have been stuttering violently immediately prior to being filmed in a video studio. However, once in the studio they were perfectly fluent throughout: . . . "with the lights and the camera I used all my controls and spoke fluently." But back outside in the hallway, all controls failed and the poor client could hardly speak. These are realities of stuttering that cause conscientious clinicians to contemplate changing professions.

Case Selection Criteria

Recently, in an attempt to lower caseloads, some school districts have been diligently working to provide qualification criteria for enrolling children in therapy. These are usually referred to as "severity rating scales" and are used both to objectify and to determine a child's candidacy for treatment. I have serious reservations about this trend for children at risk for stuttering. Some current severity rating scales have used such misleading criteria as stuttered words per minute to determine stuttering severity. Stuttered words per minute has never been a unit of measure that I could support. A shy child who is reluctant to talk may have one 20-second stuttering block during a 5-minute period of conversation. Furthermore, this may occur during a period when most utterances are telegraphic in nature. Thus, a confirmed stuttering child could receive a milder rating than a talkative child who has a number of short, effortless disfluencies in the same time period. Common sense indicates that this frequency measure has questionable validity.

Some rating scales categorize stuttering duration of 2 to 4 seconds as evidence of mild stuttering and 6 to 12 seconds as moderate stuttering. Try timing a 4-second stutter or have a silent prolongation on a word for 10 seconds and see if you consider this a moderate communication disorder! I consider such guidelines, which are intended to aid the school SLP, as inappropriate. Moreover, many rating scales assume that only the child who stutters severely should be seen for treatment. Under these guidelines, a child with a mild or moderate problem may not be eligible for therapy services. This, of course is intended to reduce the size of the school SLPs caseload, which is a common goal we all share. However, it is my contention that mild stuttering, if neglected, often becomes moderate and moderate becomes severe, etc. Stuttering can be a progressive disorder, and the longer services are withheld, the more involved the disorder frequently becomes. Gradually, sociological, environmental, and emotional ramifications of stuttering collectively take their toll on the young child and progressively derail the efficiency of his or her speech-motor system.

A final argument against using rating scales in this way is that a beginning or mild stutterer often requires less clinical expertise and has the most optimistic prognosis. There is well-documented controversy throughout the stuttering literature, but most now would agree that early intervention is of the utmost importance! So I encourage the treatment of all stuttering students regardless of severity.

In reference to the decision regarding the appropriateness of therapy, most textbooks on stuttering provide detailed charts and guidelines that differentiate normal disfluencies from stuttering; e.g., the books by Bloodstein[8] and Van Riper[9] are two good examples.

I have attempted to make you aware of the fallibility of accepting test results derived from standard tools. This doubt is unpleasant but nevertheless a reality we all must face. So let us knowingly accept this unpleasant reality of our profession rather than blindly adhering to criteria that do not consider the complex nature of stuttering in children. These aspects of the diagnostic evaluation necessitate a willingness to accept and deal with a lack of absolute certainty.

Clinical Management: The Parent Conference

Treatment begins with the parent interview following the diagnostic evaluation. In some cases this interview helps to determine whether or not to place a child in treatment. In others, a parent interview will be the first step in the treatment process.

The parent interview is no easy assignment for the school SLP. Time is limited and scheduling is often difficult when parents work. Meeting with both parents is ideal, particularly if they were the referral source. The variability of stuttering makes this important. The parents need to observe the child's speech during the diagnostic evaluation to compare it with the child's stuttering at home. This increases the validity of your diagnostic observations since many times the two are dramatically different.

Having the parents observe your diagnostic evaluation can lead into the counseling process. The parents need to observe your interactions with their child, to see the accepting way you react to stuttering, and how you and the child can discuss stuttering in an objective and unemotional manner. This may be our most valuable contribution to the parents. Having them witness this demonstration may be of more value than all the advice that we routinely provide parents.

I first ask parents, following the interview, to validate the stuttering sample that they just witnessed. Then, I quickly point out that stuttering is variable and intermittent and it would not be surprising for the child's speech during the interview to be different than it is at home.

Next, I ask historical questions about the onset and progression of the child's stuttering, family incidence of stuttering, and siblings and the child's interactions with them. I try to identify the child's daily and weekly routine of activities. Some children seem overwhelmed by all the activities that well-meaning parents provide for them. Many times, some clients have decreased their severity of stuttering just by reducing these activities (karate, piano lessons, athletic and church activities, etc.). Children need time to be children!

Talking with Parents about Cause

Although I am reluctant at times to discuss cause, clinicians should provide parents a reasonable explanation that they can understand. They are often anxious for the clinician to stop talking so they can ask about the cause of stuttering.

Over the years parents have provided me with many myths about the etiology of the child's stuttering. I usually comment that anything is possible and that their description may indeed have some bearing on the stuttering. Generally, I have felt that most parents try to absolve some feelings of guilt through these descriptions. My goal is to remove some of this parental guilt. First of all, I do not believe (in most cases) that the parents are at fault for their child's stuttering. Secondly, guilty parents are not going to be effective partners in the treatment process.

I am not saying that parents do not make mistakes with their children that may affect their child's speech. Usually parents get the blame or credit for the behavior of their children. Generally, however, I assume that stuttering occurs in spite of, not because of, something the parents have done. How else can we account for all the children growing up in miserable conditions of abuse and neglect that have normal fluency? So, one mission is to ameliorate parental guilt and help parents feel less emotionally involved with their child's stuttering.

Eventually we must speak to the question of cause. Since descriptions of cause should be individually tailored, I do not have a canned presentation that I use for all parents. Nevertheless, there are some general themes that I address with most parents. I might talk about cause in this manner:

> Although childhood trauma or emotional problems may in some cases be related to stuttering, such children are definitely in the minority of all the children I have seen during my professional career. More often, speech problems in children are caused by a slow-developing nervous system. It's interesting in this regard that girls develop faster than boys and about four times as many boys stutter as girls. These slow developers are just that! They are perfectly normal children with normal intelligence, etc. It just takes them longer to join together all the circuits of the nervous system. For instance, what would happen if we took five children and attempted to teach them how to jump rope? Probably two of the five would learn the technique in a few minutes and start jumping rope with a minimum of error. Two other children might not be so adept at first, but after some patience and practice they too would learn the necessary coordination. However, I'll bet one child out of the five would experience more difficulty. He would try hard and do his best but jumping rope at his current age and physical development may not be possible. Now this last child may be as intelligent as his playmates and be able to ride a two-wheeler as well, but for some reason jumping in rhythm to the swinging of the rope is not something his nervous system can quickly learn.
>
> Speech, like jumping rope, takes a lot of coordination and skilled nervous system functioning. Some kids take longer than others to learn the necessary skills. Perhaps your child fits into this category.

Many children who begin stuttering will outgrow their halting speech and become fluent speakers. As these children mature, they develop a nervous system that is able to handle the complexities of fluent speech. As their nervous systems develop, there is an increase in fluent speech. It is important to remember that speech is a complicated act of fine-motor coordination. It may take several years to develop the necessary skills, and some youngsters need extra time. Most children seen for stuttering probably fit into this 'need extra time' category.

Still other children may have some physical reason why that area of their nervous system responsible for speech is not functioning properly. The medical profession still does not have equipment sophisticated enough to answer these questions, but all the evidence indicates that some malfunction does indeed exist.

With most parents, I would include parts of the delayed maturation explanation of cause.

Parents do not want to hear a lecture on stuttering. They just want to be reassured that it is not *all* their fault. Aunt Martha, after all, has told them that other relatives are wondering what they have done to make little Johnny stutter so. If we can help the parents deal with the Aunt Marthas of the world, then they will be more willing to help us during the course of therapy.

When talking to parents of more severe stuttering children, I do feel it important to mention the possibility of an organic cause for stuttering, even though most of our time I stick with the delayed-maturation explanation. In the coming weeks, I may talk further about some of the research that has implied an organic component to stuttering. The possibility of continued chronic stuttering also needs to be addressed. I may provide them with Eugene Cooper's essay[10] on chronic stuttering printed by the National Stuttering Project. For many parents, awareness that an organic component may result in chronic stuttering provides a sense of relief. It is a relief for them to know that stuttering is not their fault.

Advice to Parents

In addition to questions about cause, parents want to know what they can do about stuttering at home. Typically their child's stuttering makes them feel helpless and that soon leads to frustration. They may feel that nothing they try works for long. Addressing these concerns provides an opportunity to use a "Do's and Don'ts" list. These lists can be viewed as providing support for the position that Johnny's stuttering is the result of parental errors. So I am careful about dispensing these lists and often may do so at a later date. One of the best lists I have found is *A Brochure for Parents of Children Who Stutter*, by Peter Ramig and Dorvan Brietenfeld, which is distributed by the National Stuttering Project.[5]

Rather than beginning with a guilt-enhancing list of parental advice, I prefer to ask parents to describe the intervention strategies they have used at home. Once again their answers are not ridiculed. I am attempting to discover how the parents use their beliefs about stuttering when addressing their child's problem.

Clinicians who have worked for any length of time with parents of stuttering children are quite familiar with the typical responses. Let us look at some of them and see if we can find more effective procedures that will instruct without being viewed negatively by parents.

1. *Ignore It*: The most common response I hear is: "We just try to ignore the stuttering and pretend nothing is wrong." Is there anything wrong with this attitude? Of course, the same advice is given in most of our "Do's and Don'ts" lists.

   When discussing this response with parents I begin by saying that most SLPs agree that ignoring stuttering is recommended. This information should come as a relief to parents who fear they are somehow at fault. However, I feel it is important to discuss this popular dictum further.

   First, I have never been convinced that parents can ignore stuttering and pretend nothing is wrong. Children are quite alert to nonverbal communication and although parents may not discuss stuttering, it is my belief that children both see and feel parental disapproval. There are many nonverbal cues sent out that tell a child there is something wrong with his or her speech. A look, evidences of muscular tension, and abrupt halts in activity are telltale signs that the child has done something wrong. Children recognize these signs of alarm and must wonder why their speech problem is treated differently than other inappropriate behaviors that are routinely addressed.

   Children surely know they are doing something wrong, and the parents must feel uneasy about avoiding the truth. Let us expose this great deception to the light! To this end, parents should be told it is acceptable, in fact beneficial, to discuss stuttering with the child. Stuttering can be explained in simple language, and the children need to be reassured by parents that stuttering is accepted. This mutual understanding and acceptance need not be complicated or time-consuming, and parents need not discuss stuttering every time the child is disfluent. However, by talking about stuttering they will have created a foundation from which future discussions may ensue.

2. *Just Slow Down*: Another typical response is: "Just slow down and take your time." I always compliment the parents for their insight, for it is true that slower speech does result in greater fluency, but parents need to be aware of the way children may react to this advice. No one likes to be the recipient of continual criticism. Children do not know that it is their behavior the parents are correcting and may begin to think there is something wrong with their character. This was certainly not the intention of the parents, but the result is often a child who begins to feel punished for stuttering.

   Perhaps we need to take the attitude that slowing down the child's speech is a desired goal, and then try finding ways of achieving this goal without damaging the child's self-esteem. We could advise parents that children respond to their perceptions of the environment. If the environment is relaxed and slow paced, then the child will, in all likelihood reduce the speaking rate. But if the environment is noisy and the listener is inattentive, then the stuttering child will tend to increase his or her rate at the expense of fluency. So in essence, we are telling the parents that their attempt to reduce rate is appropriate, but let us find better methods of accomplishing this goal.

3. *The Bad Times*: Concurrently, with discussions of rate reduction I like to broaden the discussion to include the "bad times." Most parents are aware

that there are certain times of the day when stuttering is most noticeable. Usually these bad times are related to some exciting or emotional antecedent event. For example, a child may come running into the house after his sister pushed him down or the neighbor's dog chased him while he was riding his bike. School children get off the bus and run breathlessly with an exciting tale of some event that happened at school. It may be that a child has misbehaved in some way and the parent immediately demands an explanation or admission of guilt. Whatever the reason, there are situations during the day when emotion and excitement are high. It is during these times that stuttering children are particularly vulnerable.

I think it is important to defuse these bad times when they arise; otherwise, they lie festering in the child's memory and foster the progressive nature of stuttering. My goal during these emotional periods is to reduce the child's rate and dampen some of the accompanying excitement that may lead to rampant stuttering. However, it may not always be possible during these episodes to reduce speech rate. There is simply too much adrenaline flowing, which inevitably overwhelms the child and prohibits his or her ability to effectively manage speech.

Therefore, my advice is to discourage speech altogether! But how can parents get this excited child to stop talking? It is really not that hard to do but somewhat more difficult to explain. Therefore, I suggest they use various monologues:

> "I see you're all excited and out of breath and have a lot to talk about. But I haven't given you a hug all day. Come here now and let me hug you! Let's be quiet a minute until we get all calmed down. Then we can talk about all the exciting things that happened today. In fact, let me get you a glass of milk and a cookie and we can sit down at the table. Here, let me turn the TV off so I can listen good to what you have to tell me."

This is just one of a number of ways parents can accomplish the goal of a "time-out" from speaking. This time-out gives the child a chance to catch a breath, slow the heart rate, and increase the odds of producing more fluent speech. It is quite predictable that without this time-out, the parents could expect to hear a barrage of stuttering. Instead, the parents have corrected the child in a nice way. In fact, the correction does not hurt the child's feelings but rather reveals the parents' love and interest in the child's daily experiences. This is the type of activity that parents can do. This is how parents can change behavior without punishing.

I always have some parents who complain that their child will not be silent during the "time-out" period. If these indirect methods do not calm the child or if the child just refuses to stop talking, then a more direct attack is needed. Once again a monologue helps clarify: "Now, now, now. Just stop a minute! I see you're all out of breath and excited and in a hurry. Talking is hard when we're so upset. So let's take a minute to catch our breath."

During this more direct approach parents can talk about speech being more susceptible to breakdown when the child is excited or feeling rushed. They may even mention stuttering as their reason for asking for this pause. Sometimes parents need to be more direct but always in a positive, nonpunitive manner. If stuttering is discussed with the child at this time, the parents should do so directly but without negative emotion. Parents will not appear critical but rather will be providing direction that is accompanied by love and caring. Children will generally react positively to such extra attention, and the parents will have successfully attained the "time-out" period that is so important.

Self-Help for Parents

Another good counseling technique that can be quickly implemented is to ask parents to make a cassette recording of the child's speech at home. Most parents have audio cassette recorders, and I usually recommend the evening meal as the best time for the recording. I ask them to bring or send the tape to the next session so we can listen to the child's speech.

Naturally, I never get the tape from the first recording session. Surely, every parent will preview the tape prior to sending it and realize some of the dynamics that take place during supper time. They often hear siblings being rude or hear themselves interrupting their child in midstutter! How much better to let parents self-correct in this manner. I am not sure to what extent the parents consider clinicians' advice, but if they do, it must by its very nature appear judgmental. Probably the less we pontificate, the better. Oh, they will sit and nod their heads and bow to our authority but the seed we are trying to sow has little fertile ground upon which to germinate. Better to let parents, children, spouses, and students self-correct if possible!

Of course, more could be said about this first parent interview, but what I have covered are the essentials. This interview is most important since the parents are such critical players in the therapy process. We need to listen to what they say as well as what they are not saying. They need our respect and understanding and this must become evident during the initial conference. Next, I will discuss some therapy ideas for children who are just beginning to show signs of stuttering.

Treatment Goals for the Beginning Stuttering Child

As I discussed earlier, there is often some indecision regarding the necessity of enrolling a mild stuttering child for therapy. Sometimes we are not sure the child needs our services. Perhaps like many children, he or she is just normally disfluent. However, I remain committed to enrolling all children who may be at risk for stuttering. Better to err on the side of being overly cautious. Early treatment also gets us acquainted with the child and the family. This is valuable if, at a later date, the child develops more severe stuttering. If after a month of therapy you are convinced that these are normal disfluencies, and the parents agree with your diagnosis, then give the client a "speech vacation," agreeing to meet with the child on a monthly basis until your services are no longer needed. How much better to document successful treatment now than to attempt therapy with a severe stutterer. Since stuttering is intermittent, variable, and often a progressive disorder, this seems the most prudent course.

Working with beginning or mild stuttering children should be enjoyable for both client and clinician. The sessions are relaxed, and the pace is slow. There are no mountains to climb, rather just a peaceful stroll through the park.

Treatment Procedures: Removing the Mystery of Stuttering

My goal with a child who is just beginning to stutter is often no more complicated than to confront and remove the mystery of stuttering. Children are often confused and embarrassed by this aberration that occurs in their speech. After all, most parents either criticize or ignore the stuttering so the child does not receive much consolation from them. Now this is not meant to imply that stuttering children brood about their broken speech. Far from it! Young children have precious little time to worry about such trivial matters. There are games to play and adventure waiting around every corner. However, there are certain, brief moments following an episode of stuttering when children must be curious. They are confused for a moment by what just happened. They feel their mouth jumping spasmodically or hear sounds that are unfamiliar. We do not know exactly what a child experiences, but it seems obvious that there are times when stuttering comes to consciousness and is acknowledged. When this occurs, there is no one to explain or demystify the experience, which in itself must be confusing. Although children may not always get appropriate answers to life's questions, they usually receive some explanation. With stuttering, a code of silence hovers over the family, and clinicians need to step in and provide guidance.

Regardless of a child's outward reaction to stuttering, the momentary interruption in the fluency of speech is recognized on some physical/psychological level. We may not react every time we stub our toe, but there is awareness at some level that some mistake has occurred. Therefore, it seems appropriate to spend time helping children understand the causes of these speech mistakes.

PSEUDOSTUTTERING

The easiest way for clinicians to begin the exploration of stuttering with a child is to demonstrate some mild stuttering in their own speech. How much easier for the child to look at someone else's stuttering rather than his or her own. I may casually introduce pseudostuttering into my speech when we are playing together. At first, I may make no comment about these disfluencies and wait to see what kind of a reaction the child will have. Generally, since my pretend stuttering is mild, most children will not make an outward reaction, but again there must be recognition at some level. Student clinicians have often found that pseudostuttering appears to make a child more relaxed and willing to talk. Many children who have shown no reaction to this pseudostuttering have been later asked about the clinician's speech. They will often matter-of-factly say, "She stutters too."

After several mild pseudostutters I may decide to become more obvious. I may start stuttering on a word and interrupt myself by saying, "Hey, I got stuck a little there. Let me try that again." Then I go back and make a fresh attempt at the word, prolonging the first sound and then moving smoothly into the transition. "There, sometimes I have trouble, but if I stop and try again a little slower it comes out easy. Does that ever happen to you?" If the child agrees that he or she has trouble too, then it gives me an opportunity to continue this direct confrontation with the child's stuttering. I might ask, "What happens when you get stuck like that?" or "What do you do when you get mixed up like that?" or "What does your Mom say or do when you have trouble like that?" Regardless of what I decide to say at the time, it is the beginning of the child's exploration of stuttering. Together we will attempt to unravel the mystery behind these glitches in his or her speech.

Removing the mystery of stuttering need not be an arduous task. In fact, there is no need for long explanations or deep probings of the child's psyche. Children at this age have little concern or seldom any deep psychological scars that need attention. Rather, I have found that the best way to understand stuttering is by stuttering. I model different stuttering behaviors and get the children to imitate me. After pretending to stutter, I talk about what my mouth felt like or how I make my mouth stutter in this fashion. I explore different core behaviors and discover how stuttering is an act of physical mistiming and miscoordination. Stuttering then becomes concrete and capable of being experienced without fear or embarrassment. Children often laugh and enjoy the "funny" way their mouth feels when stuttering. They learn that stuttering has understandable rules. "When I push my tongue too hard, this happens or when I clamp my lips together, that happens." Stuttering becomes more predictable. "After all, I am the one putting my lips together too hard." "I am squeezing the back of my throat so air cannot flow out." "There is no monster or bogeyman inside me that causes me to stutter." "If I squeeze I will get stuck." "Stuttering is something that I do with my lips, tongue, and jaw." "If I can stutter on purpose and make it sound the same, then the bogeyman no longer has control." "I can explain and feel stuttering as being the result of movements that I performed."

As I demonstrate these different stuttering behaviors, I talk about where and how I position my articulators to create a particular type of stutter. Children begin to realize that stuttering is physical behavior and, as such, it can be altered, changed, or eliminated altogether.

Another advantage of the clinician's pseudostuttering is that they can have the child imitate their stuttering, which is a nonthreatening method of revealing stuttering. Imitating stuttering does not involve the negative feelings that a child associates with the act of stuttering. Imitating starts sending a message that stuttering is something that can be touched without getting burned. "If I can stutter like you and you like me, then the awful dread that there is something negative about me as a person begins to diminish."

Imitating the stuttering of the clinician is easy and unstressful. After all, the child is not forced into a negative confrontation with his or her stuttering. The act of stuttering voluntarily does much to remove the mystery of stuttering in the child's mind. Getting the child's mouth to stutter like the clinician's demonstrates to the child that stuttering is a series of physiological events that can be varied or modified at will. Stuttering begins to lose its mystery as the child learns to stutter in different ways following the clinician's model.

The time spent imitating and discussing the clinician's stuttering provides an opportunity to point out and discuss the child's stuttering. Once the child can imitate the clinician's pseudostuttering, different core behaviors are demonstrated for him or her to imitate. Bouncing, prolonging, and getting stuck are all modeled and imitated by the child. The child comes to realize during these activities that stuttering can be manipulated and modified. He or she begins to realize that stuttering can become more voluntary. Prior to intervention, stuttering is viewed as something that happens. The mouth gets tangled and the child feels like a helpless victim trying desperately to extricate herself or himself from its clutches. But now the child is stuttering in different ways and experiencing a sense of making the involuntary, voluntary.

The mystery is becoming unraveled. We can talk for hours to children about stuttering with little or no positive effect. But when a child begins to experience voluntary stuttering, he or she begins for the first time to understand the stuttering experience. Involuntary stuttering is full of panic! The child may become so overwhelmed that he or she cannot tune into the experience of the momentary spasmodic reaction of the musculature. Since panic prevents the child from truly experiencing the stutter, he or she never objectifies or defines the moment of stuttering itself. That is precisely the mystery that clinicians must help the child uncover before moving on to other therapeutic strategies.

DESENSITIZATION

In addition to removing the mystery of stuttering, the act of imitating the clinician's stuttering is desensitizing. Desensitization is terribly important for stuttering clients of all ages. Clinicians need to be ever mindful of the abrupt transformation that takes place when individuals who stutter rehearse their speech in solitude with perfect fluency, only to discover that when they walk out into the world intent on saying those same words, they stutter severely. Fluent speech, perfectly spoken when alone, becomes a tangled, twisted, tortuous attempt to communicate when a pair of ears is present. Wendell Johnson[11] underscored the point, and rightly so, when he said that when you are desperately trying not to stutter is precisely when you do stutter. When alone we do not care if we stutter, so we don't. When out in society we are trying not to stutter and we do! By imitating the clinician's stuttering the child begins developing a mind set that he or she can accept stuttering in the presence of others. This is a key element of desensitization theory.

In addition to having the child imitate different core behaviors, I demonstrate both severe and mild forms of stuttering for the child to imitate. This instills in the child a choice of how he or she will stutter. Van Riper[12] said it best when he said that we may not always have a choice as to whether or not we will stutter, but we always have a choice as to how we are going to stutter. Children are not aware that they have this choice, so the act of voluntary stuttering becomes their teacher.

Most student clinicians need to be trained in voluntary stuttering techniques. Producing a smooth prolongation on the first phoneme is easy, but in their renditions of repetitive stuttering, they often say /tətətəteɪk/ for "take." They have inserted the improper schwa vowel during the repetitions. Clinicians need to make sure that their voluntary repetitions have the proper coarticulatory posture. In addition to improper coarticulation, many clinicians make the repetitions too abrupt or too quick. The first syllable should be slowly repeated with one repetition blending into the next, into the next, etc. There should be the sensation of continuous, uninterrupted airflow. The repetitions are spoken slowly and rhythmically, keeping each repetitive unit even, rhythmic, and uniform.

Many youngsters, once they realize that this pretend stuttering is acceptable and not a sign of failure, will be delighted to stutter in bizarre ways. It is like the ability to make funny faces. Have you ever been with a child and made a funny face? Since you initiated the play, he or she feels it is all right and makes a silly face too. The child needs you to lead this form of play, because his or her mother has said that it is not proper to make funny faces in public. When the child becomes more daring, he or she may stick fingers in the corners of the eyes and mouth and really get weird. Most clinicians have seen this phenomenon with grotesque faces, and I have had similar experiences with voluntary stuttering. After learning that stuttering is accepted by me, the child feels free to initiate grotesque stuttering behaviors. The two of us often have a great time seeing whose stuttering can become the most bizarre. And the child begins laughing about stuttering!

So what's the point? Why is it important to have children laughing about stuttering. Stuttering is a fear- and anxiety-producing stimulus. If I can insulate the child from these negative emotions, I increase his or her chances to "outgrow" the stuttering.

I remember a child who became so enthused by this "fake" stuttering that his mother called me the next day and demanded to know what I had done to her child to make him stutter so. After some initial anxiety, I quieted her enough to discover that the boy was stuttering outlandishly and not in his usual manner. She said that he laughed about it and wanted her to learn to stutter too. I attempted to reassure her that this was to be viewed as positive behavior, but I am not sure she agreed. Nonetheless, the end result for this particular child was the remission of all stuttering after 1 month of biweekly therapy.

The procedures described above can also be taught to parents and teachers. Not only do parents and teachers learn to respond more objectively around stuttering, they also learn about stuttering. At first, they are embarrassed and feel helpless around stuttering. They do not understand stuttering and feel frustrated when confronted by it. There is little difference between parents and children where stuttering treatment is concerned. I prefer teaching them to stutter rather than teaching them about stuttering. The feel of stuttering in one's own mouth is worth a thousand words. While teaching them to stutter, I wait for the "Aha" experience. That wonderful expression when a parent says, "Aha, that's what he's doing. That's what makes Billy stutter!" This experience tells me that Billy's life is about to undergo a dramatic change. Parents and teachers who are comfortable around stuttering will, in turn, relate in a more relaxed way to a child's stuttering. This relaxed atmosphere promotes fluent speech from the child.

INCREASING FLUENCY

In addition to removing the mystery of stuttering for both the child and the parents, clinicians should spend time strengthening the child's fluency. After all, the majority of the child's speech is fluent. If fluency becomes stronger, stuttering will eventually grow weaker.

The first step in working with children's fluency is to help them realize the extent of their normal speech. Many children come with many misconceptions about their speech. When asked about stuttering, children will often respond, "I stutter all the time." In reality they may stutter on 2 to 10% of their words but certainly not "all the time." Do others in the child's environment imply that he or she stutters "all the time," or does the child dwell excessively on the negative until he or she loses touch with reality? Whatever the cause, most children believe they stutter more than they do, and immediate measures should be taken to erase mistaken impressions that children have about their speech.

A simple means of rectifying this error is to have the children repeat phrases and short sentences following the clinician's model. If the sentences are not too long, most stuttering children will imitate them fluently. I then ask them, "Did you stutter on any of those words?" Since children do not usually stutter during this activity, they begin to realize that most of their speech is fluent. During this activity I do not praise children for imitating me fluently, but simply make sure they get the message that most of their speech is fluent. So, much of therapy is based on facing and accepting reality. I want children to realize that they do stutter, but not all the time. In fact, they are predominantly fluent. Children, like adults, need to make accurate appraisals regarding their behavior.

FIND THE THRESHOLD

In addition to increasing children's fluency awareness, I attempt to find each child's fluency threshold for different tasks. For instance, some children can read more fluently than they can speak conversationally. For these children I will spend time each session letting them read. Furthermore, I will be quick to point out the extent of their fluent speech. Once again I do not praise fluency but simply inform the child of its presence. Since children do not understand why they are fluent or what makes them stutter, praise seems inappropriate. If the children make no conscious change in their speaking behavior but just happen to be more fluent during a certain activity, it makes no sense to praise them for something they do not control.

GOOD DAYS

The same is true for "good days." Some children with mild stuttering are so variable that there will be days when stuttering is entirely absent, regardless of the task. On these days I encourage them to talk incessantly. Sometimes I have them cover their mouth with their hand so they can feel the fluid movements of the jaw and lips through their fingers. This increases their tactile awareness of speech. Some children imagine that their mouths are malformed or diseased, so I want them to experience how smoothly their articulators can work during certain conditions. I have discovered also that increasing tactile awareness in this manner often promotes fluency. At other times I may stop them and have them repeat a sentence that they just uttered if it was free of stuttering. When they repeat the sentence, they are to feel their mouth and tongue moving in perfect harmony with the air flowing from the lungs.

Later, if I think the chances for success are favorable, I have a child read until stuttering occurs and count how many words or sentences he or she can read fluently without stuttering. Later I use a stopwatch to determine how long the child can continue a monologue before stuttering. Then I chart the progress on a graph in order to show the child and the parents how much improvement the child is making. A word of caution here. I always make sure that I am not encouraging avoidance behavior. A child may discover that to keep fluent, he or she must avoid words or situations that he or she fears will bring on stuttering. Fluency at the price of avoidance is detrimental and cannot be tolerated.

Another task I have used is to challenge the child to speak fluently in spite of my attempts to disrupt him or her. Children often find this activity exciting. I may turn my back on the child or interrupt while he or she is talking. The child's job is to resist my efforts and continue talking fluently. I may bring a stranger into the room in an attempt to create anxiety and interfere with the child's fluency. I introduce these challenging activities when I am convinced that the child's fluency is strong enough to give him or her a good chance of winning the game.

These should be fun activities, and they can be beneficial in strengthening fluent speech as long as there is not lavish praise of fluency. In addition, clinicians need to keep a watchful eye for any evidence that the child is avoiding words or sounds in order to maintain fluency.

Therapy Goals with the Confirmed Stutterer

It would be ideal if children were identified when they first began to exhibit stuttering. The clinician's task would be significantly easier, and clinical results would be better. However, most stuttering clients are seen long after stuttering has a foothold. They have been stuttering for months or years, and the chance for quick, painless remediation has been lost. Simply demystifying stuttering by increasing awareness of the physical behavior and strengthening fluency does not seem to be enough. More involved, intensive therapy is warranted, unfortunately.

Treatment Procedures

I still begin therapy with these children in the same way outlined for a child who is just beginning to stutter. I attempt to demystify and objectify stuttering. But, in addition, I usually have to modify stuttering behavior in order to reduce severity. I do not attempt to create fluent speech but rather a milder form of stuttering. I have found that once children find ways to reduce severity, they experience a rebirth of confidence that decreases negative emotion and leads to more fluent speech. Fluency then becomes a by-product of severity reduction.

NURTURING INDEPENDENCE

Let me briefly expand that last point. Too often clinicians may feel compelled to keep children in therapy until fluency is achieved. They are, understandably, fearful and apprehensive. Perhaps the fluency that has been nurtured so carefully in the clinic or at school will crumble in the real world. So we may err on the side of keeping a client in therapy longer than necessary.

The sad reality is that fragile fluency does crumble under the pressures of the real world. This is more apt to occur if dependence has been nurtured along with fluency. Children need to experience both success and failure as independent beings. Failure is part of the life experience, and it does not destroy everything accomplished in therapy. Failure is a necessary part of stuttering, and children need to develop their *own* strategies that will help them persevere.

Another reason to discharge a child before total fluency is achieved is to let the child have the satisfaction of succeeding without our help. If the child has been helped to erase negative attitudes about speech, he or she may very well achieve normal fluency and this should be his or her accomplishment. If, on the other hand, the child feels that he or she has earned fluency, it becomes stronger. The child accomplished the goal without the clinician's help. It is ego-building "stuff" and gives a child the best chance of preventing relapse.

However, what if a child experiences failure and needs renewed intervention? When a child is reinstated in therapy, he or she will be stronger and more motivated this time around. He or she has experienced some failure and realizes the need for further remediation. Therapy this time around is less involved and ordinarily can be terminated after a few booster sessions.

After removing the mystery and objectifying stuttering, I begin actively modifying stuttering behaviors. In an earlier publication,[13] I provided a rather detailed account of possible modification techniques that I have used successfully with young stutterers. It is not my purpose here to rehash those techniques. In fact I have always felt somewhat guilty about that step-by-step "cookbook" approach to therapy. My intent was to provide school clinicians who were apprehensive about stuttering a series of procedures that I had found effective in the treatment of stuttering in the schools. My personal misgivings stem from my belief that independence must be nurtured in both SLPs and stuttering children. Activities and techniques that are successful in reducing stuttering severity need to be developed and personalized for each clinician and child. With this disclaimer in mind, let me review some modification activities that can help children achieve the primary objective of severity reduction.

SECONDARY CHARACTERISTICS

I am committed to demonstrating to children that they have a choice whenever they stutter. Stuttering children often do not realize that they have this choice. They feel helpless whenever they stutter and endure this painful experience without any idea of a reliable means of escaping their torment. When they are hopelessly "stuck" and fighting for breath, they understandably begin to involve the entire body in the struggle. If a certain movement frees the "block" and allows them to continue speaking, that behavior becomes reinforced, learned. Thus, these random body movements become learned and part of the disorder. To better understand the development of these secondary characteristics, think of someone's hands tightening around your throat. As the grip tightens, your struggling intensifies. Your struggling would be not unlike secondary characteristics that children develop trying to escape stuttering.

Secondary characteristics often appear bizarre and are certainly socially unacceptable, but in reality they are learned responses to the panic induced by stuttering. Stuttering closes the airway, and when respiration stops, panic sets in. The child begins struggling to get breathing reinstated. Although these secondary characteristics begin as random struggle behaviors, they later become learned reactions to stuttering.

It has not been my practice to identify or attempt remediation of these behaviors. They are an embarrassment and if success can be achieved without confronting them, I do so. In addition, remediation is often unnecessary since these secondary characteristics diminish once the severity of stuttering has been reduced. If stuttering no longer causes panic or struggle, then the need for secondary characteristics is negated. No struggle. . . . no tension . . . . no panic. . . . no need for escape behaviors. So my rationale has always been to reduce the struggle and tension associated with stuttering, and its secondary characteristics will take care of themselves.

TEACHING IDENTIFICATION

Now back to the primary goal of reducing the severity of stuttering. A logical starting point is to identify or learn more about stuttering itself. This is important for both the child and the clinician. I am convinced that clinicians must be able to stutter like the child. Spend time in front of a mirror practicing the child's stuttering. Until you can successfully imitate the child's stuttering, you can never "know" what your client experiences during a moment of stuttering. Nonstuttering clinicians frequently lament that it is hard for them to identify with stuttering clients. However, if you are willing to stutter like your client, you will gain insight about the feelings, both physical and emotional, that your client experiences. Take his or her stuttering out into the "world." See if you can duplicate it with a store clerk or waitress. The effort taken will give you insights that you lack as a nonstuttering speaker. Can a fluent clinician really understand and identify with a stutterer? Yes, but you must learn to stutter. Most of us have fantasized about acting, so go give your best performance and you will be able to better empathize with your client's daily experiences.

The client's task in the identification process is to discover the locus of tension. Together, you must search for the areas in the vocal tract where stuttering tension occurs. You need not be interested in the words and sounds that cause stuttering, only vocal tract tension. Word and sound fears, unfortunately, will come soon enough. Instead you and the child need to become aware of the tactile feeling of stuttering if you are eventually to find ways of modifying and reducing its severity. Get the child to focus on the tension in the larynx as well as other pressure points created by the tongue and other articulators. The child needs to experience this tension in an accepting environment so that he or she can become desensitized to the feelings of fear, confusion, and panic that are overwhelming when he or she stutters. This is a key element in stuttering therapy, and it is vitally important for the child and the clinician to experience the tension in the vocal tract that results in stuttering.

If a child clearly experiences the physical abnormality of such tension, the nervous system may self-adjust and the need to teach conscious modification will become less necessary. Athletes and coaches are aware of this self-adjusting phenomenon in their training methods. Players inundated with information about how to perform a specific athletic skill can become so overwhelmed with cognitive instructions that they cannot perform at optimum levels. They are so intent on following and monitoring procedures that their nervous system is not free to perform at maximum proficiency.

But what does this have to do with identifying the locus of tension in young stutterers? I have been experimenting in our clinic with getting stutterers to focus on areas of tension that create stuttering. What I have found is that if the client can truly focus on that tactile-kinesthetic sensation, then stuttering seems to dissipate rather quickly, and it does so without further direct intervention. If the client becomes tactilely and kinesthetically aware of tension in the vocal tract, it appears that the nervous system can, on its own, implement the necessary corrections without further "coaching." If I can get the child to experience that tension with as little emotion as possible, then the nervous system often seems to self-correct.

One logical rebuttal to this viewpoint is that stutterers are too aware of their speech. Isn't such overconcern the reason stuttering gets progressively more severe? I disagree! Stutterers are overly concerned about speech but do not know much about stuttering. They know they stutter and do not like it. Whenever stuttering occurs, they go "off" somewhere until it is over. Stutterers feel embarrassment and frustration but do not look intently at the cause. If this is true, how can children develop sufficient tactile-kinesthetic skills so that the nervous system can self-correct?

One way is to ask the child where in the mouth he or she got stuck. Once again I am not interested in the sound the child stutters, but rather the location in the vocal tract where tension is occurring. If the child cannot locate the tension, I imitate the child's stuttering in order to assist her or him. Then, I ask the child to stutter in order to familiarize herself or himself with that tension. If a child is reluctant, I use "fake" stuttering to locate tension. Since this is not "real" stuttering, the child is not embarrassed and he or she can more calmly investigate and familiarize himself or herself with the tactile-kinesthetic feedback of stuttering. Once the child is calm enough to focus on fake stutterings, he or she will more likely be able to attend to "real" stuttering.

Intimate awareness of tactile-kinesthetic feedback during stuttering is crucial to the successful treatment of confirmed stutterers regardless of chronological age. The trick is to get clients to put away all of the negative emotions related to stuttering so that they can let go and focus on the tactile-kinesthetic manifestations of stuttering. This is where a clinician's skills and experience working with people become so important. There is no one way to go about this task since all clients are unique. Nonetheless, once they begin to reduce their fear enough to experience stuttering, they will be on the road to recovery.

STUTTERING MODIFICATION

While I am teaching clients to become tactilely and kinesthetically aware of stuttering, I spend considerable effort demonstrating the variations that are possible while stuttering. Stuttering clients, for the most part, feel helpless when they stutter and believe they have no choices during any particular instance of stuttering. I demonstrate that they have choices. Many of these activities have been described elsewhere in detail,[13] and I will not repeat those here but will recommend some general guidelines to pursue.

An easy way to start the process of teaching children they have some choices when they stutter is to have them repeat phrases and short sentences following the clinician's model. This is a nonthreatening activity since they can usually be fluent while imitating a model. Next, I insert a mild stuttering on one of the words in the sentence. The child will usually not notice the stuttered word and simply repeat the sentence fluently. I demonstrate again and ask the child to repeat the sentence exactly as modeled. Once the child begins repeating my modeled sentences with the mild stuttering words, he or she begins to discover that he or she can stutter in different ways. Thus, I have quite effortlessly initiated the process of stuttering modification. The child can stutter with less effort than ever imagined.

After the child learns to imitate mild stutters, I demonstrate severe stuttering and have the child tell me where in the vocal tract the tension was located. Next, I may have the client provide examples of milder, easier ways of stuttering on the word. He or she then becomes the teacher, teaching me how to stutter in more acceptable ways. Children love to play teacher. I give them every opportunity to play this role as it is a good path to learning. Teaching a concept usually promotes more learning and understanding than receiving the information as a student.

IN BLOCK CORRECTIONS

Next, I want to tackle stuttering as it happens. This is referred to as "pullouts" or "in block corrections." I want stutterers to walk into the lion's den and face their fears head on.

This is the most difficult part of treatment and takes a good deal of courage on the child's part. The moment of stuttering is when all a child's fears and anxieties converge. Panic overwhelms the child, and he or she feels a loss of control—not only loss of emotional control but also loss of physiological control. Audiences of SLPs often laugh when I dramatize this moment of fear because I probably fail to convey the abject terror that stutterers often feel at the moment of stuttering. But groups of people who stutter do not laugh. They know that the panic is indeed real and can be deeply terrorizing at times.

Since this confrontation with stuttering is both difficult and crucial, I proceed slowly, making the first steps as easy as possible. I may start by having the child demonstrate an "easier way" after I model severe stuttering. Next, I may have the child join me in a moment of severe pseudostuttering and then demonstrate how to reduce that severity. Later, I let the child model a severe stutter while I verbally provide hints and reminders to reduce tension and struggle. Another activity is to have the child model severe stuttering and then signal me when he or she is ready to start reducing the abnormality.

All of these activities are designed to gradually work up to the moment when the child will experience and modify a "real" stuttered word. I usually start with a simple activity, such as making up sentences about objects or pictures. The child is to say one sentence at a time, and if the child feels himself or herself beginning to stutter, he or she is to keep stuttering on that sound until I give the signal to reduce tension and make a smooth transition into the second syllable. During the time before my signal, the child is to focus on the tactile-kinesthetic feeling of stuttering and seek ways of reducing that tension. This is the essence of stuttering modification, and all therapy up to this point has been an attempt to prepare the child for this moment. All stuttering clients must learn the valuable lesson that there is a less deviant, less abnormal way to stutter.

VOLUNTARY STUTTERING

Along with this "pullout" activity, I teach children to insert mild voluntary stutterings into their speech. These are short repetitions and prolongations that are hardly noticeable. At first, I signal them when to insert the voluntary stuttering during structured activities. Later, using some reinforcer, I encourage children to pick their own time to stutter "easy."

The advantages of voluntary stuttering are difficult to explain to nonstutterers. The publications by Van Riper[12] and Sheehan[14] are two excellent sources that discuss the curative properties of this method of reducing anxiety and stuttering severity.

My experience has been that voluntary stuttering reduces rate, and improves proprioceptive ability by getting the child to focus on articulatory movement. Voluntary stuttering provides a means of practicing for the "real thing." The child is teaching himself or herself concepts of "easy stuttering" or stuttering with less abnormality. Finally, voluntary stuttering reduces anxiety. People who stutter, because they are normal in appearance, typically fear revealing their abnormality to others. Trying to hide through avoidance only adds to their anxiety. Voluntary stuttering relieves some of that pressure. They are exposing little bits of themselves in a manner that is both comfortable and socially tolerated.

Expected Outcomes

I have always been uncomfortable predicting the results of treatment for stuttering. It goes back to the unpredictability and variability of this disorder. If treatment is to be deemed successful, it must be tested over time, but the discipline of collecting longitudinal data is not one I possess. In addition, how long do we collect these data and what are the criteria for success?

My own personal stuttering could not withstand the test of time. I completed what I thought was successful therapy in 1971, only to have a relapse of severe stuttering 10 years later. How then do I evaluate the treatment given to me since I am currently working on my own relapse?

Enough! Forgive my equivocating but I cannot give specific percentages for successful treatment. This should obviously cast suspicion on the treatment methodology! I have continued to be critical of the treatment outlined above but so far have been unable to find a better alternative. Of course the earlier we commence treatment, when stuttering is still mild, the better the prognosis. This is just common sense. It is also common sense that once a child reaches ages 8 to 10, has been in school for several years, and has experienced a progressive escalation in stuttering severity, the prognosis for a quick, painless recovery is less realistic.

Conclusion

Being around stuttering children for 20 years has brought me great joy, but also heartache. My young clients have tested me and have presented mysteries at times that I could not solve. I have much to learn about this puzzling disorder, and I hope that you will join me in the search for better methods of treating this enigmatic human affliction.

Acknowledgments.   I would like to thank my colleague Richard Jacques, Ph.D., for his editorial contributions.

Suggested Readings

In addition to the references cited in the text, the following may be helpful in work with stuttering children.

Conture EG: *Stuttering*, ed 2. Englewood Cliffs, NJ, Prentice-Hall, 1990.

>   Much of Conture's book is devoted to children who stutter. This is seldom the case with stuttering textbooks. Although a scholarly work, this book does present information that is relevant to the clinician in the field.

Peters TJ, Guitar B: *Stuttering: An Integration of Contemporary Therapies*. Memphis, Speech Foundation of America, 1980.

>   Peters and Guitar discuss the different approaches that are being used to treat stuttering children. They provide guidelines designed to aid the clinician in choosing the appropriate methodology for each stuttering client. An attempt is made to find an eclectic middle ground.

Peters TJ, Guitar B: *Stuttering: An Integrated Approach to Its Nature and Treatment*, Baltimore, Williams & Wilkins, 1991.

>   This is a more thorough look at the subject they began exploring in 1980 (see above).

Starkweather CW, Gottwald SR, Halfond MM: *Stuttering Prevention: A Clinical Method*. Englewood Cliffs, NJ, Prentice-Hall, 1990.

>   This is a detailed description of the work being done at Temple University with young children who are in danger of continuing the progressive cycle of stuttering.

References

1. Sheehan J, Martyn MM: Spontaneous recovery from stuttering. *J Speech Hear Res* 1966; 10:121–135.
2. Fraser J, Perkins WH (eds): *Do You Stutter: A Guide for Teens*. Memphis, Speech Foundation of America, 1987.
3. Conture EG, Fraser J (eds): *Stuttering and Your Child: Questions and Answers*. Memphis, Speech Foundation of America, 1989.
4. Ainsworth S, Fraser J (eds): *If Your Child Stutters: A Guide for Parents*. Memphis, Speech Foundation of America, 1988.
5. *A Brochure for Parents of Children Who Stutter*. San Francisco, National Stuttering Project (4601 Irving Street, San Francisco, CA 94122-1020).
6. Riley GD: A stuttering severity scale for children and adults. *Journal Speech and Hearing Disorders*. 1972; 37:314–320.
7. Johnson W, Darley FL, Spriestersbach DC: *Diagnostic Methods in Speech Pathology*. New York, Harper & Row, 1963.
8. Bloodstein O: *A Handbook on Stuttering*, ed 3. Chicago, National Easter Seal Society, 1981.
9. Van Riper C: *The Nature of Stuttering*, ed 2. Englewood Cliffs, NJ, Prentice-Hall, 1982.
10. Cooper EB: *Chronic Stuttering: Todd's Story*. San Francisco, National Stuttering Project (4601 Irving Street, San Francisco, CA 94122-1020).
11. Johnson W: *People in Quandaries*. New York, Harper & Row, 1946.
12. Van Riper C: *The Treatment of Stuttering*. Englewood Cliffs, NJ, Prentice-Hall, 1973.
13. Dell CW: *Treating the School Age Stutterer: A Guide for Clinicians*. Memphis, Speech Foundation of America, 1979.
14. Sheehan JG: *Stuttering: Research and Therapy*. New York, Harper & Row, 1970.

4

Behavioral Treatment of Stuttering Children

Janis Costello Ingham, Ph.D.

Introduction

The assessment and treatment of children who stutter have been controversial topics for decades, although behavioral techniques have become increasingly popular and accepted over the years. This may be because these are the techniques that stem most directly from known principles of human behavior and are supported most clearly by evidence obtained in laboratory and field experiments. Behavioral techniques require clinicians to rely primarily on observable phenomena in children's behavior and to resist making diagnostic and treatment decisions based on speculation or intuition. What follows is a description of the methods of assessment and treatment used in our clinic with children (aged 2 to 8 or so) who stutter. They are based upon behavioral principles and are a combination of techniques gleaned from the experimental literature and from clinical experiences.

Clinical Evaluation

In this sytem the purpose of clinical evaluation is threefold: (1) to make a judgment of whether the child is a stutterer, (2) to recommend an appropriate type of remediation program (given that the child is judged to be a stutterer), and (3) to specify and systematically measure the relevant characteristics of the child's speech to serve as a baseline against which to compare future measures.

Case History

For this kind of assessment, I have found that traditional case history information has rather limited value for the diagnosis of childhood stuttering, because young stutterers are typically free of predictive birth, developmental, and family histories. One exception is information regarding family history of stuttering. When children have immediate family members who are or have been stutterers, the possibility that those children's nonfluencies may be stutterings is enhanced.[1] However, neither the research literature nor personal experience leads to the belief that such information is useful in predicting children's ultimate response to treatment. For example, two 7-year-old twin (dizygotic) brothers treated several years ago in our clinic showed quite diverse responses to treatment. The stuttering of one changed relatively quickly and generalized broadly, while the other required much longer and more intensive treatment.

Other information of value that I seek from parents during the diagnostic interview relates to whether they consider their child to be a stutterer and, if so, how long the child's stuttering has existed. I consider longer than 6 months a hallmark. I also inquire as to whether a child's nonfluencies fluctuate across time and across situations. Such fluctuation is typical of early stuttering. The parents' report of their children's reactions to their nonfluencies is also informative. Stories of children's expressions of frustration, anger, or bewilderment regarding why words cannot be produced at certain times, or reports of children being unwilling to attempt speech in certain circumstances, are definitely influential in establishing the existence of stuttering.

A primary function of taking a case history is that it provides an opportunity for parents to air their feelings and fears regarding their children's speech. Many parents have heard the folklore that suggests that something in their relationship with their child is responsible for stuttering.[2] Or perhaps they have their own theory of the cause of stuttering for their child, and they want to have the chance to discuss their ideas with an expert. The interview used to obtain case history information affords an opportunity for parents to express these notions and for me to allay their fears (by assuring them that there is no evidence to support parental responsibility as a cause of stuttering),[3] to update them on recent theories and relevant research regarding potential etiologies of stuttering, and to inform them of the success rates associated with treatment of stuttering in young children. During this interview, as well, I discuss with the parents their role in treatment of the child's stuttering, should treatment be recommended. This is a chance to ascertain whether they are responsive to sharing the responsibility for the child's treatment.

Observation and Tests

First, the following caveat: A child's suspected fluency disorder must not be allowed to distract the clinician from noticing whether other communication difficulties exist. In fact, there is some evidence to suggest that a substantial number of stuttering children are prone to display other concomitant communication problems. Therefore, I employ standard screening procedures for the presence of hearing, language, phonology, and voice disorders to determine if further diagnostic testing is needed. If such problems exist at a clinically significant level, and the child is also determined to stutter, I will have to decide whether to design treatment that addresses those problems concurrently, or whether to concentrate on the constituent that appears most fundamental to the child's aberrant communicative status and, in the meantime, monitor the status of the other dimension(s).

In the diagnostic process of discovering and describing stuttering, the most critical information is obtained from direct observation of the child's speech and the analyses that are drawn from those observations. This process extends over a period of several weeks so that the chance of observing all variations in the child's speech is enhanced. I obtain a set of audio- and/or video-recorded standard talking samples (STSs) from each child.[4,5] These are connected speech samples taken from multiple settings with different speaking partners that are representative of common speaking situations for the child. Each is generally 10 to 15 minutes in length. (The goal is to obtain a cumulative 5 minutes of child speech from each sample.) A typical set of STSs might be (1) conversation in the clinic with the clinician, (2) conversation in the clinic with one parent, (3) reading in the clinic (for older children), (4) conversation at home with the other parent or a grandparent, and (5) conversation at home with a sibling or at school with a peer. (It is important that at least two of these samples are obtained in natural settings outside of the clinic.) These recordings are typically made once per week for a period of at least 4 weeks before a final judgment is made regarding whether the child is a stutterer and, if so, whether and what kind of treatment ought to be planned. (Beyond-clinic recordings are one example of responsibilities we expect parents to undertake.) Thus, the assessment procedures that help determine whether a child is a stutterer in the first place also serve as baseline against which to measure behavior change for those children enrolled for treatment.*

ANALYSES OF STANDARD TALKING SAMPLES

A number of relevant aspects of children's speech can be empirically evaluated from the STSs. Further, each can be compared across samples for a given sampling period (week) as well as across time for the 4 weeks of the evaluation period. Thus, the full range of variability (for which stuttering is infamous) can be observed. The dimensions of speech that are most basic to this analysis are frequency of stuttering, speech rate, and speech naturalness. Other measures that may be useful are the duration of typical and outlying stutterings, the duration of typical and outlying stutter-free utterances, and global ratings of stuttering severity.

Frequency of Stuttering. The occurrence of stuttering is, of course, the primary behavior of interest in determining whether a child is a stutterer and in gauging the severity of the disorder once it is determined to exist. However, measuring this phenomenon is not as straightforward as one might hope. To determine whether a child is, in fact, a stutterer, the occurrence of even only one genuine moment of stuttering ought to be sufficient. To gauge the severity of the disorder, in order to aid in the selection of an appropriate treatment program and to provide objective evidence of the status of stuttering prior to treatment (and thereafter), more particular information is required. Still, both of these goals require the examiner to be able to recognize the occurrence of a stutter in the speech of a child. Herein lies the rub!

Distinguishing between nonfluencies that are normal and nonfluencies that are stuttered requires perceptual judgments on the part of the listener, and there is no

---

*For the child for whom periodic monitoring is recommended before a decision regarding enrollment in treatment is made, STSs are obtained every 2 to 3 months until the data convince the child's parents and me that the child is definitely stuttering (perhaps even getting worse) or is definitely not stuttering (perhaps even showing the frequency of nonfluencies to be subsiding over time—the "spontaneous recovery" reported to occur for some children who stutter).[6]

independent way to validate the correctness of those judgments. While many nonfluencies are obvious to listeners as unusual or pathological, some nonfluencies, especially those occurring in the speech of potential incipient stutterers, may be equivocal. Some researchers have attempted to differentiate stuttered and nonstuttered nonfluencies on the basis of topography (e.g., phrase repetitions and revisions versus silent and audible part-word repetitions and prolongations)[7]; others have trusted the validity of the practiced listener's "perceptual threshold" for discerning which nonfluencies are stutters and which are normal disfluencies.[8] Neither method has produced satisfactory reliability among different listeners.[9,10]

I prefer the latter method. Assisted by a computerized program, a clinician listens to the child's speech sample (e.g., the STSs) and presses a button whenever the child is judged to stutter. The button is pressed once for each new occasion of stuttering, independent of its duration. The computer program converts these counts into the percentage of syllables spoken that are stuttered (%SS). Typically the clinician will have listened to samples of the child's speech beforehand and will be familiar with the varieties of forms of stuttering the child produces. There is no attempt, however, to designate particular topographies of nonfluencies as stuttered or not stuttered. That is, clinicians at our clinic do not make a priori definitions of stuttering and record only forms of speech that meet those definitions. Rather we listen to the child's speech and signal (by the button press) any event that surpasses our perceptual threshold of normalcy. We keep in mind that some nonfluencies are normal, and attempt to disregard those in our counts. Therefore, the computer records the number of stutters (and %SS) that are judged to occur in a particular sample.

Reliability of Judgments of Stutterings. Using the above-described method, it is important that clinicians assess their self-agreement. The value of counts of stuttering is negated if those counts are not reliable. Therefore, relistening and recounting and comparing second counts with the first set are important activities to help verify the caliber of the data collected. Clinicians who cannot agree with themselves regarding counts of stuttering from specific speech samples need self-training and practice until they have established such consistency. This will also be important for the clinician during treatment activities. Unfortunately, training programs that teach the skill of reliable identification of stutters are not currently available (although such a program is in the early stages of preparation in our laboratory).

At certain points in the use of a measurement system such as that described above, assessment of interjudge reliability is also pertinent. That is, clinicians should confirm their judgments of stuttering by asking other listeners to make the same judgments on at least some of the same samples. Certainly before the child is formally diagnosed as a stutterer, corroborating judgments of another experienced speech-language clinician should be obtained, based on that person's stuttering counts made on the STSs. Such confirmation is appropriate, as well, when decisions regarding termination of treatment are made.

Speech Rate. The speed of a child's speech is important to assess for a variety of reasons. First, of course, the clinician would like to know whether the child's speech rate is within normal ranges. The presence of stuttering typically slows down overall speech rate (e.g., the number of speech units produced per amount of speaking time); therefore, increases in speech rate are to be expected as one by-product of successful treatment. Some children (and many adults) who stutter actually speak at unusually fast rates. If this is recognized, treatment directed toward speech rate modification alone may lead to reductions in stuttering. Because of the presence of stuttering, fast speaking rates are sometimes difficult to identify unless speaking rate measures are obtained only from periods of speech that do not contain stutterings. This *articulatory rate* can be highly informative.

Another reason to measure speech rate is to ascertain whether differences in stuttering frequency across different samples (i.e., in different settings or in comparisons of pretreatment and posttreatment speech samples) might be artifacts of reductions in speech rate rather than "real" changes in the child's manner of speaking.

Our clinic measures speech rate with the computer setup mentioned above. As the clinician listens to the child's speech sample, a button is pressed as each syllable is produced. A second button is pressed for *stuttered* syllables, as described above. At the end of the speech sample, the computer calculates overall speaking rate as the average number of syllables spoken per minute of the child's talking time. The total syllable count is also used in the calculation of %SS (described above).

Speech Naturalness.   In the last decade, stuttering frequency and speech rate have become relatively common, utilitarian measures of the speech performance of people who stutter. However, clinicians and researchers have struggled to find a method to assess empirically the rather global aspect of speech production referred to as speech quality, or speech naturalness. For example, two stutterers who are similar in regard to %SS and syllables per minute still may not be perceived as equally impaired. In spite of occurrences of stuttering, one may speak in a style that listeners judge to be relatively natural, while the other may sound highly unnatural. Likewise, two stutterers may display no stuttering and speech rate within normal ranges at the end of treatment, but sound quite different in regard to the naturalness of their speech. The speech of one may be perceived as tentative, uneven, prolonged, or calculated, while the speech of the other may sound highly natural, spontaneous, and essentially indistinguishable from that of non-stutterers. The speech naturalness measure described by Martin, Haroldson, and Triden,[11] and now in frequent use in the literature, has been shown to be a valid and reliable indicator of this heretofore unmeasured aspect of speech production (although, interestingly, naturalness ratings for children's speech have only infrequently been reported in the literature).[12]

In our system,[13] a computer keeps track of the listener's periodic ratings of naturalness. While the clinician is listening to the speech sample and pressing buttons in time with the child's production of stuttered and nonstuttered syllables, every 15 seconds a signal sounds. At this time the clinician rates the perceived naturalness of the child's speech for the preceding 15 seconds by touching the appropriate number between 1 and 9 on the computer keyboard. A rating of 1 indicates the child's speech was perceived to be "highly natural"; a rating of 9 indicates the child's speech was perceived to be "highly unnatural." Research using this system with adult speakers indicates that the speech of nonstuttering speakers is typically rated between 1 and 3.[11]

Social Validity.   Before a final decision is made regarding a diagnosis of stuttering, the input of other relevant persons is sought. That is, at our clinic we attempt to confirm the validity of our diagnosis by asking others their perception of the child's speech. The viewpoint of the parents, obtained during the case history interview, is one source of social validity.[14] We usually ask at least two other sources—one familiar with the child's speech in natural settings, such as the child's teacher, and one who is unfamiliar with the child or with communication disorders in general, such as a layperson visitor to the clinic. (The layperson is asked to watch or listen to a representative sampling of the child's STSs.) We ask these independent sources simply to judge whether they consider the child to be a stutterer. These same sources are consulted again at the termination of treatment, thereby serving to confirm (or otherwise) the success of treatment. The children themselves can also provide input into whether or not they stutter. Older children can be asked directly their opinion on the subject. For younger children (who might not understand the question if it were put to them directly), inferences can be made from parental reports and examiner observations of a child's awareness or frustration regarding speech.

Other Measures.   Especially for the child who is judged in need of treatment, two other analyses of the STSs are useful: duration of stutterings and duration of stutter-free utterances. One of the first changes apparent during treatment is typically a reduction in the duration of individual moments of stuttering, especially because accessory feature components (ancillary facial and body movements, avoidance mechanisms, etc.) are virtually eliminated. This change in behavior is not necessarily reflected in %SS data, but it is revealed in measures of (1) the durations of the three longest stutters in a sample and (2) the average duration of stutters in the sample (based on a random sampling of a minimum of ten stutters). These measures add empirical information to the picture of the overall severity of a child's stuttering and are also extremely potent in the evaluation of change produced by treatment (i.e., in pretreatment-posttreatment STS comparisons).

Most of the speech sample analyses described thus far emphasize, directly or indirectly, stuttered nonfluencies. However, the aspects of the child's speech that are of primary interest during treatment are utterances that are stutter-free. For this reason, empirical information regarding the status of stutter-free utterances in a child's pretreatment speech is beneficial for treatment planning and for assessment of the progress of treatment. Therefore, from representative STSs clinicians tally the lengths of stutter-free periods (i.e., the number of syllables that occur between moments of stuttering) and then summarize the findings by reporting the average length of stutter-free speaking periods and the length of the longest stutter-free period in the sample.

Summary.   It should be obvious from the substantial number of pages allocated to this section that a diagnosis and any treatment that ensues (when appropriate) are predicated on thorough and detailed assessment procedures. The variability that may exist in the child's speech is examined through multiple speech samples obtained over time in a variety of settings with different pertinent speaking partners. Empirical descriptions of those speech samples are made, providing quantitative measurement of the dimensions of speech considered most relevant:

frequency of stuttering, speech rate, speech naturalness, durations of stutters, and durations of stutter-free utterances. This evidence serves as the basis for deciding whether the child is a stutterer, and this "objective" finding is bolstered by the more impressionistic judgments of social validity informants. Further, for the child who is diagnosed as one who stutters, these measures provide baseline data for the treatment that will follow and a standard against which to compare the child's speech performance at the termination of treatment.

CASE SELECTION CRITERIA

The crux of the issue regarding whether the child's speech is considered to contain stuttering is determined *before* most of the above-described measures are made. That is, the frequency of stuttering cannot be assessed unless and until the examiner has identified the presence of stutters in the child's repertoire. Therefore, the most fundamental part of the process is not necessarily an empirical one; it is the examiner's judgment that at least some of the child's nonfluencies are perceived to be stutters. And because the examiner, as a speech-language pathologist, has special expertise in making such judgments, I believe that the perceptions of the examiner generally hold the greatest weight. However, if an examiner's stutter counts are not reliable (i.e., in self-agreement comparisons and with another speech-language pathologist), this may indicate that the child's nonfluencies are too ambiguous to be considered bona fide stutters. Further, if an examiner's judgments are not supported by the impressions of the social validity informants (parents, teachers, laypersons, children themselves), a diagnostic label of "stutterer" would be withheld.

Another kind of reliability that should be considered in arriving at a verdict regarding whether a child's speech is indicative of stuttering is the consistency exhibited by the child in the STSs obtained across settings and over time. While a wide range of variability is expected in the speech of young children who may be incipient stutterers, substantial numbers of samples that contain little or no stuttering are not expected. If this is combined with generally low stuttering counts across samples, again, the diagnostic label of stutterer would be withheld.

For a child whose speech characteristics cannot be reliably judged as stuttering (by the examiner's measures or consistency of the child's performance across settings and time), the continuation of bimonthly STSs (often referred to as monitoring) will eventually establish the child's fluency status. If the child is, or becomes, one who stutters, moments of stuttering will become more consistent across settings and time and easier for the examiner to identify reliably. And, if periodic monitoring is carried out frequently enough, the child will be identified as one in need of treatment early enough not to have a negative effect on the outcome of that treatment or on the child's social development.

Clinical Management

A recent review of the literature related to treatment of children who stutter[15] indicates that direct, behavioral treatments, even for preschool-age children, have at last become acceptable and, in fact, even popular. This may be because these are the methods that have been derived from systematic experimentation and, therefore, have the greatest amount of evidence to support them. Or it may be simply because once tried, their effectiveness is obvious and their harm, fictional. The particular approaches to behavioral treatment that I advocate have been described previously[16-19] and will be updated and detailed with greater specificity in the pages that follow. Throughout the years the fundamental principles of this treatment have remained unchanged. The procedures rely on (1) arranging extensive talking opportunities for the child and using these to facilitate successful and progressively more realistic speaking experiences, (2) objectively recording relevant observable features of the child's behavior (the moments of stuttering, stutter-free utterances, speech rate, and speech naturalness described above) and using these records to evaluate continually the progress of treatment, (3) developing a functional feedback system and using it to decrease the frequency of stuttering and enhance stutter-free speech, and (4) assessing the generalization and maintenance of fluency change in the child's speech in the natural environment and using this information to modify treatment procedures as necessary to produce clinically significant effects.

Treatment Goals

The espoused goals of this treatment are to facilitate children's spontaneous and automatic use of natural-sounding, stutter-free speech under all talking conditions, in all settings, with all speaking partners and audiences. *Spontaneous and automatic* means that the speech used by the child at the termination of treatment should not require special attention or effort on the child's part. *Natural-sounding, stutter-free speech* refers to speech that is indistinguishable from that of a child's nonstuttering peers. In other words, the goals of this treatment are that its beneficiaries become normal speakers.

Treatment Procedures

The treatments I and my colleagues use, while based on the principles listed above and elucidated below, can be highly individualized so that they suit the speech characteristics and personalities of the children served. They are driven by continuous evaluations of their effects, so that unsuccessful treatment strategies can be modified midstream. I do not adhere to one particular treatment program, but rather to an overarching set of principles that takes various forms. These principles and some of their manifestations in terms of treatment strategies are described in what follows.

SPEAKING TASKS

Behavioral treatments gain their label by concentrating treatment directly on the behaviors considered to be "correct" and "incorrect." In the case of children who stutter, correct behaviors are periods of speech that do not contain stuttering, and incorrect behaviors are syllables or words that are perceived to be stuttered. Obviously, the occurrence of these two central response classes cannot be observed or modified unless the child is talking. Therefore, an important aspect of treatment is the use of activities that will generate lots of speech from the child. (For some children who may be particularly reticent or even uncooperative, treatment begins with procedures aimed exclusively at encouraging talking, fluent or otherwise.)

With children aged about 4 and over, I often to arrange speaking activities that control the length and complexity of children's utterances. By first building a foundation of short, simple, stutter-free utterances, the clinician can expand children's fluency gradually by facilitating stutter-free utterances that are progressively longer. I have referred to this treatment strategy as "extended length of utterance" (ELU).[16] Its forebear is Ryan's[20] "gradual increase in length and complexity of utterance" (GILCU). (A more detailed description of the ELU program appears later in this chapter.) The length of children's utterances can be controlled by the use of clinician models, written stimuli, or the presentation of pictures or topics that evoke responses of the desired length. The latter is generally preferred, but sometimes a mixture of these different forms of evoking stimuli is useful—especially for children who are not very successful at producing stutter-free spontaneous responses in early treatment steps.

ELU treatment procedures are less appropriate for very young children who stutter (e.g., 2- and 3-year-olds). Because these children are in the early stages of language development, their utterances are generally short in the first place, so controlling their length is less important. Further, because the metalinguistic awareness of very young children is not yet developed, they are generally unable to use speech for "display" purposes or to conceive of speech as a practice activity. Hence, the kinds of speech activities required in ELU procedures (e.g., naming strings of pictures, formulating short phrases and sentences to describe the content of pictures, speaking continuously for progressively longer periods from 3 seconds to 5 minutes) are difficult for very young children and, therefore, not appropriate. These younger children are generally treated via conversational speech between the child and clinician during play activities known to be of special interest to the child. Of course, the clinician needs to select play activities in which talking on the part of the child is essential and in which a variety of child speech acts are likely to occur. And, as clinicians already know, it is vital to have a range of such activities available to maintain the child's interest and spontaneity. Although clinicians necessarily shoulder a major part of the burden for maintaining conversation with very young children, the focus is on obtaining as much talking on the part of the child as possible. (This is sometimes tricky for speech-language pathologists; many of us seem to get into this business because we like to talk ourselves!)

Broadly, the bulk of treatment is conducted during children's spontaneous connected speech, although, as described above, treatment may begin with shorter, nonconversational utterances. Often monologue speaking tasks are used early in treatment, because they afford children the opportunity to produce a lot of speech without having to deal with the pragmatic, interactive components of dyadic language use, such as responding to questions, turn taking, coping with interruptions, and producing utterances that are responsive to themes introduced by the conversational partner. In addition, children who are able to read may use oral reading as a speaking task early in treatment. This is a task that is generally easier than conversation, because not only are the pragmatic requirements removed, but so are the demands of planning and executing the syntactic and semantic components of a message. However, when treatment has been initiated in reading or monologue, clinicians should move to connected conversational speech as rapidly as a child's developing fluency skills allow, because that is the style of speech used most often in the natural environment and thus the style of speech the child needs to practice under treatment conditions. It is also the most difficult style of speech for most children who stutter; so when they have mastered it, they are typically able to speak fluently in monologue and reading, even if they have not had direct treatment in those modalities. On the other hand, generalization does not usually flow in the reverse direction (i.e., from reading to connected speech).

Summary. The first step in treatment is the selection of speaking activities that meet the requirements of the treatment program, that are within the capabilities of the child, and that will sustain the child's efforts to speak so that treatment methods can be applied. Speech-language pathologists are typically highly skilled at developing creative and interesting methods for getting children to talk, so this aspect of treatment presents nothing particularly new to the practicing clinician, except, perhaps, the emphasis that is placed on it in this treatment. A general rule of treatment is that the more talking produced by the child, the more likely, and the more quickly, that treatment will be effective.

MEASUREMENT

Within-Treatment Measurement. The use of measurement is inherent in our treatment, which cannot begin until target behaviors have been specified. That is, the clinician must identify observable behaviors in a given child's speech that are to be the targets of treatment. Typically, these are stutters (to be reduced or eliminated) and occasions of stutter-free speech (to be increased). The previous discussion of clinicians' perceptual judgments of stutters is pertinent here as well. Treatment depends upon the clinician's skill in immediately discriminating all occasions of stuttering in the child's speech. Although occasions of stutter-free speech are typically targeted as well, the clinician's recognition of such occasions hinges upon recognition of stutterings, because stutter-free speech is just that: speech that does not contain stuttering. The unit of stutter-free speech that is targeted varies with different treatment strategies, but it is generally defined by its duration in syllables, words, or length of talking time.

I follow the principles of programmed instruction[21] in which target behavior requirements are increased slowly and in small steps. For example, in the ELU program (see Appendix A) early steps require stutter-free production of utterances that are one, then two, then three syllables in length, and later the requirement becomes stutter-free utterances that are 3, 5, and 10 seconds in length, until late in the program stutter-free responses of 3, 4, and 5 minutes are required.*

---

*For the younger child who is unable to segment responses in a manner appropriate for the ELU program, a modified version of the concept is applied in the context of child-clinician conversations. Based on pretreatment analyses of the child's speech, the clinician selects stutter-free responses of a specific duration as a treatment target. When 90% of a child's utterances of the designated length (and shorter) are stutter-free, the target is raised to a longer utterance and so forth until the ultimate criterion of complete fluency is met.

Programmed instruction also stipulates mastery of each step as prerequisite to advancement to the next step. Mastery is operationalized by specifying a minimum level of performance required at each treatment step. For example, in the ELU program, mastery of step 14 (3-minute stutter-free monologue) requires that level of performance to be achieved five times, consecutively. Specification of such a "pass criterion" is made on the assumption that a child's successful performance implies proficiency in the skill required at that stage of the program and also establishes a base upon which to build the next level of behavior. Treatments also specify "fail criteria," the level at which a child's performance on a given step of the program is deemed unsatisfactory and change in the treatment program is sought so that the child does not continue failing. In the ELU program, for example, the fail criterion for step 14 is seven consecutive trials containing stuttering, or 50 attempts to produce the specified stutter-free behavior without meeting the pass criterion.*

In order to ascertain when a child has met the pass criterion (or fallen to the level of the fail criterion), performance data must be obtained on-line during treatment. This means that the clinician scores each trial as correct or incorrect on a data sheet so that it is apparent when either criterion has been reached. This simple kind of event recording also allows calculation of the number of trials required to meet the criterion and the percentage of correct trials for each step of the program. These numbers reflect the ease with which children progress through treatment and highlight program steps that are difficult, and therefore might be revised before the treatment program is used with another child.

Beyond-Treatment Measurement.   The first section of this chapter described measurement procedures used during the pretreatment assessment period, especially data collected from weekly STSs. STSs continue to be obtained throughout the duration of a child's treatment (about once monthly) and at follow-up (at progressively longer intervals) in a time-series fashion. Thus, information regarding the effects of treatment on the child's speech beyond the confines of the treatment setting (i.e., across-settings generalization) is readily available to the clinician and aids decisions of when to terminate treatment or when to modify treatment to enhance its effectiveness.

Summary.   A prominent component of this treatment is continuous measurement of the child's stuttering and stutter-free behaviors. STSs continue to be obtained and analyzed as described earlier, and on-line performance data are collected for every speech attempt during treatment sessions. Thus, decisions regarding moving ahead to more advanced stages of treatment, modifying aspects of the treat-

---

*While the concept of "pass criteria" is quite logical, the *particular* pass criterion specified for any treatment step within any treatment program (including the ELU program) is basically arbitrary. That is, clinicians or program designers simply use their best judgment and their clinical experience to suggest the level at which a response should be produced to meet the assumption of mastery. This is clearly an area in need of research. In actuality, a treatment program may be unnecessarily long because unduly high pass criteria are specified for every step; other programs may be unsuccessful in producing substantial and durable behavior change because they do not establish sufficient mastery of the responses required for individual program steps. Fail criteria are equally arbitrary. Nonetheless, specification of pass and fail criteria lends consistency to the administration of the treatment program and prevents capricious judgments of how and when to move children forward in the treatment program.

ment that are not productive, and terminating treatment are all made on the basis of evidence regarding the status of a child's speech in and out of the clinic setting.

FEEDBACK

The most crucial ingredient of the behavioral treatments used in our clinic is the response-contingent feedback system. Our treatments rely heavily on the principles of positive reinforcement and negative feedback (sometimes referred to as punishment, although I find the connotations associated with that term to be unduly punitive). As was mentioned above, two response classes are of primary interest in the treatment of the speech of children who stutter: moments of stuttering and periods of stutter-free speech. In a simplistic sense, stuttering and fluency are reciprocals, with changes in the frequency of occurrence of one producing covariations in the other. Therefore, procedures that reduce or eliminate moments of stuttering leave speech that is stutter-free; procedures that increase the amount of stutter-free speech necessarily reduce occurrences of stuttering. Thus, the appropriateness of the use of response-contingent feedback in treatment becomes obvious. The presentation of positive reinforcers contingent upon stutter-free speech increases the amount of stutter-free speech produced by the child; the presentation of negative feedback contingent upon occasions of stuttering reduces the frequency of stuttering produced by the child.

In theory, treatment ought to be able to be approached from either direction. However, it has been our practice to use a "double-barreled" approach that combines both procedures. That is, occasions of stutter-free speech are followed immediately by presentation of functional positive reinforcers, and occasions of stuttering are followed immediately by negative feedback. Both of these contingencies play an important role in the ultimate effects of treatment. Interestingly, it is my impression, bolstered by some experimental findings,[17,22] that reductions in stuttering frequency are dependent upon the provision of stuttering-contingent negative feedback. The tactic of reinforcing stutter-free utterances to "drive out" stutterings is not particularly powerful.* On the other hand, positive reinforcement of stutter-free utterances appears to sustain children's participation in treatment activities and give children the opportunity to discover enjoyment and self-satisfaction in talking. Further, when positive reinforcement and negative feedback are combined, milder forms of negative feedback can be used, and a positive relationship between the child and the clinician can be maintained (and even enhanced), because the clinician is associated with the presentation of reinforcement. The use of programmed instruction concepts in the design of treatment ensures that the balance between reinforcement and negative feedback always weighs heavily in favor of reinforcement.

Selection of Positive and Negative Feedback Stimuli.   Given that positive reinforcement and negative feedback are crucial components of treatment, discovery of

---

*The case for reinforcement may be different for older children whose stuttering is more severe and for adults. That is, if treatment is designed to teach a new or different speech pattern—for example, one that emanates from prolonged speech—the role of reinforcement in the acquisition of this response may be more important. However, for young children, the implicit assumption is that the segments of their speech that are stutter-free are essentially normal speech. Therefore, treatment is designed to rid that normal speech of occasions of stuttering.

functional positive and negative stimuli becomes a significant issue. It is well known that stimuli that function as positive reinforcers (or negative stimuli) for one child do not necessarily work in the same way for all children. While clinicians can often make good guesses based on their clinical experience with children, those guesses must be tested in order to ensure that the selected stimuli actually do have the power to affect behavior in the predicted direction.

In our clinic, we conduct tests of the function of selected feedback stimuli during early stages of treatment using a simple within-subject time-series design (basically, ABA).[23] The first three or four sessions are divided into eight, equal time-periods, and relevant aspects of the child's speech are measured in the same way throughout all periods. Table 4-1 illustrates the manipulations that are made in each period and the outcomes that would be expected if the selected positive and negative feedback stimuli were functional. Each stimulus is tested alone and compared to the child's baseline performance. Finally, the combination of positive and negative stimuli is tested and evaluated against baseline performance and then replicated to ensure that it is reliable. This "mini-experiment," then, indicates whether the stimuli selected for feedback during treatment are functional for the particular child to be treated. The same procedure is used later in treatment if the clinician suspects (or the data indicate) that one or both of the stimuli may be "wearing out" and need replacement or adjustment.

Several factors influence the selection of particular stimuli for feedback procedures. Generally, positive reinforcers should be able to be dispensed quickly, be relatively inexpensive (typically parents are asked to supply the reinforcers),

Table 4-1. Method of Testing Function of Positive and Negative Stimuli Selected for Use in Treatment

Period	Procedure	Expected Outcome
1	All feedback regarding occasions of stuttering and stutter-free speech withheld	Stuttering and stutter-free speech at baseline rates
2	Stuttering-contingent negative stimulus presented following all occasions of stuttering (feedback for stutter-free speech withheld)	Frequency of stuttering decreases in comparison to period 1 (and number of stutter-free utterances increases)
3	Same as period 1	Stuttering and stutter-free utterances similar to baseline
4	Positive stimulus presented contingent on every stutter-free utterance of predetermined length (and feedback regarding stuttering withheld)	Number of stutter-free utterances increases in comparison to period 3 (and frequency of stutters decreases)
5	Same as period 1	Stuttering and stutter-free utterances similar to baseline
6	Both negative and positive stimuli applied to stuttered and nonstuttered utterances, respectively	Stuttering decreases in frequency and stutter-free utterances increase in comparison to period 5
7	Same as period 1	Stuttering and stutter-free utterances similar to baseline
8	Same as period 6	Same as period 6

and of course, be of value to the child being treated. Negative stimuli should also be capable of being administered quickly and conveniently. Because they are used in conjunction with positive stimuli, mild (relatively nonaversive) negative stimuli are all that is necessary. Table 4-2 lists a few positive and negative stimuli that are oftentimes functional for young children. Ideas for positive and negative stimuli are limited only by the clinician's creativity and an individual child's preferences.

For older children (over age 4 or 5 years), token reinforcement systems are quite useful. In such systems, the reinforcer given to the child immediately following a stutter-free response (and, perhaps, withdrawn immediately following a stuttered response) is simply a token—that is, a token of the reinforcement that will eventually be earned. Tokens are stimuli that have no inherent value for the child until they have been paired with functional backup reinforcers. Our clinic uses ordinary white beans or Styrofoam "squiggles" (packing materials) as tokens. Prior to treatment, the token system is established by systematically pairing the neutral stimuli with functional positive reinforcers. (See Appendix B for an example of how this is accomplished.) The token system is held together by the power of backup reinforcers that are periodically awarded in exchange for a given number of tokens. It is important that backup reinforcers are earned often enough that the tokens do not lose their reinforcing properties through lack of pairing with functional reinforcers. We typically use a "reinforcement menu" (see Appendix C) to determine the backup reinforcers for a particular child.

Feedback Schedules.   The well-known principles of schedules of reinforcement are applied throughout the course of this treatment. Thus, in the early stages, during the establishment of new behavior in children's repertoires, feedback (both social and material) is provided for every correct (fluent) and incorrect (stuttered) response. However, as treatment progresses, reinforcement schedules are gradually "thinned" so that a reinforcer is earned after the occurrence of two fluent responses, then three, and so on. The goal is to achieve, by the end of treatment, a reinforcement schedule that approximates that of the natural environment (a schedule that may be extremely sparse).

In the spirit of altering treatment so that it becomes progressively more similar to the contingencies that exist in the natural environment, the kinds of stimuli used as positive reinforcers also change. In the beginning, "contrived" reinforcers (such as toys, prizes, opportunities to play a game, etc.), usually paired with clinician praise, are used as positive stimuli. However, as early as possible, clinicians should

Table 4-2.   Sample Positive and Negative Feedback Stimuli
for Use with Children during Treatment of Stuttering

Positive Stimuli	Negative Stimuli
Clinician praise "Good talking!", "That's right!", etc.)	Clinician highlighting ("Uh oh," "Oops," "That's one")
Plus (+) mark on data sheet	Minus (−) mark on data sheet
Receive puzzle part or lego for building	Request to repeat word
Sticker	Time-out from talking and teacher attention
Presentation of token	Loss of previously earned token

fade out these kinds of reinforcers and rely more and more on clinician praise and on the child's recognition of and self-satisfaction in the production of stutter-free responses. The clinician often can judge that this shift has occurred when children begin attending more to the "plus" marks on the clinician's data sheet than to the tokens and stickers they earn, or when they begin commenting favorably about their own responses during treatment.

In my experience, this stage of treatment is one of the most difficult—for clinicians. Once they observe directly the power of positive (and negative) feedback to facilitate change in a child's speech, some clinicians become reluctant to reduce the density of those stimuli. The use of these procedures becomes reinforcing to the clinician and, therefore, is likely to be maintained by the clinician! However, extensive research has established that behavior that has been maintained on intermittent schedules of feedback is more durable and more likely to generalize than behavior maintained on a continuous reinforcement schedule. Therefore, when the last steps of a treatment program still rely on frequently presented, contrived reinforcers, it should be no surprise if a child's newly acquired behaviors do not generalize to the natural environment. Children's natural environments typically are not replete with tokens dropped into a cup every time a fluent utterance is heard!

In regard to negative feedback provided following the occurrence of stutterings, clinicians should retain a one-to-one relationship between occurrences of stuttering and presentation of negative feedback (even while reinforcement is becoming intermittent) until quite late in the program. This is because of the earlier reported finding that negative feedback seems to be primarily responsible for producing reductions in the frequency of stutters. Nonetheless, as treatment nears completion, explicit negative feedback is removed. It is the goal of treatment that at termination a child's stutter-free behavior is completely under its own control—that is, that production of stutter-free, natural-sounding speech does not rely on feedback controlled by such external sources as the child's clinician.

Summary.   The behavioral treatments described herein rely heavily on the use of functional positive and negative forms of feedback contingent on the occurrence of stutter-free and stuttered utterances, respectively. Such feedback is applied frequently early in treatment and is faded in amount and form as treatment progresses.

EXAMPLE OF A BEHAVIORAL TREATMENT PROGRAM FOR USE WITH YOUNG CHILDREN WHO STUTTER: EXTENDED LENGTH OF UTTERANCE

One example of how the above-described features come together in a behavioral treatment program is the ELU strategy. I have found this strategy to be a good starting place for treatment. For many children, it has been the only treatment required, with or without the addition of transfer activities. Appendix A describes the ELU treatment. Highlights of the program are discussed below through explanations of each of the column headings.

Step.   The first column simply numbers each step in the treatment sequence. Not all children need to begin at step 1. If analysis of pretreatment STSs suggests, for example, that a child is regularly able to produce stutter-free utterances of say, three syllables, I would begin the program at step 2 (two-syllable response). Prior to treatment clinicians should also "probe" children's performance on the first few treatment steps, as another way of determining where treatment should begin. In these probes, children are presented with five trials of a treatment step to determine whether the required response level is already within their ability. No feedback regarding stutter-free speech or stuttering is provided in these probes. Five consecutive stutter-free trials are accepted as evidence, so that if the child is able to pass, for example, step 1 (one-syllable fluent), step 2 is probed in the same way. Probes for each consecutive step of the program are continued until a child is unable to produce five consecutive stutter-free trials. Treatment then begins on the *preceding* step so as to ensure that the program begins at a level at which the child will be able to earn lots of positive feedback. Probes of succeeding steps are also administered whenever a given step is completed. Oftentimes it is possible to skip steps in the treatment sequence. In this way, treatment can take advantage of generalization across steps to accelerate a child's progress through the program.

Discriminative Stimuli.   Information contained in this column describes, for each step of the program, the stimuli (materials and clinician instructions) used to evoke responses from children. Initially, a substantial stack of picture cards is used. It is not important that children learn to say *particular* words (or sentences), just *lots of different* words (and sentences). Therefore, a minimum of 50 picture cards is used, and this number is increased and changed throughout the course of treatment. Perusal of the items described in this column of the treatment protocol illustrates that treatment begins by evoking motorically and linguistically simple responses and gradually changes so that responses are eventually evoked by more naturally occurring kinds of stimuli.

Response.   The programmed nature of this treatment is evident by the specifications given in this column. The behavior that is required of the child to earn reinforcement at each step of the program is described. No other form of response produces reinforcement. Responses systematically increase in length (and, thereby, in motoric and linguistic complexity) as the program continues. The first step requires stutter-free production of one-syllable words, the last step requires 5-minute stutter-free conversations with the clinician in the clinic setting, and there are 18 "gradations" of response difficulty in between.

Consequence and ± Schedules.   This column contains specifications for the application of the feedback system for stutter-free and stuttered responses. As is evident, both social and token reinforcers are used in early steps of the program on continuous (1:1) schedules. Also, brief time-out from speaking is utilized as negative feedback.* As treatment progresses, feedback schedules are thinned (see step 18 and beyond).

With young children clinicians typically do not need to explain the contingencies—

---

*Time-out from speaking is not an effective negative stimulus for very young children. It appears that their metalinguistic facility with language and communication is not developed well enough to permit them to turn their speaking on and off at will. Midsentence instructions to "Stop," or even to repeat part of an utterance (instructions that might be employed as negative stimuli contingent upon an instance of stuttering), are typically ignored by young children. In such cases, clinicians can replace time-out with the presentation of a stuttering-contingent remark such as "Uh oh" or "Oops." This serves to highlight the occurrence of stuttering but does not interrupt the ongoing flow of communication.

that is, what is required to earn a reinforcer or what behavior produces the demand to stop talking (or the presentation of a negative remark). I have found that children respond to these contingencies rather naturally without explanations, and explanations often confound the effects of the treatment. With older children, explanations are used only if they are sought by the children (e.g., "Why did you say, 'stop'?"). It quickly becomes clear by the way children change their behavior that at some level, the contingencies are "understood," even though they may not be verbalized by the children or the clinicians.

For the most part, children do not need instructions regarding *how* to be fluent. That is, clinicians do not have to tell them to use "easy" speech or slow speech or to think first about what they want to say, etc., although some children appear to find these solutions for themselves. Part of the power of these procedures may be the problem solving and hypothesis testing that children must undertake in order to discover the kind of response that will earn reinforcement and avoid negative feedback. Usually children are somehow able to generate stutter-free responses from their own behavioral reservoirs.

It is well known that feedback that *immediately* follows the occurrence of a response is most likely to influence the probability of that response occurring (or not occurring) in the future. Therefore, clinicians should deliver the request to "Stop" (talking) *as soon as the beginning of a moment of stuttering* is detected. Oftentimes, then, the stuttered syllable, and the stutter itself, are interrupted by presentation of the negative stimulus. The procedural requirement to consequate every occasion of stuttering (1:1) and to do so essentially instantly necessitates a clinician's ability to rapidly discriminate the occurrence of a stutter in the child's speech. Whether these procedures can be optimally effective if some occasions of stuttering are "missed" or if feedback regarding their occurrence is delayed has not been empirically studied. Therefore, especially in the early stages of treatment, it is important to be especially careful to provide positive and negative feedback within these constraints.

Criteria.   This column lists the pass and fail criteria that specify how well, or how poorly, children must perform the target behavior (stutter-free utterances) before advancing in the program, or before the program is altered due to failure.* When the fail criterion is met, the program usually needs to be modified in some fashion, based upon an analysis of why the step was failed. Repeating the previous step, on which the child had performed at criterion level, is not generally a solution to the

---

*Clinicians should not be confused between occasions when a child has earned the requisite number of tokens required to exchange for a backup reinforcer (which can occur in the middle of a treatment step) and occasions when a child's performance level has met the pass criterion (which signals the completion of that step). Both events are determined by the data recorded on the clinician's data sheet. When the former occurs, treatment is temporarily halted and the child immediately receives the previously selected backup reinforcer before the next trial is administered. At this time, a new backup reinforcer is selected, and the full complement of tokens is once again available for the child to earn as treatment continues. When a pass criterion is met, the clinician simply changes the stimulus and/or definition of a correct response, and/or the feedback schedule to that appropriate for the next step of the program and continues. No particular mention is made to the child unless the new step requires some kind of introduction. Clinicians should *not* say something like, "Now you've passed that step, we're going to do something even harder!" The prospects of "something even harder" may not be perceived by children as the exciting, satisfying challenge we intend!

problem. Sometimes the "behavioral space" between two steps is too large for the child to bridge, and an intermediate step needs to be inserted; sometimes the feedback system needs adjusting because the reinforcers may be weakening, or the token-backup reinforcer exchange rate is too stiff; sometimes a child may initiate a trial without obvious concentration. Whatever the nature of the "branch" step that is created when a child has failed a step, when the criterion is met on the new step, the child is returned to the regular sequence.

Measurement. In this column are described the data that are collected, response by response, during each step of the program, and the calculations that are made from those data. These calculations provide evidence of the effectiveness of the ongoing treatment.

Comments Regarding Particular Aspects of the Extended Length of Utterance Program. The first six steps of the program move the child from one-syllable through six-syllable utterances. Obviously, some very young children will be unable to produce five- and six-syllable utterances due to their lack of well-developed expressive language or memory rather than to the intrusion of stuttering. In such cases, these steps are omitted.

One tricky part of the program is the transition between utterances defined by syllable length and utterances defined by time (i.e., transition from step 6 to step 7). Because a fundamental principle of this treatment is control of length of utterance, children must learn to stop when they are signalled (by the click of the stopwatch or the clinician saying "Good") that the required response duration has been met, even though this may occur in the middle of a sentence or idea. A practice step is inserted to help a child learn this procedure.* Also at this stage, some children will have difficulty formulating their own phrases and sentences or descriptions of the picture stimuli. If this occurs, it can be useful to introduce a "story retell" task wherein the clinician models a response of the appropriate content and duration and the child then produces a similar response. In this case, of course, the child does not need to use the same words or even express the same ideas that the clinician modeled. The child needs only to produce stutter-free spontaneous speech of the required duration. As soon as a child catches on to this task, the clinician's model is faded out.

At step 9 (10-second stutter-free responses required) the program suggests that the clinician occasionally monitor children's speaking rates. This is accomplished easily by making a pencil dot on the data sheet for each syllable produced in the 10-second utterance, and then multiplying that number by six to extrapolate syllables per minute. While speaking rate is not generally a problem with very young children, older children oftentimes use speech rates that appear to be beyond their ability to manage. If this appears to be the case for a given child, reminders regarding speech rate, or even contingencies for speaking within a specified range of speech rates, can be added at this point in the program.

---

*Once again, very young children have difficulty understanding this procedure, which is why I do not use this version of the ELU program with them. Instead, positive reinforcers are presented at natural pauses in conversation following stutter-free utterances that meet the target behavior criterion (see the footnote on page 77).

Summary. The ELU program is an example of the application of established behavioral principles within a flexible framework that fosters individualized treatment and a high level of accountability. Further, the treatment program is relatively simple to administer and enjoyable for the clinician and child alike.

Expected Outcomes

The outcomes expected of this treatment are the same as the previously stated treatment goals: spontaneous and automatic use of natural-sounding, stutter-free speech under all talking conditions, in all settings, with all speaking partners and audiences. Evidence from the STSs is the primary source of information regarding whether these outcomes have been produced. Because STSs are obtained periodically throughout treatment, clinicians are able to know well before the assumed termination point of treatment whether these goals are being met. If the within-clinic treatment data or the beyond-clinic STS data indicate that the child's speech is not changing in a predictable fashion, the treatment can be altered to facilitate additional change. Sometimes "additives" are needed to strengthen the treatment.[16] One such additive, reduction in speech rate, has already been mentioned. Occasionally, broader changes in speech patterns, such as the implementation of "gentle-onset" initiations at the beginning of utterances or prolonged speech, seem appropriate. Our clinic does not incorporate such additives into the early steps of treatment because (1) they may not be needed, (2) they are difficult for young children to employ, and (3) they alter the naturalness of children's speech and must eventually be severed from the child's manner of speech production.

ACROSS-SETTINGS GENERALIZATION

Of course, an especially important aspect of treatment outcome is whether the child's newly acquired stutter-free speech generalizes to the real-life conditions in which speech is produced. Unfortunately, little information is known regarding children's proclivities in this regard or regarding the relationship between generalization and particular components of treatment. In my experience, some children do spontaneously generalize their clinic-style speech to their home, school, and other settings without benefit of additional "transfer" steps added to the end of their treatment program. The likelihood of such "spontaneous generalization" appears to be enhanced when one or more of the following components are included in the treatment procedures.

Self-Management. Many children are able to take greater responsibility for their own behavior change than clinicians typically allow. And if a child has control over components of treatment, the treatment leaves the clinic with the child. Each aspect of the treatment paradigm offers opportunities for the child to take responsibility. In regard to the stimuli used to evoke speech, the child can be responsible for bringing in pictures (e.g., family photograph album) and picking conversation topics. In regard to the feedback system, children can learn to monitor their responses and judge whether they contain stutters or are stutter-free. The children may even be encouraged to record the data regarding their responses. (Taking this sheet home to show to parents and friends is often a powerful reinforcer for high levels of stutter-free speech.) Certainly children should play a major role in determining the reinforcers to be used in treatment, and oftentimes they can learn to award both positive and negative feedback to themselves following their judgment of the correctness of their responses. Even before they are taught to do so, many children begin spontaneously to stop themselves midstutter, and it is certainly not unusual to observe young stutterers reminding the clinician when reinforcers are due! Teaching young children to take responsibility for more aspects of their treatment helps develop a treatment strategy that can be applied in the child's natural environment in the absence of the clinician—a goal of procedures aimed at producing transfer. The usefulness of self-management techniques depends partially on the child's age, but the best way to determine this issue is by gradually shifting control of various treatment components to the child and by observing the child's readiness to accept this new role.

Parent Training.   Whenever possible, parents should be taught to serve as adjunct clinicians. Sometimes this is done by training the parents to administer the program being used in the clinic. As soon as a child's performance has met criterion on a given step of the program in the clinic, the parent is taught how to administer that treatment step at home, and regular 10- to 15-minute sessions are held daily. Typically parents are taught to use social reinforcement contingencies, but not negative feedback contingencies, in case some might get carried away and make the home treatment unnecessarily aversive. In other cases, parents are informed regarding the level of stutter-free speech the child has achieved in the clinic, and are instructed to reinforce occasions of similar stutter-free speech in the child's spontaneous speech at home or elsewhere, any time it occurs. In either case, parent training is conducted systematically, by having the parents observe the clinician's sessions with the child and then having the clinician observe the parents' sessions with the child. Direct training in the recognition of targeted stutter-free responses and how to reinforce them (and how to ignore stuttered responses) is crucial to this process.

Inclusion of a Peer or Sibling in Treatment.   At some point in treatment, the earlier the better, it is useful to include someone who is in frequent contact with the child in the natural environment. The goal is for this person to become a discriminative stimulus for stutter-free speech. Such persons become salient stimuli when they are responsible for providing reinforcement for stutter-free utterances. If they have been included in the child's treatment sessions, they can be taught to recognize stutter-free speech and reinforce it. Clinicians can arrange conditions so that the peer/sib has the opportunity to earn reinforcers for correctly identifying occurrences of the child's target stutter-free speech in the clinic, with the assumption that the presence of that child in the natural environment will serve as a "reminder" to the stuttering child to use stutter-free speech.

Concurrent Treatment across Settings.   Although it is somewhat difficult for the clinician to manage, arranging for treatment to occur concurrently in more than one setting helps prevent discrimination on the part of the child. That is, the child is less likely to learn to produce stutter-free speech only in the clinic and in the presence of the clinician. One way to accomplish this is by training both a parent and a teacher in the treatment methods used in the clinic.[24] Besides preventing narrow stimulus control, this procedure multiplies the treatment and practice opportunities available to the child.

Conclusion

Many years of clinical experience in using variations of behavioral treatments with children who stutter have been very reinforcing to me. Children are not tainted when direct attention is paid to their stuttering. In fact, they oftentimes express that they are glad their speech difficulties and frustrations are being acknowledged and dealt with. On the other hand, many young children complete treatment with little awareness that they were ever in "treatment." Behavioral treatments have the advantage of being based on experimentally verified principles of behavior change and carry with them accountability factors inherent in continuous measurement. They are relatively easy for clinicians and others to administer. They address directly the behavior of primary interest: a child's stuttering. Behavioral treatments are able to be individualized for different children and modified, as needed, to produce greater behavior change. And, most important, the behavioral treatments described here are highly likely to offer beneficial treatment outcomes for children who stutter.

Suggested Readings

Costello JC, Ingham RJ: Assessment Strategies for Stuttering, in Curlee R, Perkins WH (eds): *Nature and Treatment of Stuttering: New Directions.* San Diego, College-Hill Press, 1984.

Ingham RJ, Costello JM: Stuttering Treatment Outcome Evaluation, in Costello JM (ed): *Speech Disorders in Children: Recent Advances.* San Diego, College-Hill Press, 1984.

These two chapters describe measurement procedures that facilitate judgments regarding the characteristics of a child's stuttering and how or whether those characteristics change as a function of treatment.

Costello JM: Current Behavioral Treatments for Children, in Prins D, Ingham RJ (eds): *Treatment of Stuttering in Early Childhood: Methods and Issues.* San Diego, College-Hill Press, 1983.

Ingham JC: Therapy of the Stuttering Child, in Blanken G, Dittman J, Grimm H, Marshall JC, Wallesch C-W (eds): *Linguistic Disorders and Pathologies.* Berlin, Walter De Gruyter, in press.

These two chapters present overviews of philosophies of treatment for children who stutter, with contrasts between behavioral and other styles of treatment.

Onslow M, Costa L, Rue S: Direct early intervention with stuttering: Some preliminary data. *J Speech Hear Disord* 1990; 55:405–416.

This article describes and documents experimental findings regarding a behavioral treatment of young children who stutter. The procedures described are variants of those advocated in this chapter.

References

1. Kidd KK: Stuttering as a Genetic Disorder, in Curlee RF, Perkins WH (eds): *Nature and Treatment of Stuttering: New Directions.* San Diego, College-Hill Press, 1984.
2. American Speech-Language-Hearing Association: Let's talk. *Asha* 1990; 32:63.
3. Ingham R, Ingham JC: Let's talk about stuttering. *Asha* 1990; 32:42.
4. Costello JM, Ingham RJ: Assessment Strategies for Child and Adult Stutterers, in Curlee RF, Perkins WH (eds): *Nature and Treatment of Stuttering: New Directions.* San Diego, College-Hill Press, 1984.
5. Ingham RJ, Costello, JM: Stuttering Treatment Outcome Evaluation, in Costello JM (ed): *Speech Disorders in Children: Recent Advances.* San Diego, College-Hill Press, 1984.

6. Ingham RJ: Spontaneous Remission of Stuttering: When Will the Emperor Realize He Has No Clothes On? in Prins D, Ingham RJ (eds): *Treatment of Stuttering in Early Childhood: Methods and Issues*. San Diego, College-Hill Press, 1983.
7. Wingate ME: A standard definition of stuttering. *J Speech Hear Disord* 1964; 29:484–489.
8. MacDonald JD, Martin RR: Stuttering and disfluency as two reliable response classes. *J Speech Hear Res* 1973; 17:691–699.
9. Curlee R: Observer agreement on disfluency and stuttering. *J Speech Hear Res* 1981; 24:595–600.
10. Young MA: Identification of Stuttering and Stutterers, in Curlee RF, Perkins WH (eds): *Nature and Treatment of Stuttering: New Directions*. San Diego, College-Hill Press, 1984.
11. Martin RR, Haroldson SK, Triden KA: Stuttering and speech naturalness. *J Speech Hear Disord* 1984; 49:53–58.
12. Onslow M, Costa L, Rue S: Direct early intervention with stuttering: Some preliminary data. *J Speech Hear Disord* 1990; 55:405–416.
13. Fowler SC, Ingham RJ: Stuttering Treatment Rating Recorder. Santa Barbara, University of California, 1986. Available upon request from author @ $300.00.
14. Wolf MM: Social validity: The case for subjective measurement or how applied behavior analysis is findings its heart. *J Appl Behav Anal* 1978; 11:203–214.
15. Ingham JC: Therapy of the Stuttering Child, in Blanken G, Dittman J, Grimm H, Marshall JC, Wallesch C-W (eds): *Linguistic Disorders and Pathologies*. Berlin, Walter De Gruyter, in press.
16. Costello JM: Current Behavioral Treatments for Children, in Prins D, Ingham RJ (eds): *Treatment of Stuttering in Early Childhood: Methods and Issues*. San Diego, College-Hill Press, 1983.
17. Costello JM: Time-out procedures for the modification of stuttering: Three case studies. *J Speech Hear Disord* 1975; 40:216–231.
18. Costello JM: Operant Conditioning and the Treatment of Stuttering. *Semin Speech Lang Hrng* 1980; 1:311–325.
19. Costello JM, Ingham RJ: Stuttering as an Operant Disorder, in Curlee RF, Perkins WH (eds): *Nature and Treatment of Stuttering: New Directions*. San Diego, College-Hill Press, 1984.
20. Ryan BP: *Programmed Therapy for Stuttering in Children and Adults*. Springfield, IL, Thomas, 1974.
21. Costello JM: Programmed instruction. *J Speech Hear Disord* 1977; 42:3–28.
22. Costello JM, Ferrer JS: The effects of three punishment procedures applied to programmed instruction with young children. *J Commun Disord* 1976; 9:43–61.
23. Barlow DH, Hersen M: *Single Case Experimental Designs*. New York, Pergammon, 1984.
24. Ingham JC: Measurement and facilitation of across-settings generalization. Presented at the annual meeting of the American Speech-Language-Hearing Association, Atlanta, November, 1991.

APPENDIX A: THE EXTENDED LENGTH OF UTTERANCE (ELU) PROGRAM

Step	Discriminative Stimuli	Response	Consequences and ± Schedules	Criteria	Measurement
1	Minimum of 50 cards containing monosyllabic words (or pictures) within vocabulary range of client—presented without model—one card at a time. Example: **car, leaf** Instructions: "Say each word." (added instructions regarding speaking rate as appropriate for particular clients)	Fluent word/syllable	Positive social reinforcer ("Good!," "Right!," "Excellent!," "Good talking!," "Perfect speech!," etc.). 1:1 Positive token reinforcer, 1:1 (tokens exchanged for back-up reinforcers throughout program as follows: 10:1, 20:1, 35:1, 50:1; the exchange rate may be altered backwards as responses get longer or when client's data indicate the need for increased motivation)	Pass—10 consecutive fluent responses Fail—7 consecutive stuttered responses or 100 trials without passing the step	+ Each fluent response − Each stuttered response At completion of step, calculate % correct responses and no. of trials required to meet criterion
		Stuttered word/syllable	"Stop," said by clinician during or immediately following a moment of stuttering; client must stop speaking; 1:1		
2	1. Minimum of 50 cards containing monosyllabic words or pictures (as above) presented in pairs	Fluent two-syllable utterance	As above	As above	As above
	2. List of minimum of 50 two-syllable words (presented for imitative or spontaneous response, depending on client's reading skill) Example: **mother, scissors**	Any moment of stuttering	As above		

3. List of minimum of 50 two-syllable syntactic word combinations (presented for imitative or spontaneous response, as above)

Example: **a house, run fast, tall man**

Stimuli from each of the above three categories are intermixed and presented in random order

Instructions: "Say each word," or "Say what I say."

3	Same stimuli as above except **three-syllable word strings** (continually use new words), **three-syllable single words**, and **three-syllable syntactic monosyllabic word combinations**	Fluent three-syllable utterance	As above	As above
		Any moment of stuttering	As above	As above
4	Same stimuli as above except **four-syllable word strings, four-syllable single words**, and **four-syllable syntactic monosyllabic word combinations**	Fluent four-syllable utterance	As above	As above
		Any moment of stuttering	As above	As above
5	Same as above except **five-syllable word strings and five-syllable syntactic monosyllabic word combinations only** (do not include five-syllable single words)	Fluent five-syllable utterance	As above	As above
		Any moment of stuttering	As above	As above

(Continued on next page)

Step	Discriminative Stimuli	Response	Consequences and ± Schedules	Criteria	Measurement
6	Same as above except **six-syllable word strings and six-syllable syntactic monosyllabic word combinations only**	Fluent six-syllable utterance Any moment of stuttering	As above As above	As above	As above
Practice	Minimum of 100 pictures with lots of activity in them, topic cards, objects, etc. Instructions: "Tell me about this (present one stimulus) and keep talking until you hear the watch stop, like this." (Click the stopwatch.) "I'll show you." Describe one picture in relatively slow, simple connected speech and stop at the end of **3 seconds**—stop in the middle of a sentence if necessary, and click the stopwatch at the same time. Demonstrate on two or three different stimuli. "Now it's your turn. Keep talking until I stop the watch and say 'OK'." (For some young clients it may be necessary to conduct this and some of the following steps as a "retell" task wherein clinician speaks for 3 seconds and then client repeats the same content in his or her own words for 3 seconds)	Continuous talking in connected speech for a duration of 3 seconds (stuttering allowed) Nonconnected speech, pauses, problems thinking of things to say, etc. Be sure client learns to stop as soon as the watch stops, even if utterance is not completed Be sure client does not increase speaking rate in an attempt to complete utterance before clock stops	Positive social reinforcer, 1:1 Re-explain task and/or change stimulus materials Occasionally helpful to let client watch clock second hand reach the "3"	Pass—3 consecutive correct responses Fail—continue task as practice until client meets pass criterion	Start timing with stopwatch when client begins talking Do not initiate client's response by saying "Go!" and thereby implying a fast speaking rate is appropriate

Step	Stimuli/Instructions	Response	Consequence	Criterion	Scoring
7	Same picture, topic card, and object stimuli as above presented in random order Instructions: "Tell me about this one and keep talking until you hear the watch stop, just like you've been doing." If necessary, clinician will model each utterance until the client is able to generate utterances independently.	Fluent 3-second connected speech utterance (uninterrupted by clinician: monologue)	Positive social reinforcer, 1:1 Positive token reinforcer, 1:1	Pass—10 consecutive fluent responses Fail—7 consecutive stuttered responses or 75 trials without passing step	+ Each fluent trial − Each stuttered trial At completion of step calculate: % correct trials and no. of trials required to meet criterion
		Any moment of stuttering	"Stop," said by clinician during or immediately following a moment of stuttering; client must stop speaking; 1:1 (Be sure you do **not** say stop at the end of **fluent** utterances when the clock has reached the 3-second time; say, "Good," etc.)		
8	Same stimuli and instructions as above	Fluent 5 seconds of connected speech in speech in monologue	As above	As above	As above
		Any moment of stuttering	As above		
9	Same stimuli and instructions as above	Fluent 10 seconds of connected speech in monologue	As above	As above	+ Each fluent trial − Each stuttered trial For every third or fourth trial count the number of syllables spoken in the 10-second utterance and multiply × 6 for approximate SPM speaking rate
		Any moment of stuttering	As above		
		Fluent or stuttered utterance over 160 SPM	Reminder to speak a bit more slowly, 1:1		

(Continued on next page)

APPENDIX A: THE EXTENDED LENGTH OF UTTERANCE (ELU) PROGRAM (CONTINUED)

Step	Discriminative Stimuli	Response	Consequences and ± Schedules	Criteria	Measurement
9 Cont.					At completion of step calculate: % correct trials, no. of trials required to meet criterion, and average SPM speaking rate (based on all trials upon which rate data were taken)
10	Same stimuli and instructions as above	Fluent 20-second monologue	As above	As above	As above (for rate data, multiply 20-second syllable count × 3 for approximate SPM/response)
		Any moment of stuttering	As above		
		Fluent or stuttered utterance over 160 SPM	Reminder to speak a bit more slowly, 1:1		
11	Same stimuli and instructions as above	Fluent 30-second monologue	As above	As above	As above (for rate data, multiply 30-second syllable count × 2 for approximate SPM/response)
		Any moment of stuttering	"Stop," said by clinician during or immediately following a moment of stuttering (as above)		
			For some clients it may be appropriate to increase the negative feedback for stuttered responses by adding the removal of one token for each stuttered response (response cost); this can be done here or earlier or later on, as needed		

No.	Stimulus	Response	Consequence	Criterion	Notes
		Utterance over 160 SPM	Reminder to speak a bit more slowly, 1:1		
12	Same stimuli and instructions as above	Fluent 1-minute monologue	As above	As above	As above (for rate data count syllables for 15 seconds of each 1 minute utterance and multiply $\times$ 4 for approximate SPM/response
		Any moment of stuttering	As above		
		Utterance over 160 SPM	As above		
13	Same stimuli and instructions as above	Fluent 2-minute monologue	As above	Pass—10 consecutive fluent utterances	As above (for rate data count syllables for 15 seconds of each minute of the 2-minute utterance, add, multiply $\times$ 2 for approximate SPM/response)
		Any moment of stuttering	As above	Fail—7 consecutive stuttered responses or 50 trials without passing step	
		Utterance over 160 SPM	As above		
14	Same stimuli and instructions as above	Fluent 3-minute monologue	As above	Pass—5 consecutive fluent utterances	As above (for rate data count syllables for four different 15-second intervals during the 3-minute utterance and add for approximate SPM/response
		Any moment of stuttering	As above	Fail—as above	
		Utterance over 160 SPM	As above		
15	Same stimuli and instructions as above	Fluent 4-minute monologue	As above	As above	As above
		Any moment of stuttering	As above		
		Utterance over 160 SPM	As above		
16					

(Continued on next page)

APPENDIX A: THE EXTENDED LENGTH OF UTTERANCE (ELU) PROGRAM (CONTINUED)

Step	Discriminative Stimuli	Response	Consequences and ± Schedules	Criteria	Measurement
16	Same stimuli and instructions as above	Fluent 5-minute monologue	As above	Pass—4 consecutive fluent utterances	As above
		Any moment of stuttering	As above	Fail—20 trials without passing step	
		Utterance more than 160 SPM	As above		
17	Topics introduced by clinician and client for conversational discussion	Fluency (0 %SS) during 2-minute conversation with clinician	As above	Pass—10 consecutive fluent conversations	+ Each fluent conversation − Each stuttered conversation
	Clinician's questions, interruptions, overlapping utterances, topic changes, etc., i.e., mirroring natural conversational interactions (clinician keeps her utterances as short as possible)	Any moment of stuttering		Fail—7 consecutive stuttered trials or 50 trials without passing step	Count syllables in 15-second interval of uninterrupted client talking, one time per 2-minute utterance—multiply × 4 for approximate SPM/response
		Utterance over 160 SPM	As above		At completion of step calculate: % correct trials, no. of trials required to meet criterion, and average SPM speaking rate for step

18	Stimuli as above	Fluency (0 %SS) during 3-minute conversation with clinician	Positive social reinforcer, 1:1 Positive token reinforcer, 2:1	As above	As above
		Any moment of stuttering	As above		
		Utterances over **180 SPM** (unless permanent target for client will be less than this)	As above		
19	Stimuli as above Instructions regarding new rate contingency	Fluency (0 %SS) during 4-minute conversation with clinician	Positive social reinforcer, 1:1 Positive token reinforcer, 3:1	Pass—7 consecutive fluent conversations Fail—30 trials without passing step	As above (for speaking rate count syllables in four different 15-second intervals uninterrupted by clinician talking and add for approximate SPM/response)
		Any moment of stuttering	Report to client at end of trial—do not stop client at moment of stuttering		
		Utterances over 180 SPM (unless permanent target will be less than this)	Report to client at end of trial and count as incorrect total		

(Continued on next page)

APPENDIX A: THE EXTENDED LENGTH OF UTTERANCE (ELU) PROGRAM (CONTINUED)

Step	Discriminative Stimuli	Response	Consequences and ± Schedules	Criteria	Measurement
20	Stimuli as above	Fluency (0 %SS) during 5-minute conversation with clinician	Positive social reinforcer, 1:1	Pass—6 consecutive fluent conversations	As above
		Any moment of stuttering	Report to client at end of trial and count as incorrect trial	Fail—25 trials without passing step	
		Utterances over 180 SPM (unless permanent target will be less than this)	Report to client at end of trial and count as incorrect trial		
	Measure for extraclinic generalization; begin transfer program, if necesary (usually will be)				

APPENDIX B: GUIDELINES FOR THE ESTABLISHMENT OF A TOKEN REINFORCEMENT SYSTEM

Training to establish tokens (beans) as conditioned positive reinforcers can be accomplished during assessment sessions.

1. At the beginning of the first token training session children are shown several reinforcers (small toys, crayons, picture books, etc.) selected from items rated 5 on their reinforcement menu (see Appendix C) and told to select one. It is explained that they will have the opportunity to earn that item, and it is put aside, but in sight. A clear plastic cup with a line drawn around the lower portion is shown, and children are told that they can earn beans for things such as helping the teacher line up the picture, sitting quietly, and putting materials away, and that when the cup is filled to the line (ten beans), they will have earned the item. During the session the clinician reinforces appropriate behaviors with beans and verbal praise. When the ten beans have been earned, children are given the selected item, allowed to play with it for a moment, and then told to put it aside for safe keeping and select another item to earn.

2. A second cup with a line drawn around the midportion is then shown. This time 25 beans are required to fill the cup to the line. Beans are distributed in the same way as before, and when 25 beans have been earned (the end of the session), they are exchanged for the second item.

3. At the beginning of the second session, children once again choose an item from the available backup reinforcers. It is explained that this time it is necessary to earn enough beans to completely fill the cup (50 beans). Beans are earned in the same way described above, and it is arranged that the cup will be filled and one item earned. Then the process of earning yet another reinforcer is begun. This time, however, by the end of the session, the number of beans required to fill the cup a second time will not have been earned. The cup is set aside, and the next session begins with this partially filled cup.

4. At the beginning of the third session, the partially filled cup is produced. Reinforcement procedures as described above continue for this session and the next. By the time four sessions have been completed, children have learned that a full cup of beans can be exchanged for a backup reinforcer of their choice and that a full cup might not be earned in every session. At this point it is assumed that a functional token reinforcement system has been established, but treatment data are always required to verify the function of the reinforcers. If, during treatment, the tokens appear to lose their strength as conditioned reinforcers, usually lowering the exchange rate for backup reinforcers, and/or procuring more desirable backup reinforcers will solve the problem.

APPENDIX C: SAMPLE REINFORCEMENT MENU

This is the version given to parents. Individual children rate the same items in a discussion with the clinician.

Please read over this list of toys and activities and rate each one using the following 5-point scale:

1—My child would definitely not like this.
2—My child would probably not like this.
3—My child would like this somewhat.
4—My child would probably like this.
5—My child would definitely like this.

_____ bubbles
_____ coloring books
_____ art supplies
_____ Play Doh
_____ stickers
_____ knitting kits
_____ Magic Slate
_____ doll clothes
_____ marbles
_____ sugarless gum
_____ Magic Markers
_____ erasers
_____ jewelry
_____ Slinky
_____ Superball
_____ miniature furniture
_____ squirt gun
_____ windup toys
_____ Gumby and Pokey
_____ sand toys
_____ puzzles
_____ makeup
_____ perfume
_____ nail polish
_____ play tools and tool box
_____ ball
_____ racing car
_____ Barbie clothes

_____ crayons
_____ books
_____ finger paints
_____ balloons
_____ weaving kits
_____ bead jewelry
_____ miniature dolls
_____ jump rope
_____ jacks
_____ pencils and pens
_____ tea set
_____ doctor set
_____ play baking kit
_____ Matchbox cars
_____ puppets
_____ Legos
_____ Lincoln Logs
_____ stuffed animals
_____ Go Fish cards
_____ Old Maid cards
_____ Micronauts
_____ plastic horses
_____ play trucks
_____ rocket ships
_____ bean bags
_____ baseball set
_____ pickup sticks
_____ Ninja turtles

5

Therapy for School-Age Stutterers
An Update on the Fluency Rules Program

CHARLES M. RUNYAN, PH.D.
SARA ELIZABETH RUNYAN, M.A.

Introduction

Choosing the most effective treatment procedure for the preschool and young school-age stutterer, given the constraints associated with the delivery of services in the public school setting, continues to challenge the speech-language pathologist. Public school speech-language pathologists are required to provide services to a significant number of students and the resultant caseload numbers have been high. School-based speech-language pathologists find it difficult to fulfill their responsibilities for complete assessments, intervention plans, and carryover services when nationally reported caseloads average 50. These caseloads, combined with frequent scheduling conflicts, limit the number and length of treatment sessions during a school year. Runyan and Bennett[1] reported that in Virginia, the average caseload for a public school speech-language clinician was 60 children. The effect of this caseload size and its associated problems on the delivery of services in Virginia was that, on the average, a child was enrolled in two 30-minute therapy sessions per week and was seen for a total of 25 sessions per school year. Since these studies, speech-language pathologists in Virginia and in other regions of the country have consistently reported that caseload size and scheduling conflicts remain unchanged. Therefore, based on these reports it would appear that public school speech-language pathologists still seek an effective treatment program for young stutterers that can accommodate the job constraints found in the public schools.

As a result of the initial publication of the Fluency Rules Program (FRP),[2] we received numerous requests for additional information and clinical updates. It has been gratifying over the past few years to have public school clinicians, as well as clinicians in other treatment settings, speak with us at professional meetings and share not only their results but also the adaptations used while implementing the

FRP. Unfortunately, as gratifying as these interactions have been, to our knowledge no additional data have been gathered using the FRP in public school or other clinical environments. Therefore, the changes in the FRP that are presented in this chapter reflect our experiences with young stutterers in a university clinic and private practice setting, and as consultants to public school systems. Although two of these clinical environments differ from public school environments, we are confident that the suggested changes and therapy recommendations remain applicable to public school treatment settings.

The Revised Fluency Rules

The FRP was developed in 1981 in an effort to teach young grade school children to speak fluently and naturally. The individual rules were devised to instruct young children, in language they could comprehend, about the physiological concepts associated with fluent speech production. Originally there were ten fluency rules, and through clinical trial and error, the effectiveness and utility of each rule were evaluated. Subsequently, some rules remained unchanged; still others were modified or deleted until the current seven rules evolved. The treatment paradigm has also been clinically tested and modified. At first, the FRP treatment procedure was designed to teach a stuttering child all of the fluency rules. However, with continued use of the FRP, it became apparent that this procedure was not a time-efficient means of delivering services. Teaching all of the rules consumed a significant amount of time and often required a clinician to teach skills the children already evidenced. Therefore by 1986, when the FRP was first published, the treatment program consisted of seven rules, with therapeutic instruction provided only for those rules that were violated. Continued application of the FRP has not dramatically changed the rules but has significantly altered their application.

   The remainder of this chapter will describe these fluency rules, present the revised FRP, and update our clinical results. The seven fluency rules will be presented individually starting with the two universal rules, followed by two primary rules, and finally three secondary rules. For each rule, background information will be provided followed by therapy suggestions regarding the application of each rule.

Universal Rules

Rule 1: Speak Slowly (Turtle Speech)

BACKGROUND

The intent of this rule is to allow the child additional time to develop self-monitoring skills necessary for acquisition of the physiological skills required for fluent speech production. When this rule was first considered as a component of the FRP, little information was available in the literature relative to the speaking rate of early grade school children. This lack of information made it difficult for clinicians to determine how much to reduce a stutterer's speaking rate.

   To obtain some initial data for the determination of normal speaking rates of young children, Purcell and Runyan[3] conducted a study of students who were enrolled in grades 1 through 5. Ten children, five males and five females, with no history of a communication disorder were selected from each grade. The experimental tasks required each child to repeat a story and to describe an exciting or personal experience. The authors calculated speaking rate in both words and syllables per minute for each grade and these results are presented in Table 5-1. Obtaining these normative data on speaking rate has proved helpful for implementing this rule. Although this rule is labeled "speak slowly" or "turtle speech," it was never intended to have children produce speech that was abnormally slow or to produce speech one word at a time. In fact, it has been our clinical experience that children acquiring linguistic competency are not concerned with expression rate. The message takes precedence, and attempts to manipulate rate to one sounding abnormally slow do not have the desired effect. Also, it is unlikely that a child will use a dramatically reduced speaking rate or will produce speech one word at a time outside the clinical setting.

A secondary benefit of this rule, that we have observed and that has been supported by reports of public school speech pathologists, has been that a slow rate of speech has an overall calming effect on the child and family. This calming effect appears to contribute to a life-style and speaking environment that is conducive to fluent speech development. Clinically we have often noted that following a therapy session in which the goal was reduction to a slow, normal speaking rate, the child appeared more relaxed. Interestingly, during such sessions, there was also a marked reduction in stuttering; however, speaking rate remained virtually unchanged. Therefore, we attribute the reduction in stuttering and the improvement in fluency, in part, to a general calming effect.

THERAPY SUGGESTIONS

1. *Symbolic Material*: Use symbolic therapy materials such as turtles and snails to characterize slow speech.

2. *More Symbolic Material*: Use modeling or choral speaking to contrast slow turtle speech (i.e., normal speech rate) with race horse speech, using horses to portray too fast or rapid speech.

3. *Metronome*: Use a desk-level metronome set at 60 beats per minute as background stimulus during therapy. This technique has proved successful in the past[4] and on occasion we have also found it to be useful. The intent of this

Table 5-1.   Means and Standard Deviations of Speaking Rate of Children in Words and Syllables per Minute

Grade	Words per Minute	Standard Deviation	Syllables per Minute	Standard Deviation
1	124.92	12.17	147.66	13.47
2	130.44	12.05	156.72	17.14
3	133.44	10.01	158.94	14.86
4	139.32	16.33	165.66	24.58
5	141.84	16.24	170.04	23.19

therapy technique is to create a calm atmosphere and to encourage slow speech production, not the rhythmic production of one word per beat.

4. *Old Ears*: This technique has been used with considerable success with both universal rules. Making a pair of old ears, with wrinkles and gray hair, from construction paper can enhance the teaching of this rule. Tell the child your (i.e., the clinician) ears are old and tired and if the child uses race horse speech or says a word more than once, it will confuse your ears and you will not be able to understand him or her. As a consequence, the child may miss having a speech break or a speech treat because his or her speech could not be understood. After implementing this technique, the child will often report to the parent that he or she is helping the clinician's ears by "talking better" (i.e., following the rules). There is an obvious secondary value to this technique in that it places the child in the role of helper rather than the recipient of therapy.

5. *Modeling*: Clinicians and parents should use a very relaxed, slow-motion form of speech production. We tell parents to just slow down their speech but not to prolong speech or use too many pauses because this produces speech that sounds abnormal. To prevent the parents from an excessive reduction in speech rate, which often occurs following this instruction, use a speedometer analogy and suggest that they reduce their rate by only 10 miles per hour (mph), thus allowing them to stay in better control without becoming a traffic hazard. In other words, slow down from 65 mph to 55 mph but do not slow to 25 mph because that is too slow and could cause a problem.

6. *Animal Tracks*: Clinicians can put turtle tracks (e.g., Ninja tracks work well) and race horse tracks (e.g., horse shoes) on the floor and have the children simultaneously walk and talk relative to the trail they are on. See rule 6 for additional information.

Rule 2: Say A Word Only Once

BACKGROUND

Because the dominant speech characteristic of stuttering children's speech is part-word and whole-word repetitions, a rule to help control this characteristic is vital for any treatment program designed for young stutterers. For this rule to be effective, the child must understand the concepts of "once" and "word."

THERAPY SUGGESTIONS

1. *Railroad Train*: Two different railroad trains are compared. The first train contains different cars and represents fluent speech (i.e., each car/word is different). The second train has a number of similar cars (e.g., box cars) placed in a row and represents speech that contained repetitive speech samples. This technique can also be used by comparing two different rows of coins, tokens, or zoo animals.

2. *Monitoring Clinician/Parent Speech*: Have the child detect instances of repetitions in the speech of the clinician. The clinician randomly produces speech containing repetitions and records the percentage of correct identifications made by the child. As the child's ability to correctly identify repetitions produced by the clinician increases, more therapy time is allotted to identi-

fying repetitions in the child's speech. A number of our most dramatic treatment successes have occurred after the child has used this therapy technique at home and spontaneously identified instances of repeated words in his or her parents' speech. Apparently once the concept of not repeating elements of speech is understood, a child often carries over this awareness to the home and corrects the parents' speech. Once such spontaneous generalization occurs, progress can be quite rapid, usually going from a significant number of stutterings to zero in a very short period of time.

3. *Old Ears*: Explain that a person does not have to repeat words to be understood. Then use a humorous exaggerated example of repeating a word ten times followed by asking if the repetitions helped the child better understand the message.

4. *Different Feet*: Use the turtle trail again to facilitate this technique (see rule 1: technique 6). Have the child say different words with each step while walking the turtle trail. Walking is easy and smooth when different feet are used for each step, but if the same foot is used and we start to hop, then walking becomes "hard and bumpy." And, if we use the same word over and over, our speech gets bumpy and people may have difficulty understanding our speech.

Primary Rules

Rule 3: Use Speech Breathing

BACKGROUND

During the last 5 years while implementing FRP, we became increasingly impressed with the necessity of using this rule when more direct physiological intervention was required. During this time period we were also using the Computer-Assisted Fluency Establishment Trainer (CAFET) with adolescent and adult stutterers.[5] A major component of the CAFET program is measuring chest-wall expansions and contractions and making therapeutic inferences regarding inhalation/exhalation. While using the CAFET clinically, it was noted that virtually all of our vocal abuse and stuttering clients, except the preschoolers, use the same unusual speech breathing pattern. This pattern starts with a normal-appearing exhalation (i.e., contraction of the diaphragmatic/thoracic area), but just prior to speech a rapid expansion of the diaphragmatic/thoracic area occurs. In spite of this unusual breathing pattern, positive therapeutic results have occurred using speech breathing techniques that focus on prevoiced exhalation. Usually, we explained to the child the difference between regular and speech breathing. For speech breathing, the explanation includes: breath in, slowly let your air out, speak on "out" breath, and keep the air moving (i.e., do not hold your breath).

THERAPY SUGGESTIONS

1. *The Breath Curve*: Draw a typical breath curve on a chalkboard or piece of paper, illustrating a rapid inspiration period and gradual slope for exhalation. Next, place an "X" on the line shortly after the exhalation starts to indicate where speech should begin. Have the child motorically trace the breath curve

as he or she "feels" the breathing pattern. After the child understands the feeling of speech breathing, practice initiating speech at the point on the breath curve where the "X" has been placed. At first, have the child count, recite days of the week, or say months of the year as he or she traces the breathing curve. Following this technique, therapy material consisting of four- and five-syllable phrases is used for practicing prevoiced exhalation while still tracing the breath curve.

2. *Tactile Feedback*: This activity evolved as a supplement to therapy suggestion 1. The previous activity encouraged the stutterer to visualize speech breathing and, we hope, feel the physiological components of speech breathing. This second activity emphasizes the feeling of the physiological aspects of speech breathing. To accomplish this, the clinician first places his or her palm below the child's sternum where the lower ribs flare and then places the child's hand on the clinician's. Used with the first therapy suggestion, the child can now both visualize and feel speech breathing. If needed, another clinical activity can be added. The clinician can place a hand around the child's upper arm and gently squeeze when it is time to initiate speech. Thus, as the child traces the graph of the breath cycle and feels the speech breathing cycle with a hand on the abdomen, he or she is given a squeeze on the arm as a tactile cue to begin speech. These combined therapy activities have been used successfully and usually require only a short period of time to gain the child's awareness of speech breathing and prevoiced exhalation.

3. *For Breath/Speech Holding*: Have the stutterer start a typical speech breathing cycle, and at the designated speech mark, begin counting from 1 to 20. At the count of 4, have the child pull up sharply on the sides of the chair until breathing and speech momentarily stop. Then have the child continue to count, pulling and tensing on every fourth count. Explain that if we tense the neck and airflow stops, then speech will also stop. Next, have the child repeat this procedure without pulling and feel how prevoiced exhalation and easy initiation of speech should feel.

Rule 4: Start Mr. Voice Box Running Smoothly

BACKGROUND

An important modification has been made to this rule since its first publication. The original wording, "Keep Mr. Voice Box running smoothly" was modified to "Start Mr. Voice Box running smoothly." This subtle change in the rule occurred because it is very important for young stutterers to learn the feeling of starting their vocal folds vibrating easily and smoothly. This is often referred to as a gentle onset and is used in a number of treatment programs for stutterers.[5,6] Although this is a commonly used therapeutic activity with stutterers, there does not appear to be a universally accepted definition of gentle onset. For our therapy program, it is defined as the gradual increase of intensity over time that occurs at the beginning of an utterance. This definition is modeled after the definition used in CAFET. Therapeutic success has occurred in the past using the concept of "gentle onset" with those children who identified a laryngeal problem by pointing to their neck and indicating that this is where they get "stuck."

THERAPY SUGGESTIONS

1. *Awareness*: A variety of caricatures have been used to represent "Mr. Voice Box" in order to show children that "he lives" in the neck, and when running you can feel the vibration. Have the child hum while feeling the neck area with his or her hand to demonstrate the location and existence of "Mr. Voice Box."

2. *Contrasting*: Demonstrate two distinctly different modes of initiating phonation, to illustrate the difference between a gentle and a hard onset. First, have the child feel the tension in the neck and the resulting abrupt or hard onset as he or she pulls up on the chair. Next, ask the child to feel the absence of tension in the neck area as he or she phonates without pulling up on the chair. We have also found Conture's strawman analogy[7] helpful in teaching children to relax the neck prior to attempted initiations of easy onsets.

3. *A Suggestion Changed*: Our original FRP suggested that clinicians have children use a breathy voice to learn and experience gentle onset. Once breathy voice production, and implied gentle onset, was learned, the clinician was instructed to systematically return the child's voice to one that was less breathy and more natural sounding. More recently we have occasionally experienced considerable difficulty in eliminating the newly acquired breathy component from the child's voice. Therefore, we questioned the appropriateness of teaching breathy speech production and then asking the child to reduce its use immediately. We have not experienced any substantial difficulty in teaching a school-age child easy onset without using the breathy voice model.

4. *Gentle Not Soft*: Early in our use of gentle onset, it became apparent that some children misinterpreted this therapy goal as soft onset (i.e., reduced intensity). Therefore, these children would begin talking at a very low intensity. To illustrate that the goal is a gentle not soft onset, two horizontal lines are drawn on a chalkboard or paper with a sloping line, at about a 45-degree angle connecting the lower to the upper line. The lower horizontal line is marked as zero intensity (we explain it as silence); the upper horizontal line, as the child's normal speaking intensity; and the 45-degree connecting line, as gentle onset. Using this drawing, the child is asked to begin speech with an easy onset of phonation as he or she traces the sloping line while initiating speech with an exaggerated slowness. As soon as the clinician believes the concept has been learned, the child is instructed to reduce the exaggerated slow onset to normal-sounding speech. Single-syllable, vowel-initiated words are usually used as therapeutic material for this task.

Secondary Rules

Rule 5: Touch the "Speech Helpers" Together Lightly

BACKGROUND

The "speech helpers" (i.e., lips, tongue, and teeth) have been depicted as cartoon characters that are parts of the mouth and that are important in the production of "speech sounds." A number of public school speech-language pathologists have used these cartoon "speech helpers" to decorate the walls of their therapy rooms/ offices, which also increases the awareness of most children to these anatomical structures. We explain to the children that it is necessary to touch the "speech helpers" together very lightly, because if they press them together too hard, speech breathing and speech will stop.

THERAPY SUGGESTIONS

1. *The Hard Contact*: Have the child produce a bilabial plosive (or any other stop consonant) by pressing the lips together tightly "until a word pops out." A number of the older children we have treated have been instructed by their parents to "just try harder" and their speech will improve. Therefore, we frequently need to spend clinical time to explain and demonstrate that trying easier, not harder, is necessary to produce fluent speech. Often we practice these hard contacts with a great deal of animated effort in front of a mirror, to point out humorously the futility of trying to produce speech with excessive effort.

2. *Can I Hold Your Arm?*: Another treatment technique we have used effectively to illustrate the goal of light contact of the "speech helpers" involves squeezing the child's arm as he or she speaks. As the child speaks fluently, the clinician holds an arm lightly, and then when a hard contact occurs, the clinician squeezes the child's arm gently but firmly. The amount of pressure applied to the arm should be roughly proportional to the amount of tension perceived.

Rule 6: Keep the Speech Helpers Moving

BACKGROUND

This rule was originally designed to eliminate prolongations but has been expanded to include the easy movement from one speech sound to the following sound. Using this rule in conjunction with rule 5, Touch the "speech helpers" together lightly, has also proved to be clinically effective. Several examples of combining these rules are included in the therapy suggestions that follow.

THERAPY SUGGESTIONS

1. *Turtle Tracks or Lily Pads*[2]: With turtle tracks from rule 1, or lily pads, have the child move from one track or lily pad to the next smoothly and step on each one lightly. During this activity we usually use five-syllable phrases for the child to imitate. By using this phrase length, five tracks can be placed close together, indicating the syllables for each phrase, with a larger space used to represent the pause between phrases and the place for the child to start the speech breathing and gentle-onset cycle again.

2. *Piano Fingers*[2]: Moving the thumb to each finger or tapping the thumb and fingers on a table top has proved useful in teaching this speech rule. We explain that speech should be produced easily and smoothly, just as we can move our thumb to our fingers or our fingers to tap the table top. With each digit representing a speech sound or syllables, the child produces short phrases, saying them and moving smoothly from sound to sound. Next, we

demonstrate that if the thumb and finger stay together too long, or a finger remains on the table too long, a prolonged sound will be produced. In addition, we can show the child that if the fingers press together with too much force, airflow and speech will slow down and stop.

Rule 7: Use Only the "Speech Helpers" To Talk

BACKGROUND

This rule explains that fluent speech is produced by moving only the "speech helpers" and it is not necessary or helpful to move other muscles or body parts when speaking. The intent of this rule is to eliminate any secondary behaviors that may have developed.

THERAPY SUGGESTIONS

1. *The Mirror*: A mirror has often proved useful in eliminating secondary behaviors. Frequently, children may be unaware of extraneous body movements or other secondary behaviors and, once these behaviors are visually pointed out, they are often quickly eliminated

2. *Too Much of a Bad Thing*: The mirror is again used with this technique. For example, if a head turn is used as speech begins, we explain that turning the head alone does not produce speech. Standing together with the child in front of the mirror, humorously demonstrate that "we are going to turn our heads as hard and as frequently as possible until a word comes out." Obviously speech does not occur, and it is clear that turning the head to start speech should be eliminated. This therapy technique can be used to illustrate to a child that a great number of motor responses can be produced but that speech does not begin until airflow begins and the "speech helpers" are moved.

Fluency Rules Program: Revised

Since the first version of the FRP was published, we have become increasingly aware of the importance of the order of presentation of the fluency rules. Originally the therapeutic steps that were followed were:

1. Determine the fluency rule broken.
2. Teach language concepts necessary for complete understanding of instructions.
3. Develop the child's self-monitoring skills.
4. Practice fluent speech production using the fluency rules.
5. Carry over to the home and classroom.

In the current version of the FRP, step 1 has been modified to the suggested order of presentation for fluency rules in this chapter. Although the original FRP version was successful with many young children, with its continued use, however, our therapeutic paradigm steadily changed. Originally, we recommended that clinicians work only on the fluency rules that were broken and gave no suggestions regarding which rule to treat first or in what order to teach other rules that were broken. A review of our recent clinical records indicated that therapy was always started with two rules: "Speak slowly," and "Say a word only one time." Therefore, these rules are now viewed as universal. This review also revealed that when children were treated using these two universal rules simultaneously, there was often a dramatic improvement in fluency without any additional therapeutic intervention. Thus, when these two rules were appropriately used by some children, other aspects of the stuttering (e.g., struggle and/or accessory behavior) frequently disappeared, and the need for additional fluency rules was eliminated.

As effective as the universal rules have proved to be, children who struggle during speech disruptions frequently continue to stutter. Therefore, when application of the two universal rules did not result in fluent speech production, the two primary rules became the focus of therapy. These two rules were always taught as a pair with rule 3, Speech breathing, explained first followed by rule 4, Get Mr. Voice Box running smoothly. Teaching these rules concurrently not only reflects our new procedure, but also appears to be consistent with other therapeutic practices that emphasize the importance of the interaction between speech breathing and gentle onset of phonation.[5,6,8] The rationale for designating these two rules as primary rules is that a clinically significant number of young stutterers exhibit laryngeal tension and report that "words get stuck in my throat." Many of these same stutterers do not demonstrate an appropriate speech breathing pattern or consistently coordinate speech breathing with the onset of phonation. Twelve of 14 young stutterers treated during the past 3 years have exhibited these breathing/voice onset problems, the most frequent being the tendency to "push the words out." These children appeared to reverse the direction of movement of their thoracic/abdominal wall, particularly when about to stutter, and occasionally when they were fluent. Thus, as they began to exhale, their thoracic/abdominal wall contracted, but immediately prior to initiating speech production, they reversed the direction of these movements and expanded the thoracic/abdominal area as if they were inhaling. It was our impression that these stutterers were using this type of physiological maneuver in an attempt to push words out. Those children old enough to understand our questions regarding such behavior verified that they were, in fact, trying to "push the words out."

The three secondary rules are used only if needed. Although we now use these rules less frequently, rule 5, Touch the "speech helpers" together lightly, has been used more frequently than the others. These secondary rules are used in the FRP as needed when aberrant behavior first occurs. For example, if the therapeutic goal is to teach the universal rules and a secondary behavior is observed, the clinician should immediately stop instructing the universal rules and teach the appropriate secondary fluency rule. When satisfied that the child understands the new rule, the clinician should return to teaching the universal rules.

Carryover and Transfer

The final phase of the FRP involves the carryover or transfer of the fluency rules that have been taught to the home and classroom. Obviously, to accomplish transfer, it is essential that the child remembers the rules in new speaking environments. The most effective procedure we have found to facilitate such carryover has been to place a discriminative stimulus in each environment. In school the speech-language pathologist, the classroom teacher, subject teacher, and the student meet to select a small unobtrusive item that will be placed in each room as a reminder of the fluency rule (e.g., stickers on notebooks or refrigerator magnets on the edge of chalkboards). Only the teacher and the student need be aware of the item and its significance. Then, if the child forgets to use a fluency rule, the teacher can provide a reminder by glancing in the direction of or touching the stimulus item. At home, the same procedure can be used. We place the stimulus items—we use symbolic elephants because elephants never forget—in conversation areas (e.g., the family room, kitchen, bedroom, and dining room) and have family members use these stimuli with the stutterer as needed. The subtle nature of these stimuli and their use also provides a secondary benefit. Eliminating the need for direct confrontations when fluency rules are not used can reduce family conflicts that may arise from reminding children of their fluency rules, particularly during the early stages of transfer. Ideally the transfer segment of therapy will result in the fluency rules being generalized to areas away from the therapy room and ultimately will lead to fluent speech in all environments.

A new and more effective discriminative stimulus that we have begun to use clinically involves video games. Nintendo and other video games provide an opportunity of using materials that have considerable motivational appeal with children. These games can be used to motivate children to use the fluency rules during therapy, at home, and at school. During a scheduled therapy session, Nintendo breaks are a regularly scheduled aspect of therapy and are used to reinforce correct application of the fluency rules. To facilitate carryover of fluency rules to the home, a lending library arrangement allows children to check out one game until the next therapy session. In order to check out a game, the child must agree to use their fluency rules at home and at school, particularly when playing the game. An additional positive effect that the lending library creates is that it stimulates more parental involvement in the therapeutic process. Because these games can be played competitively, parents are encouraged to find the time to play these games with their children. This leads to enjoyable times together and allows the parents to remind the child of the fluency rules, if needed, and to monitor how well the child is using the rules. We have been pleasantly surprised with the feedback received from both parents and children about using this procedure at home. Equally impressive is the motivational value of these games in the clinic with children. When our lending library was started, there were two difficult children on the caseload. Their renewed interest and subsequent increased cooperation in therapy were impressive. Both successfully completed therapy, which we feel was due in part to the implementation of the library and the interest that the use of these games brought to the therapy process.

Finally, telephone calls have also been used as a discriminative stimulus to help with carryover of fluency to the home environment. This technique has been used near the end of therapy, when the child is effectively using the fluency rules in therapy sessions. At this point, we encourage more awareness and use of the rules at home. To assist in keeping awareness high, the child is called at home and asked how his or her speech is doing and if he or she is remembering to use the rules. At first, with the parents' permission, these calls are frequent, about five calls a night. This frequency level is used for about a week, then calls are systematically reduced until they occur infrequently, about twice a week. Periodically, we again call five times on randomly selected nights. The intended outcome of this procedure is that after a short period of time, the child thinks that every time the phone rings "the crazy therapist is calling again," which serves as a reminder to use the fluency rules. Since the creation of the lending library, calls are now longer and more effective, because conversations can also be directed toward the use of the video games and not just checking up on speech. Such calls also provide an excellent opportunity to evaluate the child's fluency in different settings than the clinic.

Therapy Outcome

In our first description of the FRP, therapeutic results based on nine children were reported. The children consisted of five males and four females with an average age of 5 years, 5 months. Based on Riley's severity scale[9] three were rated mild, four as moderate, and two as severe stutterers. Five of these children were followed for 2 years after therapy while four were followed for 1 year after therapy. All had been treated in a public school setting, receiving therapy two or three times a week for 30 or 40 minutes. The data indicated that all of the children evidenced a significant improvement in fluency while maintaining normal speaking rate and eliminating all secondary behaviors. Further inspection of the data revealed that the improvement in fluent speech production that occurred in the first year of therapy was maintained during follow-up. However, a lingering concern remained. Although each child demonstrated marked improvement in fluent speech production, each child's speech also contained slight, residual signs of the stuttering. These residual effects were mild part-word repetitions of two or less iterations and no secondary behaviors. Unfortunately, these children could not be followed for longer periods of time and no additional data are available.

During the past few years, we have consulted with numerous public school systems regarding the implementation of the fluency rules program and have supervised a number of students as they used the program. Most recently we have personally treated 14 young stutterers, and it is the information from these stutterers that follows. This group consisted of 1 female and 13 male stutterers whose ages averaged 7 years, 1 month (Table 5-2). Based on the Stuttering Prediction Instrument,[10] there were 2 severe, 8 moderate, and 4 mild stutterers. Nine of these children demonstrated secondary behaviors. The mild stutterers and 1 moderate stutterer did not exhibit accessory behavior. Ten of the 14 children are currently fluent and have been so for the following periods: 4 subjects, 3 to 5 years; 2 subjects, 2 to 3 years; 2 subjects, more than 1 year; and 2 subjects, less than 1 year. All 10 children's speech was judged to be within the acceptable range on the naturalness scale at the termination of therapy.[11] Average length of therapy was 9 months, with a range of 3 to 20 months. At the beginning of therapy, most of the children attended twice a week for an hour session and then once a week for an hour session near the end of therapy. The 4 remaining children continue to stutter and are still enrolled in therapy.

Efficiency and adaptability were important factors in the design of the FRP

Table 5-2. Subjects Identified by Age, Severity Based on the Riley Prediction Instrument (RPI), Current Therapy Status, and Follow-up Period

Subject Age (y = mo.)	RPI Severity	Therapy Status	Follow-up (y)
8-2	Moderate	In	N/A
2-3	Moderate	In	N/A
8-1	Moderate	In	N/A
6-11	Moderae	Released	1
5-6	Mild	Released	1
11-0*	Moderate	Released	1
7-0	Severe	In	N/A
8-10	Moderate	Released	3
7-1	Mild	Released	5
10-1†	Mild	Released	4
9-8	Mild	Released	2
9-4	Moderate	Released	1
3-10	Severe	Released	4
8-1	Moderate	Released	2

*Female.
†Learning disability.
N/A = not applicable.

because of the typical public school treatment format. Results of the first group of children treated using this program demonstrated that it was effective in reducing stuttering when treatment was conducted in the public schools. Of the clinical outcomes just described, six of the ten children received services in the public schools in addition to private practice therapy. Therefore it appears that the FRP can be implemented successfully in combined effort between the public school and the private sector.

Finally, we again encourage clinicians in all therapeutic environments to use the FRP and to share their results, techniques, and experiences with us and their colleagues at professional meetings. The FRP's ultimate effectiveness and utility can only be demonstrated when larger and more diverse groups of stuttering children are treated by different therapists in different settings and followed over longer periods of time.

Suggested Reading

Conture EG: *Stuttering*, ed 2. Englewood Cliffs, NJ, Prentice-Hall, 1990.

References

1. Runyan CM, Bennett CW: Results of a survey of public school speech language pathologists in Virginia. *J Speech Hear Assoc Va* 1982; 23:91–95.
2. Runyan CM, Runyan SE: Fluency rules therapy program for young children in the public schools. *Lang Speech Hear Serv Schools* 1986; 17:276–284.
3. Purcell R, Runyan CM: Normative study of speech rates of children. *J Speech Hear Assoc Va* 1980; 21:6–14.
4. Greenberg JB: The effects of a metronome on the speech of young stutterers. *J Behav Ther* 1970; 1:240–244.

5. Goebel MD: A Computer-Aided Fluency Treatment Program for Adolescents and Adults. ASHA, miniseminar, November 1984, San Francisco.
6. Webster RL: *Precision Fluency Shaping*, 1. Roanoke, Va, Communication Development Corp, 1974.
7. Conture EG: *Stuttering*, ed 2. Englewood Cliffs, NJ, Prentice-Hall, 1990.
8. Costello J: Treatment of the Young Chronic Stutterer: Managing Fluency, in Curlee RF, Perkins WH (eds): *Nature and Treatment of Stuttering: New Directions*. San Diego, College-Hill Press, 1984.
9. Riley GD: A stuttering severity scale for children and adults. *J Speech Hear Disord* 1972; 37:314–320.
10. Riley GD: *Stuttering Prediction Instrument*. Tigard, OR, CC Publications, 1981.
11. Martin RR, Haroldson SK, Triden KS: Stuttering and speech naturalness. *J Speech Hear Disord* 1984; 49:23–58.

6

Management of Stuttering
Treatment of Adolescents and Adults

DAVID PRINS, PH.D.

Introduction

Typical adolescents or adults who stutter have difficulty remembering a sustained period when their speech was not punctuated by stuttering episodes, those moments when they perceive imminent or ongoing interruptions of fluency and try urgently to prevent or escape their consequences. They may also harbor handicapping attitudes about their ineffectuality as speakers and as individuals. If present, these attitudes are likely to have a negative effect on their personal adjustment and feelings of self-esteem. This chapter concerns the treatment of stuttering in such individuals. It emphasizes an approach called the "management of stuttering,"[1] which uses the stutter event as a focal point for resolving the disorder.

Nature of the Problem and Its Treatment

As a disorder of human behavior, stuttering consists of essential features at three levels: impairment, disability, and handicap.[2] Impairment refers to deficit conditions that may underlie a disability. Disability refers to the observable breakdown in behavior, and handicap concerns the effect of disability on social, educational, and vocational adjustment. When faced with treatment decisions for an adolescent or adult who stutters, the clinician chooses from approaches that focus on one or more of these levels. In recent years, treatment has emphasized the level of disability, that is, helping stutterers eliminate or ameliorate the occurrence of stutter events. Two general approaches have been used: 1) the management of fluency, and 2) the management of stuttering. Although employing different points of attack, both approaches share a similar ultimate objective: to help the person who stutters "learn to speak as fluently as he is able and has the will and the motivation to do."[3]

In essence, the first approach seeks this outcome by helping the stutterer learn to *enhance the fluency parameters* of his speech, thereby *preventing the occurrence of stutter events*. Seeking a similar end, the second approach helps the stutterer learn to *respond fluently to the cues that signal these events*. This chapter will emphasize the latter approach; however, the two can, and in many cases should, co-exist in a single treatment program. In fact, Peters and Guitar[4] have recently emphasized this idea.

Inherently, neither of these approaches is more "behavioral" than the other. Depending upon manner of implementation, both may or may not adhere to behavior modification principles. Frequently overlooked, this point was made earlier by Ingham.[5]

STUTTERING AS DISABILITY

According to contemporary theory and practice, two components constitute the stutter event: 1) an interruption of fluency and 2) the speaker's reaction thereto.[6,7,8] By and large, in the typical adolescent or adult stutterer, the behavior that *most debilitates* the perceptible normality of speech is associated with the second component; that is, the defensive, coping maneuvers that the stutterer mobilizes in an effort to prevent or escape perceived or anticipated fluency interruptions and their associated consequences. These emergency reactions include neuromuscular tensing and related struggle responses that contribute to rapid, multiple sound repetitions; sustained postural fixations; facial tremors, grimaces, and loss of eye contact; extraneous bodily movements; and the like. Also, included here are the elaborate devices that stutterers sometimes use to postpone or avoid anticipated stutter events; for example, interjections, word substitutions, and circumlocution. Even authors who express quite diverse opinions concerning the original sources of fluency interruption in stuttering generally agree about the nature of the reactive components.[6,8,9,10]

Social learning and self-efficacy theories provide useful conceptual models for understanding the nature of this type of defensive behavior and its resolution through treatment.[11,12,13] In the social learning view (also called "social cognitive theory"[13]) activation of defensive behavior occurs when an individual perceives cues that signal the likelihood of an aversive event unless protective actions are taken. The *cognitive nature of the cue* that forecasts the aversive consequence is essential to this idea. This *cue* has an internal representation, *a "meaning"* for the individual, *which serves not only to motivate the defensive reactions but also as an internal source for their perpetuation*.[13] Concerning treatment, self-efficacy theory states that various approaches succeed because individuals become convinced they can successfully execute (i.e., control) the behavior required for a desired outcome. The *emphasis*, here, is not upon the level of skills, but *on the conviction* about their adequacy.[11,13]

As applied to stuttering, social learning theory suggests that an adolescent or adult comes to perceive various cues during speech (for example, brief timing lags in one of several motor control processes, degrees of tension in the vocal tract, slight postural variations, etc.) as predictive of stutter events. These cues are represented cognitively, and at the instant of awareness, the stutterer engages in emergency reactions to prevent or escape the predicted outcome. An analog from daily living, the "crystal goblet phenomenon," helps to illustrate how cognition mediates such instantaneous, defensive reactions. This phenomenon occurs when, while gesturing, a diner inadvertently brushes a liquid-filled goblet. Abruptly, and with a sense of considerable urgency, he retracts his hand. He does so because the cue of the moist glass has a meaning all its own. Though the diner's reaction is instantaneous (and may actually topple the goblet); it is mediated by the stored images of liquid cascading onto the table, people leaping from their seats, disapproving stares, vocal rebukes, etc. As Bandura explains, such "transitory experiences leave lasting effects by being coded and retained in symbols for memory representation."[11,p.192] Similarly, we believe, the cognitive content associated with interruptions in speech fluency mediates the reactive components of the stutter event.

The rationale for focusing treatment on these reactive components (rather than on eliminating the occurrence of stutter events altogether) rests on the assumptions that cues which trigger stuttering reactions 1) have become an integral part of speech production processes; and 2) are likely to retain, at least under circumstances associated with communicative pressure, some of their cognitively mediated stimulus value. Unless a stutterer is convinced he can respond "normally" to these cues, he is apt, when they occur, to recoil instinctively with self-protective reactions.

STUTTERING AS HANDICAP

In terms of self-efficacy theory,[11,12] adolescent and adult stutterers harbor, to varying degrees, a sense of futility about stutter events, a *belief* that they cannot cope with them successfully. This occurs in part because the very actions they take to defend against predicted outcomes further debilitate speech production processes, thus becoming an integral part of what they are trying to defend against. As viewed in this way, the nature of the reactive behavior in stutter events illustrates their handicapping potential. That is, stutterers' seeming helplessness to achieve successful outcomes in response to cues that predict stutter events results in self-doubt about their ability to speak. In turn, this may generalize into an overall loss of self-esteem and lead to use of the disability as an explanation for perceived inadequacies.

If handicapping features are major components of the disorder, they are likely to be especially significant in determining treatment outcome. In recent years, behaviorally designed programs have paid relatively little attention to this idea.

THE MANAGEMENT OF STUTTERING

Currently, social learning and self-efficacy theories provide a conceptual foundation for treatment that emphasizes behavioral management of stutter events. According to these theories, *cognitive processes are crucial in mediating behavior change which occurs when successful performance leads to an internalized sense of mastery.*[11,13]

It is worth recalling, however, that these theories did not exist when approaches to stuttering treatment that focus on cognition and self-mastery originated. Grounded in the principles of general semantics, Wendell Johnson[14,15] pioneered, and Dean Williams[16,17,18] later refined, an approach which seeks to alter the way a stutterer thinks about his speaking behavior. Somewhat later, based on psychotherapeutic and learning principles, Van Riper[19] described treatment procedures which stress the stutterer's behavioral mastery of the stuttering moment. The ideas and approaches of these clinicians, once very popular, fell out of favor during the 1960s and 1970s, a period of so-called "radical behaviorism."[5] The techniques appeared too subjectively applied to be replicable, and measures of outcome seemed too ambiguous. Now, with the advent of social learning and self-efficacy theories, a new framework exists for developing and evaluating these approaches.

Pretreatment Evaluation

Evaluation is essentially a process which describes problem components at the three levels mentioned earlier: impairment, disability, and handicap. At the level of *impairment*, procedures attempt to identify possible factors that may underlie the occurrence of fluency interruptions. Most measures at this level evaluate speech production processes such as facility in word retrieval, speech and related timing abilities, and ability to execute speech and other coordinated movements. As part of pretreatment protocols, these measures are generally used in research settings for the purpose of determining factors that might predict outcome or be differentially related to the selection of treatment procedures. Papers by Boberg,[20] Ludlow,[21] and Peters[22] provide examples of specific tests that may be used in this way. Rigorous attempts to relate such tests to the selection of treatment procedures and to outcome are just beginning.[20,23,24,25] In the future, work of this type may have enormously important implications for treatment. At present, however, there is insufficient evidence to guide the meaningful use of such tests as a basis for planning treatment or predicting outcome.

The principal emphases of pretreatment evaluations concern the levels of *disability* and *handicap*; that is, describing perceptible deviations in speech fluency and their effects on the person's overall adjustment and the way he thinks about himself as a speaker. The purposes are:

1. To understand a client's strategies and style of coping a) during stutter events, b) in anticipation of such events, and c) in communicative situations of daily living.
2. To determine the initial targets for treatment—not only the overt features of behavior that debilitate the speaking process, but also the belief systems that appear to mediate them.
3. To obtain baseline measures of severity against which outcomes can be assessed.
4. To estimate prognosis.
5. To determine whether referrals should be made to other professionals.

The Case History

The literature contains examples of various case history forms.[4,26] Rather than duplicate a similar form, this section will concentrate on the *type* of information wanted and *why*. When completing a case history, a client records what he can remember about the origins and development of the problem, its presence in other family members, and the nature and outcomes of previous treatment. He also describes the problem currently, its effects on his educational, social, and vocational adjustment, and his reasons and objectives for seeking treatment. When provided by a preliminary questionnaire, this information serves as a guide for related questions that may be asked during an initial interview. For example:

- Tell me about the therapy assistance you have had in the past. What were its goals and how did it help, or fail to help?
- What is your speech like now compared with earlier?
- Do you know when you stutter? What are you aware of? How does it feel or sound?
- What is it about speaking situations or listeners that makes talking easy or difficult?
- How serious a problem is your stuttering?
- Does stuttering interfere with your life on a day-to-day basis? What's the worst thing about it?
- How do others feel about your stuttering? Is it important to them? Does stuttering affect how others view you? Do you view yourself in the same way others do?
- Tell me about your job (school, social activities).
- How would you describe yourself? For example, are you easy going or tense? Are you a confident person or do you often worry about failing? Do you often see yourself as inadequate to meet the demands of various situations or are you usually self-confident?
- What made you decide to seek treatment now? What do you want to achieve? How do you think we can help?

Responses to questions of this type help establish focal points early in treatment when clinician and client begin to explore speaking and related attitudes and feelings.

Observations and Tests

SPEECH

Whenever possible, video recordings should be obtained of monologue, reading, and conversational speech samples of three to five minutes each. Shortly after treatment has been initiated, video recordings should also be made of several brief telephone conversations. In addition to these in-clinic samples, audiorecordings of selected outside speaking situations are usually secured. Included here are telephone calls from home or office; short conversations with friends, spouse, and/or other family members at home or in other settings. Ordinarily, these samples are collected after treatment has begun.

Speech samples provide data for characterizing stutter events: their *frequency* and typical *duration*, and the *physical concomitants* that accompany them. The latter include audible signs of struggle and tension, facial grimaces and tremor-like movements, bodily movements, etc. The Riley Stuttering Severity Instrument[27] is useful for quantifying these observations.

In addition, the speech samples enable identification of other speech characteristics that could be associated with the problem. These include the use of interjections, revisions, word substitutions, and circumlocution at times when stutter events are anticipated. This behavior not only provides the clinician with important clues concerning the client's coping strategies and adaptive style; it will also be important later for the client and clinician to explore together. Different speech characteristics in stutterers have been associated with defense preferences,[28] giving credence to the usefulness of these observations in planning treatment. For example, a stutterer who uses elaborate verbal devices to avoid the occurrence of stutter events, and in whom such events occur infrequently, has a substantially different problem to overcome than a person whose stuttering instances occur often and who struggles openly with these instances—almost never avoiding or postponing their occurrence.

It is also useful to measure syllable rate and its regularity during nonstuttered speech. If rate is particularly erratic and syllabic stress arrhythmic, it suggests that the stutterer may not have a solid base of fluent, nonstuttered speech upon which to build, and that he may also have difficulty monitoring ongoing speech and detecting the occurrence of stutter events (see Case Selection).

ATTITUDES, FEELINGS, AND PERSONAL EFFICACY

Clinicians need to understand a stutterer's beliefs about himself and his capabilities as a speaker in order to determine the extent of handicap. It may range from little more than a circumscribed sense of futility in speaking situations to a belief that the speaking disability colors adjustment to all aspects of daily living. Questions asked during the pretreatment interview, and subsequently during the course of treatment, help provide this information. More formally, the client can be asked to respond to statements that 1) other stutterers have used to describe themselves and 2) describe various speaking situations (see Appendices A & B). For the former, the stutterer rates the extent to which such statements as, "Feeling that my speech is uncontrollable" or "Feeling that I am socially inadequate" hold true for him. For the latter, he rates speaking situations in terms of how often he encounters them, their level of difficulty, and his confidence in speaking ability.

Responses to these questionnaires help determine components of the disorder that will require special attention, as well as speaking situation hierarchies for treatment. They also provide the basis for assessing change as the program progresses. Other published questionnaires that afford similar types of information include: The Iowa Scale of Attitude Toward Stuttering and Stutterer's Self-Ratings of Reactions to Speech Situations;[29] The Modified Erickson Scale;[30] Perceptions of Stuttering Inventory;[31] Locus of Control of Behavior.[32]

Case Selection and Initial Emphases of Treatment

To achieve enduring success, treatment which focuses on managing stutter events affirms that the stutterer must 1) understand his behavior during stuttering episodes and 2) experience, and develop confidence in, alternative responses that restore speech fluency. Whether the moment of stuttering is the principal focus at the *outset* of treatment, however, may depend upon certain characteristics of the disorder as well as the client's initial needs and personal objectives.

DISABILITY CHARACTERISTICS

When stutter events are longer than fleeting gaps or facial tics and are clearly distinctive from nonstuttered speech, treatment usually begins by focusing on those events. However, if stuttering episodes are very brief and nonstuttered speech is erratic in its rate and rhythmic structure, stuttering occurrences may be difficult for the client to distinguish. In such cases, when speech may be characterized as much by cluttering as by stuttering, procedures associated with fluency management may serve as a better starting point in treatment. Similarly, if stuttering moments are extremely frequent and severe in terms of duration and physical concomitants, it may be necessary to begin with procedures that directly enhance fluency, if for no other reason than to provide sufficient relief from stuttering to permit communication during treatment sessions.

The nature of other associated speech characteristics also may serve as keys in helping to determine the initial emphases of treatment. When devices to postpone or avoid anticipated stuttering are a predominant feature of the disability, they suggest that the stutterer not only has vivid signals that he or she uses to forecast stutter events, but that their occurrence is a serious threat. In comparison to a stutterer who openly forges ahead and struggles through these events, the former may be more apt to resist direct confrontation with stuttering. At the outset, he or she may require approaches that focus chiefly on exploring attitudes and feelings that underlie the extensive use of avoidance behavior.

Guitar and Peters recommend that a management of stuttering approach is best used when speech avoidance aspects of the problem are high, whereas fluency management is indicated when there is minimal avoidance and the person responds well to prolonged speech procedures.[33]

HANDICAP CHARACTERISTICS

Results from the pretreatment interview and questionnaires help the clinician discover the extent to which the stutterer 1) regards his disability as the foundation for life adjustment and 2) leans on the disability as an explanation for perceived inadequacies or personal failures. When these handicapping features are a major part of the problem, they do not foretell the most effective approaches in treatment so much as they do prognosis. Though it does not always appear so at the outset of treatment, when the degree of handicap is high, the course of treatment is apt to be slow and erratic. Moreover, relapse following treatment will have many reasons to occur. If degree of handicap is extraordinarily high, and the stutterer's sense of adequacy and self-esteem sufficiently low, other professional assistance may be needed, usually in addition to, not as a replacement for, speech therapy.

PROGNOSIS

No known pretreatment measures can assure the best selection among treatment approaches for a given stutterer or predict the likelihood of a successful outcome. Although Boberg,[20] for example, has recently initiated a project with these purposes in mind, the clinician must currently rely upon his experience to make such judgments. In terms of client characteristics, the following are negative predictors:

- A long history of unsuccessful treatment after participation in a variety of different treatment programs.
- Extensive use of the disability to explain perceived shortcomings and the reactions of others.
- Evidence of a need to blame others for the disability.
- Limited sources of strength including family support, educational and vocational achievements.
- Unrealistic expectations concerning the ultimate effects on life adjustment of resolving the speech difficulty.

Clinical Management

In this chapter the management of stuttering approach is described as a type of cognitive behavior therapy. A basic tenet is that "to alter how people behave one must alter how they think."[13,p.519] In this approach the *processes* of change *are* viewed as *cognitive* while the *means* of change are *through performance mastery*. Emerick,[34] Maxwell,[35] and Cooper[36] describe similar approaches to treatment which emphasize cognitive restructuring and the client's feeling of behavioral control.

The treatment program described here provides the stutterer with increasingly challenging experiences in which he performs successfully and develops the conviction that he is able to do so. From the clinician's perspective, treatment is an "experiment." The clinician states hypotheses, selects procedures to test them, collects data to evaluate outcome, and makes revisions accordingly. From the client's perspective, treatment is an adventure in self-discovery and change. Its pathway involves risks but has potential for high payoff.

Treatment Goals

As mentioned earlier, treatment helps the stutterer speak as fluently as he is able and has the will and motivation to do. The following *principal goals* lead to this objective. They are stated from the client's point of view.

- Understand the nature of the problem—my responsibility for what I do and feel and for making change.
- Identify and become less reactive during occasions when I experience stuttering episodes.
- Develop a sense that I can gain control over the most significant aspects of my behavior while speaking.
- Change my behavior so that I react and act appropriately at the point when stutter events occur, as well as minimize the occurrence of such events.
- Internalize a sense of self-efficacy regarding my ability to speak.

To provide an overview of the program a written summary of these goals is given to, and discussed with, the client. Throughout the program the clinician emphasizes the co-development of more specific objectives and the client's understanding of their rationale.[35,37]

Treatment Procedures

The procedures described below concern individual (vis-à-vis group) therapy. They assume a nonintensive schedule consisting of approximately two clinical sessions per week.

Four principal phases of treatment are identified; however, they are less distinctive than the labels imply. Progress in each phase lays a foundation for the one that follows, but progress in all phases continues in parallel throughout treatment, each phase interacting with and helping to determine success in the others. Although modified substantially, these phases derive their essential character from the work of Van Riper.[38]

Elsewhere, Prins has described procedures applicable to each phase and illustrated their use within a behavior modification framework.[3] Rather than repeating such illustrations, this chapter will emphasize the importance of modeling, self-reinforcement and self-regulation of behavior, motivation, and cognitive awareness for achieving behavior change and feelings of self-efficacy.

Each treatment phase will highlight modeling procedures. Whether vicarious (through observation of others) or participatory (through client performance) they facilitate the following *component processes in observational learning*:[12]

- *Attention*: People must attend to the significant features of modeled behavior in order to learn from it. To aid this process, models should command interest and admiration.
- *Retention*: To profit from modeled behavior, people must remember it. For this purpose, clinician and client label the significant features of behavior; observe and rehearse it in slow motion and real time.
- *Motor Reproduction*: Symbolically stored images of behavior need to be translated to specific actions. Video recordings help to enable this outcome. They provide feedback to the client, enabling him to refine new responses and identify the tactual, kinesthetic, and cognitive cues to guide them.
- *Motivation*: Positive outcomes motivate the client to adopt new responses. The clinician uses reinforcement to accomplish this end, but the client's self-reinforcement is even more important as he verbalizes what he has done and analyzes why it has been successful.

The principal phases of treatment are described below. An introduction to each phase summarizes its essential character after which three separate segments review procedures for client/clinician sessions, client self-regulation of behavior, and determining achievement landmarks.

PHASE I—EXPLORATION

The initial phase of treatment helps the client understand what he does and feels as he speaks and stutters; it brings behavior and thought processes to new levels of consciousness. The client's objective is to experience and realize responsibility for doing most of the things that truly debilitate fluency; to understand that accompanying feelings need not have a cause-effect relationship with his actions.[12,18,34] That which once seemed uncontrollable comes to be perceived as controllable.

These concepts and their importance to the treatment of stuttering originated principally with Johnson[14] and Williams.[16,17,18] Although many important insights remain to be gained in other phases of treatment, significant discoveries in this phase set the stage for subsequent behavior change.

Client/Clinician Sessions (Phase I).   Clinician: "I'd like to begin by helping you learn to explore what you do and how you feel when you stutter. To give you an idea of what we are trying to achieve, I'm going to show you a videotape of another stutterer who is describing his speech while he observes himself in a mirror." As this tape is played and replayed, clinician and client note and discuss what the stutterer is describing, what he is learning, and why it is important. Clinician: "Next, I want to show you the videotape you made earlier, and we will begin to describe and catalogue what you do as you talk that interferes with fluency and communication." The tape is played in real time and in slow motion to isolate moments of stuttering. Behavioral accompaniments are studied and modeled. This is accomplished as the clinician periodically duplicates a stuttering moment from the tape and then asks the client to duplicate it as well. The purpose is to have the client discover, and internalize the perception, that his reactions are primarily responsible for the observable stuttering behavior and that these reactions are not necessary. The stutterer also tries to identify fluency arresting postures that trigger stuttering reactions. . . . things he perceives that serve as cues to feeling "blocked." He then tries to induce these cues and to trigger actual stutter events. At the same time, he attends to his emotional reactions and observes how they may vary independently of motor performance.

Next, the client may observe himself speaking before a mirror while being video recorded. Clinician: "Now I want you to observe and describe your speaking while you are doing it . . . much the same way the person did whom we observed earlier on videotape. First, as you talk, *I'll* signal you to stop and *you* describe what you are doing. Later, I want you to *stop on your own* when you observe a stutter event, and then proceed to describe what you are doing." After making these observations, the client also describes how he *feels* at the instant of stuttering.

Clinician: "Now, let's move away from the mirror and do the same thing during a conversation. This time you won't have the mirror to provide feedback, so you will need to "feel" the signals of your stutter events in order to stop and describe what you are doing. If you have difficulty with this, we'll move back and forth, with and without the mirror."

Client Self-Regulation of Behavior (Phase I).   For many years, self-therapy, or having the stutterer become his own clinician, has been an important feature of treatment.[38] More recently, self-regulation and self-evaluation procedures have illustrated their positive effects on sustaining fluency following the termination of treatment.[39] In fact, they may be among the most crucial ingredients in treatment to help assure retention of change.

According to Bandura, three constituent processes lead to effective self-regulation: self-observation, -judgment, and -reaction.[13] *Self-observation* allows cause-effect relationships to be discovered. *Self-judgment* leads to internalization of performance standards which are the bases for evaluation. *Self-reactions* influence behavior by creating motivational incentives and internal reinforcement of performance.

Self-regulation begins at the outset of the program. The client observes his speaking behavior during *activities of daily living*: at home, school, work, shopping, social gatherings, and the like. Based on discoveries made earlier during tape and mirror observations, the client uses structured formats to report the situation, level of difficulty, date/time of observation, and notations concerning stuttering, personal and listener reactions. Figure 6-1 shows a sample outline for self-observation. The client makes audio recordings of selected situations, and uses these to verify written observations. For this purpose, each client provides his own cassette tape recorder.

Concurrently, using facilities in a *"clinical laboratory"* room, the client begins independently to observe, monitor, and evaluate his speaking in greater depth. Initially, he may describe a video speech sample of another stutterer. In so doing, he becomes more familiar with observational techniques and with the complexities of stuttering reactions before he begins to study his own behavior. Next, the client reviews the video samples made earlier of his own speech; those which were initially reviewed during client/clinician sessions. Using an observational framework adapted to his stuttering characteristics, he describes his behavior in more detail. He then videotapes his imitations of stuttering instances and studies them in real time and slow motion. His objective is to make these "faked" stutters as close in appearance to his "actual" stutters as possible and to begin gaining a sense of voluntary control over the behavior. After each session, the client records on the observation sheet his comments concerning what he has "learned" about his stuttering, its characteristics and controllability, his feelings, etc. The video samples and written observations, along with the written report from outside activities, begin what will be an ongoing *record of treatment activities and progress* that clinician and client review weekly.

Date/Time	Speaking Situation	Level of Difficulty*	Speech Character-istics**	Personal Feelings***	Listener(s) Reactions

   *   Five-point scale
  **   Specifically what I did while speaking or stuttering: e.g., repeated sounds, interjected words, closed my eyes, etc.
***   In terms of emotionality, fear, tension, self-defeating thoughts, etc.

Figure 6-1. Self-observation log—daily activities.

Achievement Landmarks (Phase I). Progression to the next phase begins when the treatment record shows evidence that the client:

- Engages and observes himself in a variety of outside speaking situations;
- Describes and duplicates accurately various components of stutter events;
- Recognizes and senses his responsibility for speech actions;
- Discovers actions and feelings during speech that he was unaware of before and reveals insights concerning their function;
- Begins to show attitude shifts from self-protection to self-discovery in approaching speaking situations.

These kinds of achievements concern changes in both performance and thinking. They mark the onset of self-discovery which will continue throughout the treatment program and beyond. They also provide the necessary foundation for advancing to the next phase of treatment and form the basis for "learning" (vs. "performance") contingent progress. This distinction, according to social learning theory, *differentiates performance from acquisition of behavioral change.*[12] In this, as in subsequent phases of treatment, client progress requires evidence of cognitive, as well as surface-level, changes in *self-regulated* situations. Speech performance during client-clinician sessions suggests the client's potential for learning. However, it is insufficient evidence upon which to judge that a foundation exists for advancing to subsequent phases of treatment or for the acquisition, generalization, and retention of change (see Bandura[13]).

PHASE II: DESENSITIZATION

The purpose of this phase is to help the stutterer learn to remain emotionally and physically calm during stutter events and to recognize thought processes that inhibit his ability to do so. Van Riper developed this concept and many associated procedures.[38]

According to social learning theory, behavior results from a reciprocal determinism among performance, cognitive, and environmental factors. Based on this model, desensitization focuses on reducing the intensity of motoric and emotional reactions during stuttering while fostering self-enhancing images and a more realistic appraisal of environmental circumstances.

Client/Clinician Sessions (Phase II).

Clinician: "When a moment of stuttering takes place, or when you think it might take place, you usually have a sense of emergency, even panic, along with feelings and thoughts of helplessness. At that instant, you become desperate to prevent or escape the event, and you over-react. If you can learn to respond calmly at that point, you will have gone a long way toward removing the basis for much of what you do that makes your speech abnormal when you stutter. As you sense that you can react calmly, you reduce tension, you slow down your movements, and you focus on more positive thoughts about what you are doing. Before we begin, I want to show you a tape of another stutterer who is demonstrating the difference between emergency and calm stutter reactions."

Using a model on videotape, the clinician points out and discusses differences in the extent, duration, and speed of movement, the overall amount of effort, the apparent comfortableness of the speaker, and other factors that serve to contrast desensitized and ordinary stutter events.

> Clinician: "Now, I'd like you to experiment with making the same changes in your stuttering. Read this (or talk about a selected topic) and we'll try to collect some stuttering episodes. While you're doing this, the video camera will record your responses so that we can review them later. Each time you stutter on a word, I'll ask you to stop and stutter again on the same word. Your objective is to experience the cues that trigger the stutter event and to react calmly, while developing the sense that it's not necessary to suddenly retreat or to barge forward. Be aware that as you lessen the tension of your muscular reactions, the movements become slower and smoother, and you feel calmer. In other words, be aware of both your feelings and your performance."

This, or a similar activity, is repeated with periodic reviews of the videotape to observe and discuss performance, feelings, and thought processes. At this point in treatment, the client also identifies verbal postponement or avoidance devices. As needed, work concentrates on discovering these devices in accompaniment with becoming calm during stuttering episodes. Another principal feature of this phase is the development of eye contact during stutter events. This is an integral part of calm stuttering reactions as the client observes listener feedback and becomes aware that "looking" can serve the dual function of calming both self and listener.

Next, stuttering episodes are rated. Using a five-point scale, the stutterer signals, immediately after each instance of stuttering, whether the feeling and/or performance was a "1" (calm/relaxed) or a "5" (emotional/tense). He does this by raising the appropriate number of fingers without verbal comment. The videotape provides verification of judgment accuracy. Earlier, Prins[3] described a small step sequence of activities for this purpose. Activities are done first with the clinician only, and then with other listeners in the room.

A mirror may also be helpful in similar activities. Following each stutter event and the client's rating, the clinician provides feedback concerning his observations about performance change, including comments about less apparent tension and effort, slower movements, reduced range of movement, better eye contact, etc. This description helps the client attend to key changes and to internalize their effect.

Another modeling experience occurs when client and clinician (or another stutterer who has successfully completed this phase of treatment) enter outside speaking situations together. While the client observes, the clinician or other stutterer executes the motor features of calm stuttering, retains eye contact with the listener, and reports low levels of emotional arousal. Through discussion, the client realizes that maintaining eye contact and calm feelings during these episodes represents a challenge for the clinician which is similar to that which the client faces. The client then participates until he can achieve the established goal.

Client self-regulation of behavior (phase II).   Using the rating system developed during client/clinician sessions, the client evaluates his performance in a variety of *daily living activities*. Activities done at home, for example, talking with family members, friends, or on the telephone, can be audiorecorded for self-evaluation. The client records the ratings (1–5) of his performance and emotionality during each stuttering instance. These ratings and accompanying audio samples are then discussed and verified at subsequent clinical sessions. For speaking situations outside the home, the client plans in advance which encounters he will rate and, afterward, writes down his mean ratings for each situation.

The *clinical laboratory* room is used to videorecord and play back various conditions that the client and clinician plan, including telephone calls and conversations with other listeners. After each call or conversation, the client reviews the videotape and rates his reactions for each stutter event. The clinical laboratory experience is particularly valuable for this and subsequent phases, since it allows the client to see, as well as hear, the changes he is making; literally, to view himself behaving in a new way and to internalize the self-concept. His written report of these and outside-clinic observations becomes a part of the treatment record.

ACHIEVEMENT LANDMARKS (PHASE II)

Before moving to the next phase of treatment, the client demonstrates calm ratings (1–2) during stutter events in a variety of speaking situations, including client/ clinician sessions and self-regulated activities. The clinician must agree with these ratings which are verified by video and audiotape samples. In situations which the client considers most difficult, calm ratings (1–2) are unlikely until completion of the program. What the client must illustrate for himself, however, is that in some situations where stuttering episodes used to be characterized by emergency-type reactions, he can and does respond calmly, and is aware of the relationship of changes in feeling, thought processes, and performance. To help amplify this awareness, he takes frequent opportunities to explain to the clinician and others what he is working to accomplish and what insights he has gained. Through questions and discussions, in this and subsequent phases of therapy, *the stutterer's attention is focused on the meaning of treatment experiences* in relation to the nature of his problem and the objectives of the program (see Maxwell[35]).

PHASE III—REPLACEMENT OF STUTTERING REACTIONS

In this phase of the program the stutterer learns to respond with slow, smooth, effortless movements to cues which formerly triggered stuttering reactions. To do so, he must be able to detect the occurrence of these cues and shift to actions which have the utterance of the syllable or word as their goal. Furthermore, he must be able to do this *automatically*, with virtually no requirement for conscious thought. This phase has three initial substages (detection, interruption, and variation) which provide the foundation for replacing stuttering reactions.

Client/Clinician Sessions (Phase III). Clinician: "In order to replace stuttering reactions effectively, you need to be able to *detect*, as soon as possible, the cues that serve to trigger them. To give you an example, I'll try to detect the onset of stutter events while you speak. As you begin talking, my job will be to signal, by using this counter, every time a stuttering instance occurs. I'll try to signal as soon as possible after it begins, and we'll see if I can be at least 90% accurate." Here again, video recordings verify the clinician's accuracy. After the clinician models accurate identification, the client assumes the role of detector by using the counter while being videorecorded. In order to progress, he must achieve approximately 90% accuracy; that is, detect accurately 9/10ths of the stutter events.

Clinician: "Now, I want to change the detection task. Instead of clicking the counter, I want to see if you can *interrupt* each stuttering occurrence by stopping as soon as possible after the onset of the event and briefly freezing your position. Then, after you have held that position for about a second, finish the word and continue talking until the next episode occurs, etc. When you can do this, you will be in a position to vary what you do during stutter events."

This task proceeds until the client can achieve about 90% accuracy in a selected range of speaking tasks. Video feedback provides opportunities to evaluate and highlight performance.

Clinician: "Again, we're going to change the objective a little bit. This time, after you have interrupted the stutter event, I want to see if you can *vary* the pattern of the stuttering as you continue to say the word."

Depending upon the habitual pattern of stuttering, the clinician demonstrates the kinds of changes he would like the client to practice. Such changes should contrast with the stutterer's usual pattern. For example, if stutter events usually consist of fixed postures, with or without sound, the stutterer might be asked to change to a pattern of slow repetitions. This stage continues until it is clear that the stutterer can introduce planned variations during a substantial fraction of stutter events. As before, video feedback demonstrates and reinforces what is being learned.

Clinician: "You're in a position now to *replace* what you customarily do during stutter events with purposeful actions that lead to an effortless production of the word. The replacement response is *simple*. It consists of *clearly identifiable actions that contrast* with your habitual stuttering reactions and with what you would have done had you simply uttered the word without stuttering. I'll demonstrate for you:

- assume the appropriate articulatory positions for the intended sound of the syllable/ word;
- use easy voice onset and light articulatory contacts, and briefly sustain the sound (or vowel following a stop consonant);
- make a slow, smooth, deliberate transition to the following sound and complete the syllable effortlessly, without any forcing."

The client practices this response on isolated words. Initially, to emphasize cognitive rehearsal of the response, the client visualizes his production as a replacement for stuttering reactions. The concurrent use of video feedback helps to build a self-efficacy percept as well as performance skill. It is common in the perfection of athletic skills to use this type of cognitive re-enactment as part of practice.[13] In the treatment of stuttering, Frick in 1965[40] highlighted previsualization as a technique, but it has not received much attention since that time.

Next, the clinician demonstrates the replacement response on two or three underlined words in each of several sentences. The clinician should model this response smoothly and naturally in order to illustrate normal inflection, stress patterns, and speaking rate. As with any new response, the client will feel and sound awkward at first. It is crucial that he observe the smooth and effortless integration of the replacement response into ongoing speech. After the clinician serves as a model, videotapes of other stutterers help to *emphasize how automatically and effortlessly* the response can be produced.

The client then practices the response using printed material with underlined words. He gradually moves to material that contains no underlining and then to self-formulated speech, using the replacement response on a selected percentage of nonstuttered words. Modeling by the clinician, and by other stutterers on videotape, should precede each of these steps. In using this response periodically on *nonstuttered* words, the client is:

- Performing under easy conditions (nonstuttered) what later will be performed under pressure (stuttered);
- Giving stimulus value to the response, priming it for replacement of instinctively strong stuttering reactions;
- Losing sensitivity to doing something which, initially, calls attention to itself;
- Automatizing the response so that ultimately it can be done effortlessly, allowing thought processes to focus on speech content, not performance.

> Clinician: "Next, we're going to begin using this new response to replace your typical reactions during actual instances of stuttering. At the same time, however, and for the reasons we discussed earlier, you will also continue to use the response on selected nonstuttered words. We'll begin with these sentences. Each has one underlined word. Use the new response on that word whether or not it is stuttered. If moments of stuttering are triggered on any other words, your task is to use the new response to replace stuttering reactions."

At this point, the client proceeds through tasks of graduated difficulty from sentences with no underlined words, to paragraphs, short spontaneous responses, conversations, etc., with the clinician and other listeners. Progression from one task to the next is performance contingent (see Prins[3]).

The clinician points out that it is important for the client to attend to, and *believe* in, what he is *doing* and its successful outcome; that what he "feels" need not have a cause-effect relationship with what he does. Williams[18] and Emerick[34] emphasized the importance of these ideas in treatment, and research has shown that as perceived self-efficacy increases, it serves to reduce psychophysiological arousal.[13]

Client Self-Regulation of Behavior (Phase III).   At the outset of this phase of treatment, the client will report his success *outside the clinic* in detecting, interrupting, and varying stuttering reactions in selected situations that are appropriate for practicing these skills. Using percentages, he records for each situation the accuracy with which he detects, interrupts, and varies his behavior during stutter events. Whenever possible, audiotapes, reviewed by clinician and client, help verify his reports.

When the client begins to use the replacement response on nonstuttered and stuttered words, he sets up a sequence of outside situations for self-monitoring. He indicates his objectives and evaluates both performance and self-perception using a form similar to that shown in Figure 6-2. The client rates his *performance* of the replacement response using the scale values shown in the figure. Descriptors for scale values are usually specified for each client. The client practices rating his performance during therapy sessions, and reviews video recordings to verify his accuracy on individual stutter events. Then, for each outside situation he

Situation_____   Date_____

	Performance			Self-Perception**		
	No. Stutt. Events	X̄ Repl. Rating*	% Repl. Non-Stutt. Words	Confident	Comfortable	In Control
Objective:						
Actual:						

* 1 = extreme effort and forced release
2 = much effort; some forcing at release
3 = moderate effort; release quite smooth
4 = slight effort, release smooth
5 = effortless and smooth

** 1 = not at all
2 = slightly
3 = somewhat
4 = substantially
5 = completely

Figure 6-2.   Self-evaluation form—stuttering replacement response.

records his average rating across all stuttering instances that occurred. When appropriate, audio recordings of these situations provide verification. As part of performance evaluation, the client also estimates the percentage of words uttered on which he used the replacement response on nonstuttered words. He also monitors and evaluates his *self-perceptions* as shown in Figure 6-2. When completed, this form becomes a part of the treatment record.

In the *clinical laboratory* the client sets up a variety of speaking tasks including reading, conversations, and telephone calls which he videorecords after setting objectives for each activity. After reviewing the videotape, he evaluates his performance and self-perceptions using the form illustrated in Figure 6-2.

Concerning the *automatization* of new skills, three principal subprocesses underlie the procedures used in this phase of treatment:

- *Mergerization*: Initially, the client directs his thought and attention to specific elements of the response which at first he achieves slowly and awkwardly. Gradually, through familiarization, he executes the response as a whole, effortlessly and with little thought or attention.

- *Linkage to specific contexts*: The client uses the response in specific events (stuttering episodes) and situations (telephone, talking to friends, strangers, etc.).

- *Shifting the locus of attention*: The client directs his attention from the elements of the response to its effects, in this case on effortless movements of speech, internal perceptions of comfort and confidence, and listener reactions.

According to Bandura, these processes result in fully-developed complex skills that "are typically executed without much conscious deliberation."[13,p.461]

Achievement Landmarks (Phase III).   Across a full range of speaking situations, client ratings of 4 to 5 (see Figure 6-2) on stuttering replacement performance and self-perception signify successful completion of this phase of treatment. Several procedures help to verify ratings: 1) periodic videotapes of selected difficult situations such as speaking to small groups or before a class; 2) outside situations with other individuals who also rate the clients' performance; 3) unexpected telephone calls which are rated by the caller as well as the client.

The successful management of stutter events, not their frequency of occurrence, is the principal measure of progress. Usually, by the time a stutterer progresses successfully through this phase of treatment (and often, long before that) stuttering instances have decreased substantially, sometimes completely, in their frequency of occurrence.

There are instances, however, in which this does not occur and when the residual frequency of stutter events is sufficiently high that it impedes effortless, smooth speech. The frequency level at which this occurs varies with the individual and is obviously related to stuttering frequency prior to treatment. As a rule of thumb, if stuttering frequency *persists* above 3% of words uttered, treatment continues to the next phase, which focuses on enhancing speech fluency.

PHASE IV—RECEIVING STIMULUS VALUE FROM SMOOTH FLOWING SPEECH

Procedures associated with this phase are as old as the recorded history of stuttering's treatment.[38] In essence, they focus the stutterer's attention on, and initially require his exaggerated production of, selected parameters that characterize the speech of normally fluent individuals.

Although in 1943 Hahn[41] outlined a treatment sequence using many of these procedures, their organization into systematic programs is generally regarded as one of the principal contributions of behaviorism as applied to the treatment of stuttering over the past two decades.[5] Chapters that focus on these programs appear elsewhere in this volume. It is worth noting here, however, that the *motor targets* for both fluency enhancement and stuttering replacement responses are remarkably similar, a point made recently by Peters and Guitar.[4] This may suggest that a common factor accounts for their positive effects.

Expected Outcomes

All treatment programs for stuttering concern themselves with the acquisition, generalization, and stabilization of speech change. They differ, however, in what they consider to be the key experiences that enable change, what they measure as an index of change, and when and how they obtain the measurements.

Behaviorism's emphasis on accountability, the use of objective, replicable procedures and criteria for continuous outcome evaluation, has been one of its principal contributions to treatment.[5] While positive in essence, this contribution can result in negative fallout when applied too rigorously. For example, the effort to obtain unambiguous measures to gage the success of stuttering therapy has led to the frequent adoption of a single criterion: "total primacy to the achievement of stutter-free fluency."[5,p.9] As a performance-based criterion, this measure may be substantially misleading, particularly when obtained from samples taken during client/clinician sessions. It may reflect performance change only and not the "learning" required to assure stability of change. According to social cognitive theory, learning depends upon the cognitive regulation and control of behavior.[13] Thus, measurement of stutter-free fluency alone may forecast little about the kinds of change necessary for generalization and maintenance. Recently, this has been recognized by behaviorally oriented programs.[42]

More serious than mistaking performance change for learning is the effect the stutter-free speech criterion may have had on the nature of treatment itself. As an outcome criterion stutter-free speech can begin to dictate what is taught, as so often happens when outcome measurement is applied to any learning environment. Under such conditions, treatment can become a kind of "teaching to the test" enterprise, a single dimensional experience that ignores the complexity of internal and external changes that successful outcome requires. From this point of view, measures of progress and outcome should assess cognitive events (thought processes), as well as performance events (speech), and sample from self-regulated conditions rather than from client/clinician sessions.

Our overall objective for the stutterer is perceptual and performance self-efficacy. More specifically, the client should *believe* that *he controls* his speaking behavior, *feel confident* in his ability to speak effectively, and *be comfortable* in speaking situations. In these situations his speaking *performance should be effortless, smooth, and natural*. Admittedly, these are relative, not absolute, expectations. To determine their achievement, both the client and independent observers need to assess outcome. Some procedures for accomplishing this are described below.

In addition to the self-rating sheets that become a part of the treatment record, clients complete periodic ratings of selected speaking situations such as day-to-day social, business, and school encounters; telephone conversations; etc. As appropriate, independent listeners also observe some of these situations. The format for reporting is the same one used for treatment record self-assessments. Telephone calls, other speaking opportunities in the clinic when the clinician is not present, and outside situations are selectively video- or audiotaped. Using a format similar to that shown in Figure 6-3, the client and independent observers rate these samples and the samples made at the outset of treatment. The stutterer tries to achieve two things: 1) ratings that agree (plus or minus one scale value) with the average of independent observers; and 2) ratings that meet his and the clinician's objectives for treatment. There are no absolute values for all clients. In general, the benchmark rating by client and observers is from 5-7 (seven-point scale) on the following performance and self-perception dimensions: effort, smoothness, continuity, and naturalness; confidence, comfort, and calmness.

After the client begins to use replacement responses during Phase III, he and independent observers use the format in Figure 6-3 at about two-to-three week intervals to assess selected speaking situations. This serves not only to evaluate progress, but is used as a powerful motivational tool as well. Periodically, after Phase III of the program has been initiated, the client also retakes the questionnaires given at the outset of treatment concerning attitudes and reactions to speaking situations.

Client and clinician spend substantial time reviewing self- and others' ratings. In most cases, prior to termination and establishing a maintenance program, both

Situation_____   Date_____   Speaker_____

(MY) SPEECH IS

Effortful:___:___:___:___:___:___:___	:Effortless
Rough:___:___:___:___:___:___:___	:Smooth
Broken:___:___:___:___:___:___:___	:Continuous
Monotonous:___:___:___:___:___:___:___	:Melodic
Fast:___:___:___:___:___:___:___	:Slow
Loud:___:___:___:___:___:___:___	:Soft
Unnatural:___:___:___:___:___:___:___	:Natural

SPEAKER (I) APPEARS (AM)

Uncertain:___:___:___:___:___:___:___	:Confident
Uncomfortable:___:___:___:___:___:___:___	:Comfortable
Nervous:___:___:___:___:___:___:___	:Calm

Figure 6-3. Outcome evaluation form for use with videotaped and audiotaped speech samples.

parties should be satisfied with the extent of performance and cognitive change and should agree that further gains will most likely result from the client's continuing independent efforts.

Conclusion

Whatever approaches a clinician decides to use in working with an adolescent or adult stutterer, generalization and retention of speech changes are almost always the greatest hurdle. This chapter takes the position that the most crucial factors in surmounting this hurdle are likely to be the cognitive changes the client makes in his expectations of self-efficacy. If true, this means that the specific speech modification techniques the clinician uses are less important than the opportunities he gives the client to change cognitively and to adopt the conviction of his self-efficacy as a speaker.

Suggested Readings

Bandura A: *Social Learning Theory.* Englewood Cliffs, NJ, Prentice-Hall, 1977.
This is a very readable, concise description of social learning theory, its principles, relation to behavior theory, and applications to behavior change.

Bandura A: *Social Foundations of Thought and Action*. Englewood Cliffs, NJ, Prentice-Hall, 1986.
Bandura provides a thorough review of literature concerning the nature of learning and behavior change, particularly from the social learning and self-efficacy perspectives.
Emerick L: Counseling adults who stutter: A cognitive approach. *Semin Speech Lang* 1988; 9:257–267.
Emerick provides a brief, readable account of cognitive restructuring strategies and their origins.
Ingham RJ: *Stuttering and Behavior Therapy: Current Status and Experimental Foundations*. San Diego, College-Hill Press, 1984.
The evolution and characteristics of different therapy approaches are described and a thorough review is provided of literature concerning the modification and treatment of stuttering.
Johnson W: *Stuttering and What You Can Do about It*. Minneapolis, University of Minnesota Press, 1961.
Johnson provides a very readable account of his ideas concerning the nature and resolution of stuttering. It is written for stutterers and will give them many ideas to ponder and discuss.
Maxwell D: Cognitive and behavioral self-control strategies: Applications for the clinical management of adult stutterers. *J Fluency Disord* 1982; 7:403–432.
This article describes a treatment program that utilizes the principles of cognitive learning and self-efficacy theories.
Prins D: Treatment of Adults—Managing Stuttering, in Curlee RF, Perkins WH (eds): *Nature and Treatment of Stuttering: New Directions*. San Diego, College-Hill Press, 1984.
The "management of stuttering" approach is described and procedures outlined, particularly in terms of behavioral modification principles.
Van Riper C: Symptomatic Therapy for Stuttering, in Travis LE (ed): *Handbook of Speech Pathology*. New York, Appleton-Century-Crofts, 1957.
Now more than 30 years old, this chapter provides an excellent foundation for understanding Van Riper's approaches to helping the stutterer gain mastery over the stutter event.
Williams DE: A Perspective on Approaches to Stuttering Therapy, in Gregory HH (ed): *Controversies about Stuttering Therapy*. Baltimore, University Park Press, 1979.
Here, Williams provides a nice comparison of his treatment philosophy and procedures with other approaches.

References

1. Curlee RF, Perkins WH (eds): *Nature and Treatment of Stuttering: New Directions*. San Diego, College-Hill Press, 1984.
2. Frey W: Functional Assessment in the '80s, in Halpern A, Fuhrer M (eds): *Functional Assessment in Rehabilitation*. Baltimore, Paul H. Brookes, 1984.
3. Prins D: Treatment of Adults—Managing Stuttering, in Curlee RF, Perkins WH (eds): *Nature and Treatment of Stuttering: New Directions*. San Diego, College-Hill Press, 1984.
4. Peters TJ, Guitar B: *Stuttering: An Integrated Approach to Its Nature and Treatment*. Baltimore, Williams & Wilkins, 1991.
5. Ingham RJ: *Stuttering and Behavior Therapy: Current Status and Experimental Foundations*. San Diego, College-Hill Press, 1984.
6. Bloodstein O: *A Handbook on Stuttering*. Chicago, National Easter Seal Society, 1987.
7. Rosenfield D, Nudelman H: Neuropsychological Models of Speech Disfluency, in Rustin L, Purser H, Rowley D (eds): *Progress in the Treatment of Fluency Disorders*. New York, Taylor & Francis, 1987.
8. Van Riper C: *The Nature of Stuttering*. Englewood Cliffs, NJ, Prentice-Hall, 1971.
9. Wingate W: *The Structure of Stuttering: A Psycholinguistic Analysis*. New York, Springer-Verlag, 1988.
10. Brutten EJ, Shoemaker DJ: *The Modification of Stuttering*. Englewood Cliffs, NJ, Prentice-Hall, 1967.
11. Bandura A: Self-efficacy: Toward a unifying theory of behavioral change. *Psychol Rev* 1977; 84:191–215.
12. Bandura A: *Social Learning Theory*. Englewood Cliffs, NJ, Prentice-Hall, 1977.
13. Bandura A: *Social Foundations of Thought and Action*. Englewood Cliffs, NJ, Prentice-Hall, 1986.
14. Johnson W: The treatment of stuttering. *J Speech Disord* 1939; 4:170–172.
15. Johnson W: The Descriptional Principle and the Principle of Static Analysis, in Johnson W (ed): *Stuttering in Children and Adults*. Minneapolis, University of Minnesota Press, 1955.
16. Williams DE: A point of view about stuttering. *J Speech Hear Disord* 1957; 22:390–397.
17. Williams DE: A Perspective on Approaches to Stuttering Therapy, in Gregory HH (ed): *Controversies about Stuttering Therapy*. Baltimore, University Park Press, 1979.
18. Williams DE: Stuttering therapy: Where are we going—and why? *J Fluency Disord* 1982; 7:159–170.
19. Van Riper C: Symptomatic Therapy for Stutterers, in Travis LE (ed): *Handbook of Speech Pathology*. New York, Appleton-Century-Crofts, 1957.

20. Boberg E, et al: An Investigation of Central Nervous System Differences in Stutterers. Presented at the annual meeting of the American Speech-Language-Hearing Association, Seattle, November, 1990.
21. Ludlow CL: Measurement of Speech Motor Processes in Stuttering, in Peters HFM, Hulstijn W (eds): *Speech Motor Control and Stuttering*. Amsterdam, Elsevier Science, 1991.
22. Peters HFM: A Composite Motor Task for the Assessment of Speech Motor Control in Stuttering, in Peters HFM, Hulstijn W (eds): *Speech Motor Control and Stuttering*. Amsterdam, Elsevier Science, 1991.
23. Riley G, Riley J: Treatment Implications of Oral Motor Discoordination, in Peters HFM, Hulstijn W (eds): *Speech Motor Control and Stuttering*. Amsterdam, Elsevier Science, 1991.
24. Alfonso PJ: The Effect of Speech Motor Training on Stutterers' Speech Physiology, in Peters HFM, Hulstijn W (eds): *Speech Motor Control and Stuttering*. Amsterdam, Elsevier Science, 1991.
25. Watson BC, Dembowski J: Instrumentation in the Evaluation and Modification of Speech Motor Control during Stuttering Therapy, in Peters HFM, Hulstijn W (eds): *Speech Motor Control and Stuttering*. Amsterdam, Elsevier Science, 1991.
26. Boberg E, Kully D: *Comprehensive Stuttering Program: Clinical Manual*. San Diego, College-Hill Press, 1985.
27. Riley G: *Stuttering Severity Instrument for Children and Adults*. Tigard, OR, CC Publications, 1980.
28. Prins D, Beaudet R: Defense preference and stutterers' speech disfluencies: Implications for the nature of the disorder. *J Speech Hear Res* 1980; 23:757–768.
29. Johnson W, Darley FL, Spriestersbach DC: *Diagnostic Methods in Speech Pathology*. New York, Harper & Row, 1963.
30. Andrews G, Cutler J: Stuttering therapy: The relation between changes in symptom level and attitudes. *J Speech Hear Disord* 1974; 39:312–319.
31. Woolf G: The assessment of stuttering as struggle, avoidance and expectancy. *Br J Disord Commun* 1967; 2:158–171.
32. Craig AR, Franklin JA, Andrews G: A scale to measure locus of control of behavior. *Br J Med Psychol* 1984; 57:173–180.
33. Guitar B, Peters TJ: *Stuttering: An Integration of Contemporary Therapies*. Memphis, Speech Foundation of America, 1980.
34. Emerick L: Counseling adults who stutter: A cognitive approach. *Semin Speech Lang* 1988; 9: 257–267.
35. Maxwell D: Cognitive and behavioral self-control strategies: Applications for the clinical management of adult stutterers. *J Fluency Disord* 1982; 7:403–432.
36. Cooper E: A therapy process for the adult stutterer. *J Speech Hear Disord* 1968; 33:246–260.
37. Butler G: Issues in the application of cognitive and behavioral strategies to the treatment of social phobia. *Clin Psychol Rev* 1989; 9:91–106.
38. Van Riper C: *The Treatment of Stuttering*. Englewood Cliffs, NJ, Prentice-Hall, 1973.
39. Ingham RJ: The effects of self-evaluation training on maintenance and generalization during stuttering treatment. *J Speech Hear Disord* 1982; 47:271–280.
40. Frick JV: *Evaluation of Motor Planning Techniques for the Treatment of Stuttering*. Unpublished research report. University Park, PA, 1965.
41. Hahn EF: *Stuttering: Significant Theories and Therapies*. Palo Alto, Stanford University Press, 1943.
42. Craig AR, Calver P: Followup on treated stutterers: Studies of perceptions of fluency and job status. *J Speech Hear Res* 1991; 34:279–284.

APPENDIX A: REACTION TO SELF-DESCRIPTIVE STATEMENTS

By placing an "X" in the appropriate space, indicate the extent to which each of the following statements holds true for you. (The actual questionnaire format shows the scale values after each statement.)

Statements:

Feeling embarrassed about my speech.

Fear of a word I can't say fluently.

Avoiding words and sounds I have trouble with.

Fear of talking before a group.

Feelings of nervousness and tension before speaking.

Fear of being asked my name.

Feeling that I should be able to speak better.

Fear of talking on the telephone.

Not talking because I may have trouble.

Feeling helpless about the way I speak.

Hiding the fact that I have a speech problem.

Feeling that stuttering is the most significant factor in my life.

Not being able to say what I feel.

Inability to talk to strangers.

Feeling that my speech is uncontrollable.

Feeling that people react to the way I talk, not the way I am.

Feeling that if I didn't stutter, my other problems would be insignificant.

Feeling ill at ease with people.

Unwillingness to assume responsibility.

Worrying about the impression I will make.

Feeling that I am socially inadequate.

Feeling that I am less capable than other people.

Feeling that other people have more important things to say than I do.

Scale:

| :_____ | :_____ | :_____ | :_____ | :_____ | : |
| Never or rarely true | Seldom true | Some- times true | Usually true | Almost always or always true | |

APPENDIX B: REACTIONS TO SELECTED SPEAKING SITUATIONS*

Situation	Frequency[†]	Level of Difficulty[†]	Level of Confidence[†]
Talking on the telephone to a friend or family member.			
Talking on the telephone to a stranger.			
Using the telephone to purchase a ticket.			
Talking to a stranger in a social situation.			
Introducing myself.			
Placing an order in a restaurant.			
Talking to a close friend.			
Talking with parents.			
Talking with a sales clerk.			
Meeting someone for the first time.			
Asking for information.			
Being interviewed for a job.			
Talking with teachers.			
Making an appointment.			
Making introductions.			
Speaking before a group.			
Asking a question or making a comment in class.			
Giving my name in a classroom situation.			
Giving a prepared speech.			
Talking to someone of the opposite sex.			
Participating at a meeting.			
Reading aloud to others.			
Conversation at a dinner table:			
with family.			
with friends.			
with strangers.			

[†]Scale Values:

Frequency	Level of Difficulty	Level of Confidence
I encounter this situation:	This situation is:	In this situation I have:
1. More than once per day	1. Not difficult	1. Total lack of confidence
2. Daily	2. Slightly difficult	2. Very little confidence
3. Several times per week	3. Somewhat difficult	3. Some confidence
4. Less than once per week	4. Very difficult	4. Considerable confidence
5. Rarely	5. Almost impossible	5. Complete confidence

*Patterned after the Iowa Stutterer's Self-Ratings of Reactions to Speech Situations.[29]

7

Intensive Fluency Training of Chronic Stutterers

Megan Neilson, Ph.D.
Gavin Andrews, M.D.

Introduction

Treating adults who stutter presumes several things. It presumes that they will have had the disorder for a number of years[1] and, despite earlier attempts at treatment, the disorder will have remained chronic. Further, despite this chronic disability, they will mostly have managed to achieve such life goals as education, occupation, and marriage, even if some compromises have been made. Adult stutterers usually come for treatment for one of three reasons. Some come because they have only just discovered that effective treatment is available. Many of them would like to be fluent but do not give it a sufficiently high priority to justify their continual hard work and expense and so, after inquiring, do not proceed with therapy, preferring to live with their stuttering until some magical or effortless cure arrives. A second group includes those who have failed to achieve their desired occupations or relationships, or both, and who believe that if they did not stutter and were fluent, these other issues in their lives would be resolved. Treatment is onerous, and both they and their clinicians need to realize that precisely the deficits in persistence and hard work that prevent their success in other walks of life will likely preclude their achieving long-term control of their stuttering. The third group comes because they realize that stuttering constitutes an unacceptable handicap in their occupation or private life, and that the time, effort, and cost of treatment will be justified if they are able to speak more fluently, or more importantly, to communicate more effectively.

When deciding which treatments are of benefit we have argued[2] that while results from placebo-controlled research trials are preferred, other designs are acceptable, provided there is independent evidence that treatment results are not invalidated by natural remission, regression to the mean, or response to good, nonspecific clinical care. As with placebo-controlled trials, five further criteria should be satisfied before concluding that the treatment was responsible for any observed improvement. They are: (1) The treatment should be standardized and described so that its procedures can be replicated by others, (2) treatment effects should be nontrivial, (3) results should not be compromised by high dropout rates, (4) there should be evidence of a dose-response relationship, and (5) improvements should remain evident at follow-up evaluations. In fact, the latter two criteria together practically guarantee treatment benefits, whatever other threats to validity are inherent in the research design.

The treatment to be described in this chapter has a long pedigree. Initially treatment was conducted in small groups and was intensive during the first weeks when fluency was instated, then shaped to resemble normal speech, and finally systematically transferred from the clinic into the community. The principal aim of therapy was reduction of the handicap to communication; hence, the primary measures of improvement were frequency of stuttering and rate of speech. As measures of communication attitudes became available,[3] they were incorporated, and as it became clear that internalization of locus of control was a prognostic factor,[4] that too was measured and techniques to hasten this change were systematically incorporated. Treatment results that satisfy the above-described requirements for demonstrating a treatment effect have been discussed in detail.[5] More recently, it has been found that clients who have stutter-free speech, normal communication attitudes, and increased internalization of locus of control by the end of treatment have a very low probability of relapse.[6] This finding has led to active intervention in normalizing attitudes and internalizing locus of control during the final week of treatment in the program now offered. This is but one of a number of pragmatic modifications made since the program moved in 1986 from suburban Prince Henry Hospital to St. Vincent's Hospital in inner-city Sydney, Australia. Since some readers may be acquainted with the format of the Prince Henry program,[7,8] a brief overview of the development of the current St. Vincent's program will be provided.

Between 1971 and 1985 the Prince Henry unit treated some 50 clients a year, the large majority in an intensive treatment format consisting of 1 week of fluency training followed by 2 weeks of transfer and maintenance work. Initially, admission to the hospital as an inpatient was required for the duration of the program. Later, our experience with stutterers' weekend leaves suggested that generalization would be aided if transfer and maintenance were completed on a day-patient basis. At St. Vincent's Hospital all 3 weeks of the program are completed on a day-patient basis. When commuting is impractical, clients are encouraged to stay locally with family or friends, or nearby paid accommodations are arranged.

Treatment programs based, sometimes closely sometimes loosely, on ours are now available throughout Australia, and our waiting list, once 2 years long, is a more reasonable 4 to 6 months. We currently offer six programs a year, rather than the former nine, and a wider range of cognitive-behavioral treatments. Our facility, The Clinical Research Unit for Anxiety Disorders, offers intensive programs for treatment of agoraphobia, panic, social phobia, generalized anxiety disorder, and obsessive compulsive disorder[9] as well as for stuttering which, of course, is *not* an anxiety disorder. Nevertheless, the structure of the stuttering treatment program served as the model for the other treatment programs, and it now utilizes the expertise of the other programs in cognitive restructuring with stuttering clients where appropriate.

Prior to 1986, the schedule for week 1 of fluency instatement ran from 8 A.M. to 8 P.M. With ten speech-rating sessions scheduled daily, group members were often unable to meet the same fluency criterion each day. Those who had difficulty mastering fluency skills fell behind and had to start behind the others the next morning. Although such problems often evened out over the week within the group, the prospect of starting behind others in the group was never welcomed by clients or clinicians. Consequently, we continue to start at 8 A.M. but now require every group member to reach the same fluency goal before leaving. Thus, departure time now depends on each client's performance. With a group of six, earliest departure was 6 P.M., some working until 9 P.M., and on occasion, until midnight to achieve that day's fluency target. This format can be extremely demanding for both clients and clinicians, but it results in extra practice and more individual attention for those who need it most. Since 1990, we have limited groups to four people, which allows some clients to finish by 5 P.M. and has cut the latest finish to 10 P.M.

The techniques for fluency instatement, now termed "smooth speech," remain a derivative of the prolonged speech originally used except that continuous vocalization is no longer called for. We have refined our teaching of these techniques and provide extensive audio material, which clients use individually as an adjunct to group work. We have also added instruction on respiratory control and increased our focus on normalizing prosody. From the start we emphasize the need to achieve natural-sounding speech at normal speech rates without sacrificing the essentials of smooth speech.

A final change has been the introduction of a therapy fee. Fee for service has not emerged as a factor in successful treatment and for many years only a nominal charge of $A50 was used to subsidize consumable therapy supplies. The current fee of $A600 is a meaningful but acceptable amount for most clients, and those whose only income is from government or social security benefits pay $A100. The clinic is nonprofit, and these fees are used to employ a part-time therapist to assist the salaried therapist in charge.

Clinical Evaluation

Clients are referred by a health professional, most frequently their family practitioner or a speech pathologist. To minimize capricious inquiries, we ask that those hearing of the program by other means discuss their interest in treatment with their physician who will refer if appropriate. Our case selection evaluation takes approximately 2 hours and consists of completing a questionnaire, a speech assessment, and an interview. The goal is to determine first if the client stutters and second if the intensive treatment format is appropriate for this person at this time. Additional information is collected immediately prior to treatment.

Case History Information

In most instances, we obtain only a brief case history, which is taken subsequent to the normal fluency assessment discussed in the next section and is predicated on having established that the client stutters. During an interview, we establish the likely age of onset and note any circumstances that the client sees as contributory. We then seek information about short-term and long-term variability of the client's stutter and the nature and outcome of any previous treatment. We next document family history of stuttering or other speech/language disorders, endeavoring to establish the general extent of family knowledge the client can draw on. A brief personal history follows, with special note taken of educational and work records. We then probe carefully as to why treatment is being sought at this particular time.

We routinely screen for history of possible brain trauma and of injury or disease involving the central nervous system or the speech/hearing systems. The client is asked to report any knowledge or suspicion of hearing loss and if dentures are worn. We occasionally encounter a client who appears to have adult-onset stuttering without apparent physical cause and who is adamant that there is no developmental history. In this circumstance we refer promptly for full neurological investigation because neurological disease can first manifest itself as atypical stuttering. When questionnaire profiles point to psychological difficulties, or when they are suspected from the interview,[10] we try to identify any possible treatment limitations; however, the psychological difficulties usually encountered stem from high trait anxiety or a personality disorder.

Observations and Tests

Prior to the interview a client completes a set of questionnaires: the S24 Modified Erickson Scale of communication attitudes[3]; an Australian derivative[11] of the Iowa Stutterer's Self-Ratings of Reactions to Speech Situations[12]; the Locus of Control of Behavior Scale (LCB)[13]; the Eysenck Personality Inventory,[14] a measure of personality traits; and the General Health Questionnaire (GHQ-12)[15], a measure of current psychiatric casedness. Clients also list ten speaking situations, from easiest to hardest, and complete a brief form eliciting relevant medical history.

After reviewing the completed questionnaires, the clinician proceeds straight to a fluency assessment. The standard task is a 3-minute monologue on the topics of dogs, plastics, politics, and oceans. Using a double event counter with built-in timer, this sample of speech is rated live for the percentage of syllables stuttered (%SS) and the rate of speech in syllables per minute (SPM).

In this clinic our benchmark for rating fluency is the Prince Henry Yardstick.[16] All therapists train on this material and must achieve accuracy within 5% of the established values for the numerous speech samples. Intrarater reliability is checked regularly, as is interrater reliability between cotherapists. These also should remain within 5%. In assessing stuttered speech, all types of disfluencies are counted: sound, syllable and word repetitions, prolongations, blocks, unnatural hesitations, interjections, restarted or incomplete phrases, and unfinished or broken words, including pitch changes. Visual concomitants of stuttering, some of which may pass undetected audibly, are counted on all live and videotaped ratings. We count all stuttering behaviors associated with a particular syllable only once. Thus, regardless of the number of repetitions, hesitations, restarts, etc., involved in the attempt to say the syllable, it counts as only one stutter. In establishing the total number of syllables in the sample for calculating %SS and

SPM, we count only message syllables. We ignore those syllables that recur in the course of repetitions or restarts as well as interjected syllables that do not convey information (e.g., "um," "ah"). Therefore, we count only the syllables that would have been said if there were no stuttering. Timing commences as the speaker begins and includes all pauses for breath and/or language formulation. Timing ceases when the speaker is finished, with the inclusion of a brief terminal pause. Thus, SPM reflects the rate of information flow,[17] an appropriate measure of speech rate for estimating communication handicap,[11] but is distinct from articulatory rate,[18] which eliminates both pauses and disfluencies and is also reported in SPM. The %SS and SPM measures described are used in rating a client's speech throughout the program.

On completion of the monologue speech rating, we review the resulting measures of disfluency with the client and indicate how they compare with normally fluent speech. We consider disfluency rates up to 2%SS to be within normal limits,[19] while an information transfer rate of 200 SPM is well within documented ranges for fluent speakers.[19,20] We then ask the client to what extent the assessed sample is typical of current difficulties. If little stuttering has occurred and avoidance is acknowledged or suspected, we test under further conditions, such as reading. We may also observe further if a client indicates that a special condition, such as talking on the telephone, is a principal problem area. For the most part, however, a monologue sample demanded at the outset of the interview gives us adequate indication of whether or not the client is a stutterer. We then proceed to the case history, which allows opportunity for extended informal assessment of conversational speech. In this context we also informally appraise a client's comprehension and production of language and look for evidence of a coexisting articulation defect, voice disorder, or cluttering.

Case Selection Criteria

Over the past 25 years this unit has treated some 1000 stutterers in an intensive group behavioral format. The results of the program are well documented,[6,21] and we believe this to be the treatment of choice for a majority of adult stutterers. At the same time, this long experience reveals that there are some for whom our program is inappropriate. Earlier, we sketched the characteristics of three groups of adult stutterers who may seek treatment. Those in the first group, who view 3 weeks of intensive work on their speech as too great an investment, usually decline treatment and do not present a problem in case selection. The second group of people, who do not manage well in other aspects of their lives, will have similar difficulty in managing the rigors of a demanding treatment program and the ensuing self-care during maintenance. When this is apparent, we choose not to offer treatment. Although the program may bring short-term gains to such clients, there is little chance of long-term success and this attempt at change may become yet another example of personal failure. The best chance for such people is individual therapy. The program we run today is aimed firmly at those stutterers in the third group, who manage life well but who find their stutter has become an unacceptable handicap in reaching otherwise feasible goals. These clients come well motivated and well prepared for the long hours of hard work that are required by our treatment. When offered a place in the treatment program, they accept readily and begin treatment as soon as logistically possible.

Of course, life is not always simple, and there are some people who make treatment decisions difficult for even an astute clinician. When we really do not know whether or not someone is suitable, he or she is given the benefit of the doubt. This means that we inevitably take into treatment clients who should not have been accepted. Some elect to drop from the program, and we do not try to dissuade them. Others stay but do not apply themselves, thereby ensuring their failure or, despite seemingly earnest attempts, appear to be unable to apply themselves adequately, yet again confirming their more general adjustment difficulties. Vary rarely does a client's behavior (e.g., coming to sessions affected by alcohol) jeopardize the progress of the rest of the group, but in such cases we withdraw him or her from the program and arrange for alternative individual treatment.

Sometimes we assess a client as being suitable for treatment, but not at that time. Ours is an adult program that makes strong demands on resilience and maturity. With rare exceptions we do not accept teenagers. Rather, we point out that they have survived tolerably despite their stuttering and should continue to do so, and agree to reconsider them for treatment at a later time. Likewise, we insist that young adults in tertiary education defer treatment until the summer vacation, or preferably until graduation when the pressure of studies has passed and the prospect of a job search fires motivation. We also defer treatment for clients who are psychologically stable but whose generalization of fluency skills is likely to be hampered by high trait anxiety. These we refer for stress management, emphasizing their need to consolidate that learning and lower their trait anxiety levels before attempting fluency treatment. We never offer treatment to a client who is experiencing serious loss or continuing chaos. Such circumstances do not allow the client to focus fully on the task at hand and we advise them to wait for a more propitious time. Clients who have English as a second language are increasingly common in multicultural Australia, and we have treated many who have achieved good outcomes in both English and their native tongue. Since the treatment process depends on instruction and conversation in English, we ask those with an inadequate command of English to return after further study and assimilation of the language.

Stutterers who acquired their fluency difficulties as a result of cerebral insult or disease are usually seen as a special group. Market and colleagues[22] recently presented data suggesting that acquired stutterers respond well to mainstream therapeutic procedures. We too offer treatment to such stutterers if they appear to have the motivation and mental and physical capacity to meet the demands of treatment. We expect them to have the same goals as the rest of the group but are prepared, if necessary, to lower the final speech rate target. Occasionally it is unclear from the case history whether or not stuttering is developmental or acquired, e.g., where onset is reported to have occurred after serious head injury in childhood, in the context of no previous developmental stuttering but a positive family history. Again, if the client meets other criteria, we treat as usual but remain alert for possible limitations. If clients have insufficient stamina, concentration span, or intellectual functioning to undertake 3 intensive weeks of learning and application, we look carefully at their motivation and likely gains from fluency training. If they are keen, have something to work for, and seem prepared to do their best, we refer them for consideration in a less-demanding group program or for individual therapy.

Coexistence of stuttering with other disorders of speech and language has been long recognized in children[2] and may be more common than previously reported.[23] Among adult stutterers we also observe such coexisting problems but usually the client's principal concern is stuttering. If coexisting disorders are severe, we arrange further assessment and individual treatment. If they are mild and clients are otherwise suitable for the program, we proceed without special attention to the other problems. Frequently the smooth speech technique seems to benefit mild voice disorders and clients regard this as a bonus. Sometimes a long-standing phonological disorder, which previously caused the client little concern, comes to the forefront once fluency is achieved. We do not intervene and advise such clients to concentrate on consolidating their new fluency skills before seeking further therapy. Coexistence of stuttering and cluttering presents additional difficulties and when treating a client with both disorders, we also seek to modify the cluttering, principally using the rate control elements of the program. These clients often have difficulty in monitoring their speech performance and, while improvement of this skill is a cornerstone of the treatment process, the gains they make are hard won. In our experience, they need exceptional persistence to achieve an enduring, good result, and we emphasize this to the client from the outset.

Before accepting any client for treatment, we supply the following information. We give a brief account of the nature of stuttering as a disorder of speech motor control,[5] rather than a psychological or learned disorder as many in the community still believe. We explain that a "cure" of chronic stuttering is not available, but that treatment offers a means of control that will gradually become straightforward to use and maintain if they invest the time and effort required. This commitment is necessary not only during treatment but also as part of the client's continuing long-term self-management. We indicate that anyone who completes treatment can expect to get excellent short-term benefits, while long-term gains can be expected by approximately four of five clients. We then outline our treatment procedures, giving examples of how the smooth speech technique sounds at various stages and stressing that natural-sounding speech is both crucial and achievable. Finally, we re-emphasize the amount of effort and application involved in becoming and remaining fluent and stress the need for the client to be free of outside concerns and commitments for the 3-week duration of the program. With that understood, we assess the client's reaction to this information and if he or she wants to undertake our therapy program.

In summary, our selection process depends essentially on three criteria if the client is an adult who stutters. Firstly, the client must evidence strong personal motivation to achieve fluency. There is little prospect of lasting gain for those who undertake the program principally to please their family, their employer, or a lover. Secondly, the client must identify a significant goal tied to the achievement of fluent speech. Fluency simply for fluency's sake is not sufficient. There must be something to work for, such as job effectiveness, a career change or promotion, or a parent's desire to talk fluently to his or her young child. Thirdly, the client must appear to be capable of the concentrated effort and extended application that will be needed and have the resilience to cope with temporary frustrations. As Calvin Coolidge is reputed to have said, "Nothing in the world can take the place of persistence. Talent will not; nothing is more common than unsuccessful men with talent. Genius will not, unrewarded genius is almost a proverb. Education will not; the world is full of educated derelicts. Persistence and determination alone are omnipotent."

Clinical Management

Treatment Goals

We can state our broad treatment goals simply. We aim to equip clients with the skills to achieve fluency, to mediate the generalization of that fluency, and to ensure that they leave with the armory of skills necessary to maintain fluency. We use both cognitive and behavioral techniques to achieve these goals. As indicated earlier, we have established that long-term maintenance of fluency is associated with three end-of-treatment accomplishments: perfect fluency control, normal communication attitudes, and an internalized locus of control.[6] Thus, our cognitive-behavioral interventions focus on helping clients achieve these specific objectives.

Treatment Procedures

Treatment takes place over 3 consecutive weeks, and clients attend on a day-patient basis. It commences on a Sunday, when we conduct a half-day introduction and reassessment session, and then runs Monday through Friday, with weekends free. The program is staffed by a senior therapist, with full-time responsibilities for treatment and research in stuttering, and a part-time therapist who contributes 4 hours per day.

The first week of treatment is devoted to the instatement and shaping of fluency. Procedures involve instruction in the smooth speech technique and group conversations, or rating sessions, in which clients practice their fluency at gradually increasing speeds. Rating sessions also provide a forum for improving pragmatic aspects of communication. In addition, some sessions are videotaped so that clients progressively learn to appraise and enhance their fluency skills and interactional behavior. The group starts at 8:00 each morning and concludes when every client has attained a goal of stutter-free speech at a specified speaking rate. Normal speech rates are reached on Thursday evening. With a group of four clients, the median duration of these daily sessions the first week is 11 hours, with a range of 9 to 14 hours.

The second week of treatment focuses on the transfer of fluency skills to everyday environments beyond the clinic. Clients complete a graded set of assignments that require smooth speech to be practiced in real-life situations of increasing difficulty. They continue to refine and consolidate their fluency skills during morning and evening rating sessions, and they learn cognitive and behavioral coping strategies to be used when fluency becomes unstable. Again, there is an 8

A.M. start, with days lasting a median of 10 hours, although those whose assignment completion is on target leave earlier.

The third week of treatment allows clients to generalize their fluency skills to circumstances dictated by their own needs and life-styles. They also complete tasks that are challenging to normal speakers, such as giving a formal presentation to an unknown audience and speaking on call-in radio shows. Rating sessions emphasize melding smooth speech skills into natural-sounding speech, while instruction focuses on cognitive and behavioral strategies for self-management during maintenance. An evening meeting with family and friends allows discussion of the changes that have occurred and of important concerns and expectations that group members and their families may have about the future. By formally assessing fluency skill, attitudes, and locus of control early in week 3, we evaluate each client's risk of relapse and intervene accordingly with an individual remedial program for the client's remaining time in therapy. Treatment days during week 3 last a median of 9 hours.

We expect clients to return for follow-up sessions at 1, 2, 3, 6, and 12 months after treatment so that their current functioning can be assessed and discussed. These follow-up sessions run once a month and are open to all who have completed the program at any time. They provide a forum for clients at various stages in their maintenance program to interact, exchange experiences, report on progress, and seek advice.

INTRODUCTORY PROCEDURES

One month before a new group begins, we send each client a brief outline of the 3 weeks of treatment. This recaps information given at the initial interview, sketches what to expect at each stage, and sets out the daily treatment schedules. We remind them to free themselves of any external commitments during that time. We also suggest purchasing a compact cassette recorder with a built-in microphone and pause button. This type of recorder is used throughout the program and, while the clinic will supply one on loan, we encourage clients to purchase their own as they will need to continue using it when treatment concludes. This preliminary letter also asks the client to bring a household member to the Sunday introduction session.

The Sunday session runs from 10 A.M. to 2 P.M. The first hour and a half consists of an introductory meeting among the four group members, their companions, and the two therapists. This session has two purposes. It allows us to review the coming 3 weeks and ensure that each client's household is aware of both the treatment schedule and the pressures involved. We also take this opportunity to demonstrate the speech patterns that clients will be using at the various stages and emphasize that we require their speech beyond the clinic to be the same as that utilized during that day's final rating session. In addition, during the first week, overnight bonds are used to promote clients' use of smooth speech techniques beyond the clinic. Clients' compliance with this requirement relies on an honor system, and each client determines the amount of his or her bond. This program has always operated on the principle that once fluency training begins, it is counterproductive for the client to return to old patterns of (stuttered) spontaneous speech. Moreover, it is important for both client and family to understand that freedom from stuttering will depend on the client's permanent use of these techniques. We also make it clear that the early, very abnormal-sounding speech of the instatement phase will be short-lived and that achievement of speech that is not only fluent, but natural-sounding, will potentiate its routine use. We encourage and answer questions throughout. The meeting also includes information on clinic rules and logistics such as lunch, which is delivered to the clinic or brought from home for the first few days.

We conclude this portion of the session with a discussion of the therapist-client relationship as a collaborative endeavor, although we make it clear that we will be extremely strict in insisting that clients achieve demanding criteria. We emphasize that we work within a well-researched framework that brings proven success and that what may seem unreasonable at times in fact reflects strict adherence to the framework of the treatment process. Finally, we try to assure all concerned that while treatment can be demanding, exhausting, and often frustrating, there will also be light moments and camaraderie throughout.

After a break, during which time companions leave, we conduct pretreatment assessments of each client. Two speech samples are obtained. The first is a videotaped sample recorded with the group gathered around the treatment table. Each client is recorded for approximately 2 minutes while giving his or her full name, address, occupation, some details of family and/or special interests, and expectations of treatment. If a client seems to be avoiding or circumlocuting, the therapist may ask additional questions. We seek to obtain a record containing representative examples of the range of behaviors that constitute the client's stuttering. The videotape is retained for clinic records and is reviewed by the client later in treatment.

The second sample is an audio recording of the client speaking on the telephone to strangers. We require 3 minutes of speech recorded while calling about goods, services, rentals, etc. from weekend classified advertisements. The audiotape is rated and the measures recorded for later comparisons with measures on similar telephone samples during transfer and maintenance. We also review these recordings before meeting again with the clients in order to become more familiar with their characteristic speech patterns. Respiratory, phonatory, and articulatory components of each client's stuttering are detailed, as are observations of prosody and language, especially any use of avoidance devices and fillers. Secondary behaviors are also noted from the videotape. After obtaining these samples, each client is given the program's treatment manual, which contains a fact sheet on stuttering,[24] detailed information on treatment procedures,[25] transcripts of three audio teaching tapes,[26–28] forms for recording the results of rating sessions and assignments, local street maps, and paper for taking notes and keeping a diary of progress and personal reactions during treatment. Clients also receive a smooth speech training tape[26] and a set of questionnaires. The questionnaires include the scales previously administered at the initial assessment, usually 4 to 6 months earlier, plus the Defense Style Questionnaire,[29] which yields measures of emotion-focused coping styles that are currently under study in the unit. Clients are asked to read the manual overnight and to complete the questionnaires. We also ask them to listen to the training tape at least once, using the transcript as a guide.

This tape previews the smooth speech instruction that will be given the next morning and allows clients to experiment individually with the technique before group fluency instatement.

FLUENCY INSTATEMENT

Preinstatement Session.   After dealing with questions that have arisen overnight, we begin Monday morning with a group discussion of stuttering. We point out that we expect people to stutter during this session, and we urge them to speak without avoidance. Then, we initiate discussions of the information from the treatment manual fact sheet,[24] which describes stuttering as a genetically mediated or acquired disorder of speech motor control and gives basic information on epidemiology, inheritance, and stutterer/nonstutterer similarities and differences. Clients are encouraged to react to this information in terms of how it may apply to them and their beliefs about stuttering. We discuss and demonstrate how well-known fluency-inducing conditions operate and introduce the concept of fluency versus disfluency in terms of neurophysiological capacity and demand.[5,30] Clients are asked about variations they notice in their own stuttering, and we also discuss avoidance of situations, avoidance of words, and maneuvers that they use to increase their fluency.

We next introduce anatomical models, diagrams, and analogies to emphasize the complexity of the central and peripheral processes that underlie speech and language functions and their vulnerability to disruption. This leads to discussion of stuttering behaviors, and we focus individually on each client's pattern of stuttering, which usually has been well exhibited by this time. Again using demonstration material, we show how repetitions and blocks depend on laryngeal and/or articulatory constriction and stress the importance of airflow and respiratory patterns in controlling this behavior. This leads naturally to the teaching of the smooth speech technique, which we describe as a simplified form of speech that allows stutterers to operate within lowered capacities for reliable speech motor control. We acknowledge that smooth speech may seem more difficult initially because of their long-established patterns of speech behavior. We explain that its simplification comes from a lessening of precision and the slow rate initially used, and link this with sleepy or intoxicated speech patterns that also reflect lowered capacity for speech motor control. Knowing that some clients may feel uneasy about proceeding at this stage, since stuttering often differs dramatically among the group, we assure them that the same technique is appropriate, whatever the severity or nature of one's stuttering. This discussion lasts about 2 hours, and we take a short break before starting fluency instatement.

The Smooth Speech Technique.   Smooth speech is a derivative of prolonged speech. It is refined gradually so that it sounds sufficiently natural at normal speeds for a naive listener to remain unaware that a speaker is using a "technique." We teach four fundamentals in introducing smooth speech.

1. *Rate Control*: We achieve rate reduction by extending the duration of sounds and syllables and teach this skill by modeling.
2. *Breathing*: We demonstrate easy, relaxed, diaphragmatic breathing during

speech, contrasting it with some of the maladaptive patterns often observed in stutterers, such as breath holding, overextension, interruption of expiration by inspiration, and clavicular breathing. There should be comfortable expiration and inspiration before attempting to speak. Breath must not be held before initiating speech and must not be suddenly chopped off midphrase if a speaker is interrupted or looking for a word. Rather, it should be released gently and a new breath taken before starting again. Care should be taken never to overextend and to avoid inspiratory gasps if running out of air. We also teach breath-stream management when introducing smooth speech at 50 SPM, by instructing clients to say only two to three syllables per breath, which leads to appropriate prolongation. As rate increases, the syllables per breath increase accordingly.

3. *Easy Phrase Initiation*: Each breath phrase should be initiated easily and smoothly with airflow established before phonation. We precede phrase initial vowels with aspiration to potentiate gentle vocal onset. Phrase initial consonants are also "breathy" with soft articulatory contact and gentle vocal onset.

4. *Phrase Continuity*: Each breath phrase should be characterized by continuity of (a) airflow, (b) articulatory movement, and (c) sound. This continuity fosters gentle vocal onsets and offsets and soft articulatory contacts throughout the phrase. There is not continuous phonation/vocalization; phrases must sound joined, without gaps at syllable or word junctures, but unvoiced sounds remain unvoiced. Thinking of a multiword phrase as simply one big word often helps clients to achieve continuity skills.

Once these fundamentals are established, we help clients identify, differentiate, and understand the physical bases of behaviors that compromise easy phrase initiation and phrase continuity. When skills are imperfect, we expect clients to pinpoint the underlying problems in terms of either:

5. *Gentle Vocal Onset/Offset*, or

6. *Soft Articulatory Contact*.

When clients have progressed through the rating sessions to a target speed of 100 SPM, we introduce three additional features:

7. *Phrasing and Pausing*: Appropriate phrasing and pausing involve breaking a linguistic message into units dictated by its syntax. Thus, pauses for breath should occur at phrase or clause junctures, and always at a period when reading. These are the normal locations for linguistic formulation,[31] and stuttering clients have to learn to pause so as to minimize difficulties in lexical retrieval and the like, where there is also an increased risk of disfluency. Skill in phrasing and pausing necessarily overlaps with skill in breath-stream management.

8. *Prosody*: Smooth speech incorporates appropriate prosody, apart from rate, at an early stage. We address problems of intonation, rhythm, and loudness and the need for words to retain their proper stress pattern.

9. *Presentation*: The development of good communication style is fostered throughout the program. In assessing their smooth speech, clients learn to

judge presentation skills and interactional behavior, targeting difficulties such as lack of eye contact, alienating body language, and disconcerting mannerisms.

Instatement Procedures.   Fluency instatement takes approximately 2 hours. We begin with a brief history of the program and of smooth speech, using demonstrations of syllable-timed speech to make sure that everyone knows what is meant by a syllable. We then demonstrate the four fundamentals: rate control, breathing, easy phrase initiation, and phrase continuity. At this stage it is important to remind the group that their speech is meant to sound very abnormal, that these exaggerated patterns will help them establish the skills that will lead to natural-sounding speech at normal speeds. We also assure them that we do not expect them to change their accent or their idiom, that we want them to end up sounding like themselves, not the clinicians.

We first model vowels and diphthongs with initial /h/, which clients imitate individually and as a group. Then, we model consonants and have clients imitate single sounds or an appropriate consonant (C)-vowel (V) syllable using the vowel /a/. We start with nasals, followed by glides/semivowels, fricatives and affricatives, and finally stops, in each case discussing and comparing place of articulation and voicing. Next, we introduce example VCs, VCVs, and CVCVs, building to words and short phrases. A second training tape[27] contains example words and phrases designed to provide practice in the full range of phonetic blending. We select utterances from the tape transcript for modeling at 50 SPM, and ask clients to review the complete tape as homework. As the group becomes more comfortable and confident with the modeled material, we begin simple question-and-answer responses, such as "How are you?," "I'm okay," imposing a strict limit of three syllables per breath. Finer points of juncturing at word boundaries are modeled but are not addressed directly at this stage to avoid information overload. Later, as examples arise in rating sessions, and through homework exercises, we emphasize points such as the blending of word terminal and word initial consonants using identical or cognate phonemes, and interpolating glides/semivowels at vowel/vowel junctures; e.g., "you are" becomes /juwa/, "he is" becomes /hijIz/.

This concludes fluency instatement, and if correct speech patterns are used, stuttering is virtually impossible, and accessory behaviors almost always disappear as well.

FLUENCY SHAPING

Rating Sessions.   Rating sessions consist of interactive conversations in which each client's speech is evaluated on-line by the clinician. Each client has a target speaking rate and must keep within 20 SPM of that rate while generating a set number of fluent syllables within the session's time limit. Speech rate, number of syllables generated, and the elapsed time for each client are displayed throughout the session on computer monitors visible to both clients and clinician. The number of fluent syllables required corresponds to 7 minutes of speech at the target rate. Thus, for the initial rating session at 50 SPM, each client must generate 350 syllables of speech without stuttering. A session's time limit is based on the number of clients, allowing 7.5 minutes per person. With a group of four, the session limit is 30 minutes; with a group of six, 45 minutes. Once this limit is reached, rating ceases, and anyone not achieving his or her targets must begin the next session with the same targets. Thus, to progress to the next level a client must generate the required number of syllables within 20 SPM of the target rate, averaged over the session. If a client stutters, his or her syllable count is returned to zero and participation in the session usually ceases. If someone stutters with sufficient time remaining in the session to attain the targets, he or she may try to do so if the clinician approves. Since this could be at the expense of someone else's time, we usually make this a group decision.

All clients have the same target rate for the initial rating session of each day but as the day progresses, some fall behind. At subsequent sessions each partici-pant can speak at a different rate, with those who are speaking slower required to say less in their allocated 7 minutes. A master clock displays the total time elapsed in the session and the half-minute extra time per person allows speech rates to be slightly below target and time for brief corrections and modeling by the clinician. If lengthy instructions are needed, the master clock is stopped. With four people in the group, we schedule rating sessions at 45-minute intervals; with a group of six, at hourly intervals. This gives 15 minutes between sessions so that the clinician can give clients feedback and extra teaching, and clients can record their performance on rating sheets and receive any payments due (see below). Our current therapy timetable for four is given in Table 7-1 and shows the progression of speech rate targets in SPM.

Table 7-1. Rating Session Schedule

	Monday	*Tuesday*	*Wednesday*	*Thursday*	*Friday*
8:00–8:45 8:45–9:45	Introduction to smooth speech	50 50/V	90 100/V	160 165/V	200/1 200/V
		Break			
10:00–10:45 10:45–11:30	Fluency instatement Fluency instatement	50/B 55	110 120	170 175	200/3 Weekend briefing
11:30–12:15 12:15–1:00	Fluency instatement Practice rating session	60 65	130 140	180 185	200/4 Assignment briefing
		Lunch			
2:00–2:45 2:45–3:45	50/1 50/2	70 75/V	145 150/V	190 195/V	200/C
		Break			
4:00–4:45 4:45–5:30	50/3 50/4	80	155	200	
		Evening Briefing			
	Extra sessions until goal for the day is achieved				
Goal	50/4	80	155	200	200/C

V = video assessment session; B = barrier session <3 errors in technique; C = coping session.

This schedule allows smooth speech skills to be established at a very slow speed, after which they are shaped and consolidated at gradually increasing speeds. When skill is insufficient for a client to remain stutter-free, the procedure requires as much further practice as is necessary to achieve the skill to stay fluent at the target speaking rate. Only then does the client progress to the next speed. We encourage clients not to look on stuttering as a failure but rather as an indicator that their level of skill is inadequate. Likewise, they should not regard needing several rating sessions to achieve their targets as a punishment but as an opportunity to consolidate their skill at the current rate rather than moving to a faster rate and becoming even more vulnerable. The token-reward system that was used in early programs has been abandoned, but clients do earn small monetary payments on a schedule[25] that reinforces good performance and consistency.[32] The principal reward, however, is being able to leave for home on schedule rather than staying late.

We introduce clients to rating session procedures with a practice session at 50 SPM following fluency instatement. We review what we will count as a stutter and make clear that this will include fillers, unfinished words, restarts, etc., which most do not think of as stuttering. We insist on conversation using simple vocabulary, given the fragility of the skill and the three syllable per breath limit imposed. We usually require only 3 minutes of conversation each, rather than 7, in this familiarization session, since the purpose is to show how a session works and to demonstrate the computer rating system. The current computer system[33] provides cumulative syllable, time, and speed measures for each client throughout the session, and a graphic "speedometer," which varies according to the client's speech rate during the last 45 seconds of speech. The speedometer is easy to check at a glance, is centered on the SPM target, and provides clients additional feedback by beeping if speech is above or below the 20-SPM range limit. The number of such speed violations is also displayed, as is a count of any other errors that the clinician identified.

Video Assessment Sessions.   Beginning on Tuesday we schedule two sessions a day in which each client's speech is video recorded and played back. These sessions allow clients to improve their ability to identify and evaluate the elements of smooth speech. Self-assessment is given a strong emphasis, and when skill is lacking, video playbacks assist clients in recognizing the aspects of smooth speech technique that need attention. When skill has improved, the playback validates the progress that has been made.

Each client is taped for at least 1 minute while speaking to the rest of the group. Both speaker and audience evaluate the live performance in terms of smooth speech criteria, which consist of an estimate of speech rate and an assessment of errors in the (sometimes overlapping) categories of breathing, phrase initiation, continuity, onsets/offsets, contacts, and phrasing and pausing, and beginning on Wednesday, an overall appraisal of prosody and presentation. After all recordings are complete, each client's performance is played back. If clients wish to alter their assessments at this time, they may do so, after which they report their judgments and compare them with those of the clinician. Because these sessions are intended to teach assessment skills, clients receive monetary rewards[25] for good judgments, rather than for the quality of their performance. Irrespective of their judgment, however, clients advance to the next speech rate only if they fulfilled the usual criteria of no stutters and speaking rate within range.

Progress through the First Week.   After a Monday lunch break, we begin the first of four scheduled rating sessions at 50 SPM. Conversation is kept extremely simple, and we usually make session time limits more generous while clients are settling. By the time clients have completed four successful rating sessions, they have the rudiments of the smooth speech technique, although their skill may not be reliable. In these early sessions we often find it helpful to have clients monitor and remind each other when they notice lapses in someone's technique. This keeps clients observant, reduces the clinician's interruptions, and gives the monitoring client an opportunity to generate target syllables.

We require three further sessions at 50 SPM on Tuesday, the first a normal session, the second a video session, and the third a special barrier session. The barrier session precedes the transition to higher speech rates and requires sufficient syllables not only at the correct rate without stuttering, but also with no more than two errors in performing the fundamentals of the smooth speech technique. Errors in breathing, smooth phrase initiation, and continuity are rated and displayed on a single counter. If three are counted, the client's clock is zeroed, and he or she can begin again. There is no session time limit and the session runs until everyone is successful. Session targets increase by 5 SPM throughout Tuesday to 80 SPM, at which time clients are using four to five syllables per breath. This is still very slow speech with few linguistic formulation demands. On Wednesday, morning sessions increase by 10 SPM, and some stutterers find concentration on both what to say and how to say it difficult. For others such difficulty may not be encountered until Thursday, for others not at all, but it is not unusual for clients to plateau for several sessions, much to their frustration, until they learn to distribute their attention appropriately. By Thursday evening all clients, sooner or later, reach 200 SPM and they consolidate their skill at this rate through four successful rating sessions at this speed on Friday.

In addition to providing the backbone for building fluency skills, rating sessions provide a forum for developing conversational skills and for restructuring inappropriate interactional behavior. Stuttering is often accompanied by difficulties in these areas,[34] and where possible we use rating sessions to address them. Some clients may become alienatingly inquisitorial, others may aggressively monopolize conversation, while others may be unassertive and unskilled in developing and shifting topics. By refusing to rate the speech during such unwanted behavior, clinicians can encourage change. Likewise, assertiveness can be fostered by encouraging interruptions and, when two people talk at once, by preferentially rating the client who needs to be more assertive. When clients unskilled in conversation are the last to leave, the clinician has ample opportunity to instruct and model conversational strategies while the final rating sessions are completed.

TRANSFER

Transfer involves gradually transferring the new speech skills into situations increasingly removed from the treatment room. In our current program, transfer begins right from the start.

Transfer during Shaping.   Throughout treatment we give constant reminders that smooth speech must be deliberately and consistently applied everywhere at all times. If not, the new skill becomes conditioned to the treatment room, and old habits remain supreme in the outside world. The treatment program today offers a less controlled environment than in earlier years, which we believe aids in generalization. While the clinician monitors and reinforces fluency within the rating session, we expect clients to assume this responsibility in situations beyond the rating sessions from the outset. Once fluency instatement is complete, we caution clients not to revert to spontaneous speech. To enhance the need for constant monitoring, we introduce fines for stutters, incorrect speed, or the use of spontaneous speech. Clients are expected to fine themselves, with the clinician and other group members sounding an alert if behaviors go unnoticed. Although the clinician is usually with the clients during short breaks, lunch is not supervised. Until Wednesday, clients eat a sack lunch in the clinic but may choose to eat elsewhere thereafter. Each evening, clients leave an overnight monetary bond and report the next morning on any deductions that should be taken for interim lapses in their use of smooth speech. These penalties rely entirely on an honor system, although we point out that those who cheat disadvantage not us but themselves. We believe that most clients respond to this procedure with due seriousness.

Each night there is a homework task, consisting of skill-building exercises on Monday, followed by recording a short fluent conversation at home on Tuesday, Wednesday, and Thursday evenings. Clients are asked to replay the tape, review their performance, and to redo the task if they have not attained the required speech targets. These conversations involve the client's household in the careful monitoring that will be necessary for good, long-term fluency and pave the way for the more demanding assignments the following week.

Weekend Briefing.   Prior to the first weekend we discuss our expectations for the client's first extended period away from the clinic. Everyone is tired, but most are also elated about their achievement and buoyed by the experience of total stutter-free speech. Those who have had a reasonably clear run through the shaping are often keen to experiment with their fluency. Others express some trepidation about the prospect of speaking away from the clinic and home and may already be concerned about the next week's assignments. Our advice to all is the same. We instruct them to have a quiet weekend and to take deliberate steps to guard their new fluency. We urge them to resist all pressure for demanding interactions with friends or extended family, especially if the gathering is "to see how you're doing with this new speech." We remind them that they have completed only one third of the program, that there is much yet to do, and that their present fluency is still fragile. Moreover, while their speech no longer sounds as excessively breathy or slurred as early in the week, it does not yet sound as normal or as natural as they can expect it to sound with further work, and this is a time when gratuitous comments from outsiders are not needed. But we also tell them that our advice for the following weekend will be very different. With a week of transfer experience outside the clinic, we will urge them to start putting their fluency to the test wherever they choose, and that any vulnerabilities they identify will form a focus for work in the final week of treatment.

While reiterating the need to use smooth speech at all times, we also discuss the fact that with the present fragility of fluency, some occasional stuttering may occur. We emphasize that neither they nor their household members should be alarmed or see this as a failure on their part or of the treatment. We then examine the sort of circumstances in which they may encounter difficulty and suggest appropriate reactions. First and foremost, they should not focus on stuttering itself but rather on what led to it. Often it will simply be due to a lack of vigilance in using the technique. Some stutters, therefore, stem from basically not taking care to use smooth speech. We also tell them that it is often possible for clients to be fluent in spontaneous speech, but that while using the technique guarantees fluency, the presence of fluency is no guarantee that the technique is being used. This is something most will have realized from fluent times prior to treatment.

Some clients may also find that they feel they are about to stutter or have indeed stuttered while doing their best to use the smooth speech technique. If we analyze what occurs in such situations, it appears that the demand of the speaking task or situation outweighs the client's present capacity to apply the new fluency skills correctly. The demand may involve having to express a complex thought or to explain oneself in an awkward circumstance. Alternatively, it may involve a word or a situation strongly associated with past stuttering. In this case, the client is likely to have become preoccupied with the expectation of stuttering so that there was insufficient concentration on technique and a consequent breakdown of skill. We find sporting skills analogies helpful here, such as facing a previously difficult opponent or approaching the location of earlier falls on the ski run. We explain that such preoccupations will diminish as strengthened technique allows fluent experiences gradually to overlay the old disfluent associations. The strongest associations will take the longest to overcome, and it may take a while to achieve reliable fluency in that situation, but perseverance will win. They should bear this in mind if they strike trouble over the weekend; they should not admonish themselves for failure but view the circumstance as one that will need work in the coming weeks. Some clients may also become excessively anxious in previously difficult situations, in which case their anxiety can interfere with their ability to perform well. If the need for anxiety management has been detected during a client's initial assessment, he or she should have acquired and consolidated stress management skills prior to treatment. In this case, we remind that these strategies, as well as their smooth speech, are needed if difficulty occurs or is anticipated. If an untreated anxiety disorder becomes salient during therapy, we attempt basic individual intervention in association with transfer tasks, but this is less than ideal.

The Coping Technique.   Before clients leave for the first weekend, we have them practice what we call the "coping technique." It is to be used whenever they feel that they are in danger of stuttering or have, in fact, stuttered and need to recover and continue. While coping involves brief, judicious use of exaggerated smooth speech, there are clear similarities with Van Riper's "pullouts" and "preparatory sets" techniques.[35] To "cope," the client stops, breathes out, then in, and, without holding the breath, initiates an utterance slowly, gently, and with ample air, carefully following through with perfect continuity. Speed should increase to normal gradually, over four to six syllables. We liken it to changing gears in an automobile. Each change should be smooth and sequential, never from low gear straight to top. Coping should also be used so that the potential trouble spot occurs while speaking slowly, rather than after reaching full speed where the coping technique will no longer be helpful. While stressing the need for a new breath if there is severe difficulty or if stuttering has actually occurred, we also demonstrate how slowing and smoothing over a potentially difficult sound can be helpful. Clients first listen to examples of coping on their training tape,[26] and then follow the therapist's model in the group before completing the final Friday rating session in which they are required to demonstrate consistent, satisfactory use of coping.

Rating Sessions.   During the second and third weeks of treatment we run morning and evening rating sessions. During these sessions each person completes 3 minutes of fluent speech at 100, 150, 180, and 200 SPM, plus an additional 3 minutes while practicing the coping technique. As before, the criteria of no stutters, sufficient syllables, and speed within 20 SPM of the target rate apply; however, there is no time limit for completing the target syllables at each speed. Rather, we advance each client to the next speed as soon as the targets for the previous speed are reached. Clients are encouraged to see these sessions as consolidating their smooth speech technique for use beyond the treatment room. We liken rating session practice to the scales and exercises that musicians use in preparation for a performance. The slower speeds enforce careful monitoring and readily reveal technical faults. At the faster speeds, clients are encouraged to shape their technique toward greater naturalness and to experiment with speech that sounds "spontaneous" but still retains the essentials of smooth speech. Working across a range of speeds allows clients to become better estimators of rate, and we expect them to be able to approximate their speed targets with minimal reliance on computer feedback from on-line ratings.

All clients participate in an 8 A.M. rating session throughout the second and third week. Completion of the evening rating session is contingent on progress. Those who complete three successful assignments per day in week 2 leave early as a reward. Likewise, in week 3, evening rating sessions are reserved for those whose skill is not yet robust in the outside world.

Standard Assignments.   During the second week we expect clients to complete 15 standard assignments. These assignments provide practice across a range of common speech situations that nonstutterers take for granted but which stutterers frequently find difficult and sometimes fear or avoid. We intend for clients to build confidence in speaking as they work through these assignments, so we have them tackle easier assignments first. Most complete the assignments in the order listed below. If a client suspects special difficulty with certain assignments, we renegotiate the order. The assignments are:

1. Conversation with a family member or close friend using coping.
2. Conversation with a family member or close friend.
3. Conversation with a stranger (male or female) using coping.
4–7. Conversations with strangers (two with males, two with females).
8–9. Telephone calls to strangers.
10. Shopping.

11. 20 inquiries.
12. 14 introductions and requests.
13. Five telephone appointments and cancellations.
14. Ten deliberate stutters with coping recovery.
15. Identifying six important points from the chapter on stabilization after therapy written by Charles Van Riper[35]

We instruct the group about what each assignment involves and how they should proceed with it. This information is also given in the client's manual[25] that can be consulted for more detail. Assignments 1 through 14 are tape-recorded and must satisfy the criteria of no stuttering, speech rate between 180 and 220 SPM, good-quality smooth speech of adequate length (assignments 1 through 10 must contain at least 1400 syllables, and 11 through 14, the correct number of items).

We ask clients not to submit tapes of assignments that contain a stutter. If they stutter during an assignment, they should rewind the tape and begin again, if necessary with another person. This encourages careful monitoring of speech during assignments. It also encourages careful assessment of the tape, as clients must be vigilant for any stutters that may have eluded them when recording. We do not give a monetary reward for each assignment completed but tally on a treatment room board the attempts at each assignment, successful and unsuccessful, for each member of the group. This reinforces progress, as does permission to leave for home early as soon as three assignments per day are accomplished. There is an overall monetary incentive, however, to work efficiently and to persevere through difficulties. We offer $A50 if all 15 assignments are completed by Friday evening. About half our clients reach this goal and, if appropriate, we announce a last-minute extension for those who have just missed, with $A50 still paid if the remainder are complete on their arrival Monday morning.

Evaluation of Assignments.   Before clients submit recordings of an assignment to the clinician, we require them to listen carefully to the tape. If they believe it meets the criteria for a successful assignment, they submit it with an assessment sheet on which they evaluate the quality of their speech using the nine assessment categories used previously for evaluating the videotaped sessions. We ask them to note problems and to suggest what steps they might take to improve aspects of their speech that do not please them. The assessment sheet also elicits comments on feelings and concerns about the assignment and asks them what they thought was best about it. The clinician then rates each tape submitted, evaluates the client's own assessment, and adds notes on missed errors, comments, and general advice. These sheets are retained by the client for reference after treatment is completed.

Progress through the Second Week.   When clients arrive on the second Monday, we debrief them about their weekend experiences and reiterate relevant information given prior to their Friday departure. After completing the morning rating session, they leave the clinic to begin their assignments. We suggest that they find strangers to talk to, firstly in the hospital waiting area, and later in the local bus or train station or city park. Downtown business and shopping areas are within walking distance for the later assignments. These assignments pressure the clients to maintain smooth speech while gaining attention and establishing rapport. They must attend to their smooth speech technique while formulating an appropriate message and communicating promptly. Listeners may be reluctant, wary, or interruptive, and the client may have to speak on cue in a busy street or shop.

Just as we address clients' interactional styles during rating sessions, so too do we offer advice if these skills are lacking in the transfer tasks. Richardson and Brutten[36] noted frequent topic shifts in dyadic conversations between stutterers and nonstutterers, seemingly in reaction to the formers' tendencies to give abbreviated responses to questions and unelaborated responses to topic initiations. While control of fluency is often enough to alter these patterns, some clients need guidance in how to converse. They may also be inexperienced using the telephone and need advice on how to communicate effectively. Some find it difficult to generate useful conversational exchanges when shopping, asking only short questions that do not obtain the information wanted. It is helpful in these cases to discuss and model alternative ways that an assignment conversation might have been handled.

The second week may also bring other problems that require individual management. In feared situations, high anxiety can degrade smooth speech skill, just as it does other sensory-motor behavior requiring control and concentration. High anxiety also leads to poor judgment and detracts from one's ability to solve problems, and the combination may lead to a client feeling helpless and abandoning the task. It takes time to implement proper management of anxiety,[37] but stopgap measures that combine a hierarchical approach and cognitive restructuring can be helpful. Similar intervention is appropriate if a client is socially anxious and fears negative evaluations from others. The prospect of the assignment to stutter deliberately and recover is especially daunting for such clients, and considerable support may be needed for it to be completed successfully. This assignment forces clients to confront the reactions of others to their stuttering, but then to take control of their speech while perhaps reacting themselves. Of all the assignments, this is the one that generates the most reluctance among clients, but from which most admit that they gained a great deal.

Some clients are not generally anxious but have unusual difficulty with a specific situation, such as the telephone. If a long history of bad experiences has sensitized a client to such an extent that successful performance of the task seems insurmountable, we break it down into a sequence of hierarchical steps. Thus, the client with telephone difficulties may first speak into a disconnected telephone during rating sessions; then move to dialing and listening to recorded information, such as the weather forecast; then to talking to the recording; then to telephoning a real person with a well-rehearsed, one-line inquiry not needing further conversation; etc. In this way, a client moves in slow steps to completion of the full assignment.

When special circumstances arise, a client usually needs much of the third week to complete the standard assignments and does not have time to undertake the full range of advanced assignments intended for that week. Such clients are usually pleased to consolidate the substantial gains they feel they have made, and we reinforce their achievement with praise and congratulations.

Assessment of Progress.   When clients have successfully completed the set of standard assignments, we assess their progress in terms of predictors of good, long-term outcome: perfect fluency control, normalization of communication attitudes, and greater internalized locus of control.[6] For most clients, this occurs on the third Monday. We obtain a 3-minute sample of the client's telephone conversation with strangers and readminister the S24 and LCB scales. If the speech sample contains no stutters, the S24 is below 10, and the LCB score is more internalized by at least 5%, we consider the client to be on track for successful, long-term maintenance of fluency. If that is not the case, we take the following action. If a client did not achieve perfect fluency, we provide extra rating session practice. If speech attitudes have not normalized, we have them repeat the five standard assignments that presented the most challenge. If a client's perceived sense of control is not enhanced, we instigate an individual self-management program similar to that described by Craig and Andrews.[4] These clients pursue these additional tasks in parallel with the usual third-week program.

Results of attitude therapy for stutterers have not been impressive,[21] yet clients' perceptions of themselves as speakers and of their responsibility for their performance appear to be highly relevant to therapy outcome. We expect these changes to be mediated principally by the behavioral changes that a client experiences during the treatment program. Predication of attitude change from behavioral change[38] comes through the resolution of cognitive dissonance.[39] We seek to enhance such dissonance through our standard treatment procedures. In addition, our third-week discussions of approaches to maintenance add cognitive components that are intended to foster positive attitudes and reality-focused coping. Where necessary, individual cognitive restructuring techniques are employed.

Friends and Relatives Evening.   On the third Monday evening, clients invite friends or family close to them for a group discussion of their progress and future expectations. We show how a rating session works and have clients demonstrate how practice of smooth speech at slower and then faster speeds allows them to focus first on technical skill and then on natural speech style. Visitors are invited to join in and are usually interested to have their own rates of speech measured. We discuss the benefits of continuing this type of practice as part of a client's daily routine at home and enlist the household's cooperation in "rating session" conversations.

We use this occasion to show the pretreatment videos, which most clients have usually not yet seen. This has two purposes. First, it allows the clinician to illustrate the particular behaviors that compromised each client's fluency, and these are tagged as "danger signals" to be watched for in the future. Second, it validates the client's progress of the past 2 weeks and endorses the worth of the effort involved for both clients and family. Many clients find it a confronting, but salutary, experience to compare their past and present ability to communicate, and this often increases their incentive to prepare well for maintenance. We discuss long-term expectations and stress the fact that what has occurred is not a cure. We explain that clients need to use smooth speech all the time on an everyday basis, in which case the conscious effort to apply it will gradually lessen. We stress that the smooth speech technique is not like a Superman suit that can be whipped out when emergency strikes. Those who regard it as such will quickly find that the suit has holes that get bigger the longer it is stored away. Those close to the client can help if they remember that support in maintaining smooth speech should be positive (encouragement, praise) rather than negative (nagging, criticism). The importance of family recognition and reward, and of self-reward, is highlighted, because clients are usually with people who are unaware of the perseverance involved and who take fluency for granted. Moreover, even though a client's effort may continue at a constant level, a ubiquitous principle, power law learning,[40] ensures that the apparent gains will lessen as performance nears its asymptote. We also discuss some of the possible behavior changes and role changes that may cause concern, such as a girlfriend whose previously reticent boyfriend now chats with other women, or a wife who has her valued role as family spokesperson usurped.

While we repeatedly stress the importance of consistent daily use of the technique, we also urge clients and their families to be realistic about everyday variations in fluency. We encourage them to analyze why stuttering has occurred, rather than feeling negative about its occurrence and reiterate the information given prior to the first weekend. We also discuss variations in the fluency of nonstutterers and show a videotape of a professional speaker who becomes markedly disfluent when placed unexpectedly in an unusually demanding circumstance. Our aim is to have the gathering realize that everyday variations in fluency are normal and can be understood in terms of capacities and demands that apply to nonstutterers and stutterers alike, although their fluency baselines are different. We add a final caution, however, about lapses and relapses. If everyday variation becomes superimposed on a clear downward trend, it is time for concern. Lapses need attention before they turn into relapses and we urge families to encourage clients to take remedial action sooner rather than later. Disappointment in oneself should not be used to assume that the clinician will also be disappointed, or angry, but such assumptions can lead clients to avoid seeking early advice.

Advanced Assignments.   In the third week, we expect clients to complete four set assignments and a range of personal assignments. The set assignments are:

1. *Work Assignment*: Clients go to their workplace, usually on Monday morning of the third week, and if possible tape-record their interactions with peers and superiors. We ask them to test themselves in typical work-related speaking tasks and to evaluate their performance on the usual assignment sheet.

2. *Introductions*: Clients formally introduce their guests to the group and the therapist on the friends and relatives evening.

3. *Prepared Speech to an Audience of Strangers*: This is a 7-minute presentation delivered in the formal environment of the clinic's lecture theater. Where appropriate, clients are encouraged to speak on work-related subjects using slides or overheads. Notes may be used, but not a text, and the client is expected to answer questions from the audience. We videotape the proceedings and review it with the group.

4. *Call-in Radio*: This task involves conversation with the host of a call-in radio talk show. Successful completion requires 1 minute of perfectly fluent speech.

There is frequently a long wait before going on the air, which puts considerable pressure on the client, who must stay prepared to speak on cue. We attach a special monetary reward to this assignment. Clients post $A10 each, which the clinic matches, and which is paid to the group, if and only if, all group members complete the assignment successfully. This ensures mutual support and encouragement in a challenging task.

In addition to these set assignments, clients undertake personal assignments that are planned in discussions with the clinician. These assignments are focused on each client's individual needs and life-style. They may involve job inquiries and interviews, ordering in restaurants, making complaints, arguing on video, answering rapid-fire questions, door-to-door inquiries, a mock trial, specifically difficult phone calls, asking directions involving difficult sounds, etc.

Progress through the Third Week.   Clients arrive at the clinic on Monday after completing their set work assignment, unless they still have second-week assignments pending. In this case, they postpone the set work assignment and bring completed tapes to the clinic. All second-week assignments must be completed before proceeding further. Monday afternoon is devoted to assessing clients' progress and assignment planning, and if assessment results warrant, the clinician provides instructions on needed consolidation and/or self-management tasks. Friends and relatives gather on Monday evening, and sometimes a group eats out together afterward. Rating sessions are scheduled the first hour of each morning for the remainder of the third week, followed by 1-hour maintenance discussion sessions on Wednesday and Thursday. The formal speech presentations are scheduled for Thursday, and Friday is devoted to a final maintenance briefing and posttreatment assessment.

Unlike the second week, in which the schedule pressures clients to work efficiently and consistently, much of the third week is left free for clients to do as much or as little as they please. This is a deliberate transition to prepare clients for the coming weeks when they will be on their own. The focus of this final week is "becoming your own therapist" and we encourage clients to manage their own personal program and to set their own goals. Other than the bonus for the call-in assignment, we offer no monetary reward. We urge clients to plan their own rewards and to continue using self-reinforcement strategies during maintenance. Preparation for maintenance sessions includes discussions of daily practice, using "rating sessions" and real-life assignments, and how to pinpoint difficulties and then set about solving them. Simply saying "I must not stutter" is not likely to be helpful. Clients should use their assessment skills to focus on a specific feature of their smooth speech technique and aim to improve that specific aspect. We discuss self-management strategies and give detailed instruction on how to set up hierarchical tasks if difficult situations are encountered. The client's manual[25] contains written advice and examples of maintenance strategies, and we also supply them an audiotape containing similar information and reminders on assessment skills.[28]

The Final Day.   During the final morning rating session, clients tape their speech to keep as a permanent record of their skills at the end of the program. Reviewing these tapes during maintenance can be helpful both as a model and as a reminder of the skill a client is capable of. We take clients individually through their plans for maintenance before a final review of their pretreatment audiotape. Client and clinician identify the previous problem areas and match these with the corresponding protective features of the smooth speech technique. A client then repeats the pretreatment task of 3 minutes of telephone conversation with strangers, for the posttreatment record. The S24 and the LCB are readministered and the group meets around the rating table for the posttreatment video recording which replicates its pretreatment counterpart. Each client gives identifying information but instead of asking for their expectations in undertaking treatment, we request their reflections on those expectations. Then, we replay the tape and ask clients for general comments on their performance, with special reference to whether they like their new speech and find it acceptably natural-sounding. Lastly, without revealing the nature of the measures involved, we inform each client of the extent to which he or she has achieved our specific therapy goals and the chances of good, long-term outcome.

MAINTENANCE

We run follow-up sessions from 4 P.M. to 8 P.M. on the second Thursday of every month. Any client who has completed the treatment course is welcome to attend without an appointment, but we expect clients to attend at 1, 2, 3, 6, and 12 months after treatment. At such times, we ask them to bring a recent tape recording of a 3-minute telephone conversation with strangers. On these occasions we assess their progress in terms of the three treatment goals and discuss their maintenance program. We also run a rating session consisting of 3 minutes of speech at 150 SPM and 180 SPM, respectively, and clients have the opportunity to interact with clients at other stages of maintenance as well as other members of their own group. We give individual advice but usually deliver it in the group forum, which gives the others present reminders about maintenance strategies that can be employed. The focus remains on self-therapy, with the clinic therapists readily available for consultation. As we tell clients, a clinician confronted with a difficult problem is wise to seek the opinion of a respected colleague but still keeps responsibility for treatment.

Expected Outcomes and Conclusions

The foregoing description of the smooth speech treatment program for adult stutterers is sufficiently detailed that experienced clinicians should be able to conduct similar programs.* The results to be expected from such a program are well documented in the literature[4-8,11,21,32] reporting changes in %SS, number of clients fluent, and in the mean effect size associated with treatment. Clinically, our experience is that five of six clients who enter this treatment program become reliably fluent by the end of treatment. Furthermore, at follow-up sessions a year later, we are becoming increasingly aware, as with many other cognitive behav-

---

*Copies of the patient treatment manual,[24,25] a videotape of fluency instatement, the audiotapes of smooth speech quality,[26-28] and the rating system software are available from the authors.

ioral interventions, that the improvement is surprisingly permanent. The importance of this result is not in the number of clients who do remain fluent but in that any at all achieve fluency. Stuttering is a genetic disorder,[41] and treatment certainly does not change the genotype. Treatment teaches clients how to cope with a genetic impairment and represents a triumph of human potential over inherent disability. That it occurs at all is a triumph. That it occurs so regularly is a tribute to the capacity of humans to persevere and achieve impossible goals. Calvin Coolidge was right: Once you know what to do, it is perseverance that makes the difference between success and failure.

Suggested Readings

Andrews G, Craig A, Feyer A-M, et al: Stuttering: A review of research findings and theories circa 1982. *J Speech Hear Disord* 1983; 48:226–246.
   A comprehensive empirical review of the known facts about the nature and treatment of stuttering. Essential reading.
Andrews G, Guitar B, Howie P: Meta-analysis of the effects of stuttering treatment. *J Speech Hear Disord* 1980; 45:287–307.
   An empirical comparison of the results of all treatments for stuttering as of 1980. The picture has not changed radically since then.
Andrews C, Craig A: Prediction of outcome after treatment for stuttering. *Br J Psychiatry* 1988; 153: 236–240.
   Detail of the progress of treated stutterers in whom end-of-treatment measures predict long-term outcome.
Andrews C, Feyer A-M: Does behavior therapy still work when the experimenters depart: An analysis of a behavioral treatment program for stuttering. *Behav Mod* 1985; 9:443–457.
   A participant observer's account of the treatment program showing that the treatment remains effective in service.
Andrews G, Neilson M, Cassar M: Informing Stutterers about Treatment, in Rustin L, Purser H, Rowley D (eds): *Progress in the Treatment of Fluency Disorders*. Progress in Clinical Science Series. London, Taylor & Francis, 1987.
   The treatment manual given to stutterers on the intensive program. Complements the present chapter precisely.

References

1. Andrews G, Harris M: *The Syndrome of Stuttering*. Clinics in Developmental Medicine, no. 17. London, Heinemann, 1964.
2. Andrews G: Evaluating treatment effectiveness. *Aust NZ J Psychiatry* 1989; 23:181–186.
3. Andrews G, Cutler J: Stuttering therapy: The relation between changes in symptom level and attitudes. *J Speech Hear Res* 1974; 39:312–319.
4. Craig A, Andrews G: The prediction and prevention of relapse in stuttering. The value of self-control techniques and locus of control measures. *Behav Mod* 1985; 9:427–442.
5. Andrews G, Craig A, Feyer A-M, et al: Stuttering: A review of research findings and theories circa 1982. *J Speech Hear Disord* 1983; 48:226–246.
6. Andrews G, Craig A: Prediction of outcome after treatment for stuttering. *Br J Psychiatry* 1988; 153:236–240.
7. Howie PM, Tanner S, Andrews G: Short and long term outcome in an intensive treatment program for adult stutterers. *J Speech Hear Disord* 1981; 46:104–109.
8. Craig A, Feyer A-M, Andrews G: An overview of a behavioural treatment for stuttering. *Aust Psychol* 1987; 22:53–62.
9. Andrews G, Crino R: Behavioural psychotherapy of anxiety disorders. *Psychiatr Ann* 1991; 21: 358–367.
10. Hunt C, Andrews G: Measuring personality disorder: The use of self-report questionnaires. *J Pers Disord* in press.
11. Andrews G: Evaluation of the Benefits of Treatment, in Perkins WH (ed): *Current Therapy of Communication Disorders: Stuttering Disorders*. San Diego, College-Hill Press, 1984.

12. Johnson W, Darley FL, Spriestersbach DC: *Diagnostic Methods in Speech Pathology*. New York, Harper & Row, 1963.
13. Craig A, Franklin J, Andrews G: A scale to measure locus of control of behaviour. *Br J Med Psychol* 1984; 57:173–180.
14. Eysenck HJ, Eysenck SBG: *Manual of the Eysenck Personality Inventory*. London, University of London Press, 1964.
15. Goldberg DP: *The Detection of Psychiatric Illness by Questionnaire*. London, Oxford University Press, 1972.
16. Burke BD: The identification and measurement of stuttering in real time: The Prince Henry Yardstick. *Aust J Human Commun Disord* 1973; 1:42–43.
17. Starkweather CW: *Fluency and Stuttering*. Englewood Cliffs, NJ, Prentice-Hall, 1987.
18. Perkins WH: Articulatory rate in the evaluation of stuttering treatments. *J Speech Hear Disord* 1975; 40:277–278.
19. Andrews G, Ingham R: Stuttering: Considerations in the evaluation of treatment. *Br J Disord Commun* 1971; 6:129–138.
20. Ingham RJ: *Stuttering and Behavior Therapy. Current Status and Experimental Foundations*. San Diego, College-Hill Press, 1984.
21. Andrews G, Guitar B, Howie P: Meta-analysis of the effects of stuttering treatment. *J Speech Hear Disord* 1980; 45:287–307.
22. Market KE, Montague JC, Buffalo MD, Drummond SS: Acquired stuttering: Descriptive data and treatment outcome. *J Fluency Disord* 1990; 15:21–33.
23. St. Louis KO, Ruscello DM, Lundeen C: Coexistence of communication disorders in school children. *ASHA Monogr*, in press.
24. Andrews G: A Tutorial on Stuttering, in Rustin L, Purser H, Rowley D (eds): *Progress in the Treatment of Fluency Disorders*. Progress in Clinical Science Series. London, Taylor & Francis, 1987.
25. Andrews G, Neilson M, Cassar M: Informing Stutterers about Treatment, in Rustin L, Purser H, Rowley D (eds): *Progress in the Treatment of Fluency Disorders*. Progress in Clinical Science Series. London, Taylor & Francis, 1987.
26. Cassar M: *Smooth Speech Training Tape* (ISBN 0 85823 740 7). Sydney, Australia, Clinical Research Unit for Anxiety Disorders, 1988.
27. Cassar M: *The 100 List Tape* (ISBN 0 85823 741 5). Sydney, Australia, Clinical Research Unit for Anxiety Disorders, 1988.
28. Cassar M: *Fluency Maintenance Tape* (ISBN 0 85823 742 3). Sydney, Australia, Clinical Research Unit for Anxiety Disorders, 1988.
29. Andrews G, Pollock C, Stewart G: The determination of defense style by questionnaire. *Arch Gen Psychiatry* 1989; 46:455–460.
30. Neilson M, Neilson PD: Speech motor control and stuttering: A computational model of adaptive sensory-motor processing. *Speech Commun* 1987; 6:325–333.
31. Grosjean F, Grosjean L, Lane H: The patterns of silence: Performance structures in sentence production. *Cogn Psychol* 1979; 11:58–81.
32. Andrews G, Feyer A-M: Does behavior therapy still work when the experimenters depart: An analysis of a behavioral treatment program for stuttering. *Behav Mod* 1985; 9:443–457.
33. Neilson M, Hand R: Rater—A fluency rating computer program for stuttering treatment and assessment. Presented at the annual convention of the Australian Association of Speech and Hearing, Sydney, 1990.
34. Guitar B, Peters TJ: *Stuttering: An Integration of Contemporary Therapies*. Memphis, Speech Foundation of America, 1980.
35. Van Riper C: *The Treatment of Stuttering*. Englewood Cliffs, NJ, Prentice-Hall, 1973.
36. Richardson CM, Brutten GJ: Topic management in the dyadic conversations of stutterers and nonstutterers. Presented at the ASHA convention, San Francisco, November, 1984.
37. Clinical Research Unit for Anxiety Disorders: *The Generalized Anxiety Disorder Program Treatment Manual 1991*. Sydney, Australia, Clinical Research Unit for Anxiety Disorders, 1991.
38. Regan DT, Fazio RH: On the consistency between attitudes and behavior: Look to the method of attitude formation. *J Exp Soc Psychol* 1977; 13:28–45.
39. Festinger L: *A Theory of Cognitive Dissonance*. Stanford, CA, Stanford University Press, 1957.
40. Newell A, Rosenbloom PS: Mechanisms of Skill Acquisition and the Law of Practice, in Anderson JR (ed): *Cognitive Skills and Their Acquisition*. Hillsdale, NJ, Lawrence Erlbaum Associates, 1981.
41. Andrews G, Morris-Yates A, Howie PM, Martin NG: Genetic factors in stuttering confirmed. *Arch Gen Psychiatry* 1991; 48:1034–1035.

8

Transfer and Maintenance of Treatment Gains of Chronic Stutterers

ROGER J. INGHAM, PH.D.

This chapter describes the procedures that are currently used in treatment studies at the University of California, Santa Barbara, to transfer and maintain therapy gains. For the most part, the procedures that will be described are the end products of experimental treatments that have been designed to improve the durability of gains from behaviorally oriented stuttering therapy procedures.[1] The treatments in which these procedures have been employed were conducted with adult and adolescent clients, but with appropriate modifications they have occasionally been used with children as young as 5 years.

The procedures employed have been integrated with therapy schedules that are designed to produce stutter-free and natural-sounding speech within clinic settings. The beyond-clinic settings have been either clinician-prescribed or client-defined in order to represent, as much as possible, the client's customary speaking environment. Both transfer and maintenance strategies are introduced after every endeavor has been made to achieve normal-sounding fluency (see below) within a clinic-based establishment phase. Some data have been reported from individual therapy,[2,3] but most have come from therapy studies that involved intensive group programs conducted in residential settings[4] where the establishment and transfer phases are completed in a 9- to 28-day period. During the course of this initial residential treatment period, the intensity of treatment (that is, monitored speaking time and practice) is systematically reduced from about 14 hours per day down to approximately 4 hours per day. Transfer procedures are introduced during the residential period of the program and are then gradually blended with maintenance procedures. Thus, maintenance procedures are actually introduced prior to the cessation of the client's residential treatment period and then continue, with scheduled decreases in frequency of contact between client and clinician, over 2 or 3 years. In short, the aim of the maintenance phase is to decrease contact between client and clinician contingent on the client demonstrating that normal-sounding speech has been sustained in routine speaking situations.

166

Most transfer and maintenance procedures now employed in stuttering therapy appear to have at least four general (though not always compatible) objectives.[5] These objectives are supposed to be reflected in therapy benefits that are sustained across situations and over time:

1. To have the client use therapy practices that reduce or eliminate stuttering in the absence of formal therapy.

2. To have the client demonstrate that factors associated with therapy (e.g., situations and/or people) are not necessary for the client to continue to evidence therapy benefits.

3. To have others regard the client as a normally fluent speaker.

4. To have the client no longer "do things with his or her speech" to sound fluent.

A principal difficulty in characterizing most current therapy procedures is that it is far from clear how it can be determined which of those objectives has been (or will be) achieved. As a result, much of my recent research has been concerned with measurement of stuttering as much as its treatment, in an attempt to ensure that any clinical validity that may exist in these procedures is not compromised by inadequate measurement methodology. Actually, present measurement methods do not appear to carry sufficient validity to make it possible to determine which objective is reached by any procedure. Perhaps objective 1 can be demonstrated satisfactorily, but attainment of the others is somewhat more difficult to demonstrate. What follows is a description of some of the methods that have been developed to reach objectives 2 through 4.

A Core Transfer-Maintenance Procedure

The core transfer and maintenance procedure that is used is a performance-contingent schedule, which formed part of a token economy therapy program that was developed some years ago.[6] That program now relies on what has been termed "hierarchy control"[4]; the token system is rarely used. The current therapy program continues to be constructed around a stepwise hierarchy of generic speaking tasks, or stages, that must be completed in a prescribed number of trials prior to progressing to another stage; otherwise the client must return to the tasks of the previous stage. This performance-contingent schedule typifies many behaviorally oriented therapies; the difference in this case is that the schedule combines task and time-completion criteria in the maintenance phase.

Increasingly, it is recognized that the setting in which therapy is conducted may also provide some essential or necessary conditions for effective therapy. These conditions are probably crucial to ensuring a client's continued participation in a demanding therapy schedule. For instance, clients are usually not admitted to therapy unless the following contractual arrangement has been agreed upon: All treatment phases must be attempted and are changed only if the client continues to fail after four attempts at a hierarchy stage, and informal sampling of the client's speech must be permitted at any time throughout the course of therapy. (All recordings made are returned for the client's decision as to whether they will be erased.) This is far less contentious than it may seem because most clients, especially adults, appreciate that informed assessment may yield very different speech performance data from that collected overtly or at times known to the subject.[7,8] Finally, most clients are admitted to intensive therapy only after it has been determined that they have not responded to less intensive therapy for their disorder.

Treatment Foundation of the Core Transfer-Maintenance Procedures

The current residential part of the treatment program[4] is briefly summarized first because it sets the foundation for the core transfer-maintenance procedures.

The initial or establishment phase trains the client to complete a hierarchy of six successive speaking stages with zero stutterings at specified speech rates and speech naturalness ratings. In the first three stages of the hierarchy, the client is required to be stutter-free throughout a schedule that requires gradual increments in speech rate; in the last three stages the speech rate targets are replaced by incremental changes in speech naturalness targets. If two successive attempts at the first step of a hierarchy stage are failed, the client returns to the beginning of the preceding step. Prolonged speech target characteristics are provided via tape-recorded models that the client and clinician practice between rating sessions.

The client talks on most any topic during rating sessions while speech is rated in real time by a clinician using an electronic button-press counter.[9] Clinicians are trained to count syllables and stutterings on previously recorded samples from stutterers and nonstutterers. The clinician's accuracy is then checked against a criterion test of unfamiliar stutterers' speech samples. Clinicians are also trained to record speech naturalness ratings at 1-minute intervals during rating sessions.

Between rating sessions, the client's speech is informally monitored by other clinicians; any stuttering observed during these intervals causes the client to repeat the preceding rating session. The client may then receive guidance or may choose self-directed practice speaking with or without the clinician.

By the completion of the establishment phase, the client is expected to speak spontaneously and stutter-free in six consecutive rating sessions of 1300 syllables with mean ratings of less than 3 (per 60 seconds) on the 9-point speech naturalness scale[10]; this is the target behavior for all subsequent therapy phases.

Applying the Core Transfer-Maintenance Procedure

The transfer procedures used are logically connected to the format of the previously described establishment phase. The principal assumption underlying the design of these transfer procedures is that if target behavior can be consistently demonstrated in settings that constitute the client's routine speaking situations, then operationally the target behavior has been transferred to those settings. Of course, the fact that the target behavior appears across speaking settings does not mean it is maintained consistently in those settings. That is the principal reason why most current transfer and maintenance procedures are necessarily integrated.

A feature of this program is the effort to ensure that each client is fully aware of the rationale for the program's structure and the purpose of each speaking task. I am also increasingly persuaded that the most powerful therapy effects might be linked to a client's judgment of self-efficacy[11]; that is, the client learns to recognize that normal-sounding speech is effectively and essentially achieved by self-managed practices. For this reason every effort is made to ensure that the client achieves the target behavior in the most personally relevant and routine speaking situations. I suspect that this feature is common to many current stuttering treatments, but one that is greatly in need of research to delineate its functional components.

The general procedures that constitute transfer and maintenance phases are summarized below:

TRANSFER PHASE

A hierarchy of six to seven speaking tasks or stages usually constitutes the core transfer procedure. Clients nominate the order in which they will complete these stages, all of which involve self-formulated conversations. Each stage requires the client to make six 1300-syllable recordings that are stutter-free and yield mean speech naturalness ratings of less than 3 (speech naturalness is rated at 1-minute intervals). Typical examples of a transfer phase might be as follows: (1) conversing with a male stranger in the institution, (2) conversing with a female stranger in the institution, (3) conversing on the telephone (we permit only two conversations with familiar persons and at least two must be calls received from strangers), (4) conversing with salespersons in a local shopping center, (5) conversing with family members, (6) conversing with peers at the client's workplace or school, and (7) making speeches before an unfamiliar audience. Recordings are made on a voice-activated microcassette recorder that is concealed during conversation with strangers. Throughout this phase, the clinician intermittently monitors the client covertly when possible; any observed stuttering means that the client must repeat that step in the hierarchy stage. By the end of the hierarchy, frequency of contact between the clinician and client is decreased, to reduce as much as possible any contact between the transfer and maintenance phases.

MAINTENANCE PHASE

After completing the transfer phase during the residential period of therapy, the maintenance phase is initiated 1 week after the client leaves the institution. The maintenance procedure schedule is shown in Table 8-1. The client must obtain six recordings, each of 1300 syllables, that contain conversational speech over occasions that are systematically separated in time, contingent on the client achieving the target behavior. These recordings are given to the clinician during scheduled visits to the clinic, at which time visual and auditory recordings are also made. It can be observed from this table that the requirement for completing the maintenance phase hierarchy is more demanding than requirements in the establishment and transfer phases. For instance, the client may reach MP32(1) and still be returned to MP1(1) if stuttering or departure from the speech naturalness target range is recorded.

Between-session monitoring of the client is conducted in several different ways. The most useful appears to be at least one unscheduled telephone conversation between each visit to the clinic. This is supplemented by "surprise" meetings arranged through the client's parents, teachers, or peers. If any stuttering is identified, the client is informed immediately and returned to MP1(1), the first step of the hierarchy.

Throughout the maintenance phase, the clinician is expected to tap relevant sources of information to estimate informally the client's beyond-clinic performance. Three sources of information are commonly used for this purpose: the office staff's contact with the client (usually through telephone conversations), the client's parents, and the client's peers or teachers. This information determines whether additional recording procedures should be integrated with core maintenance phase assessments. For example, if parents have indicated that stuttering still occurs at home, then home conditions are specified and the client must obtain at least two recordings in this setting for assessment at the next clinic session. This requirement continues, or terminates after at least two clinic visits until the target behavior is achieved on the recordings and the sources report that stuttering has ceased. At each session the client is also questioned, and if stuttering is reported, then the same procedure is followed.

The effectiveness of the maintenance phase schedule in maintaining durable improvements in speech performance has been demonstrated in a group study that was conducted with nine subjects (9 to 56 years of age).[7] A modified version of this schedule that was used with one subject was also reported by the author.[2]

Self-Managed Maintenance

More recently I reported on the development of a self-managed variation of the performance-contingent schedule which is based on self-evaluation training.[8] This variation is introduced while clients are still in residence during the last three stages of the transfer phase and requires them to estimate their speech performance during specified rating sessions. These estimates are in terms of stuttering frequency and speech naturalness, that is, above, below, or at a mean rating of 3 on the naturalness scale. If the client's scores agree with the clinician's (within ±1 unit on the naturalness scale), then the client's scores are used to score performance in the clinic. Intermittent checks ensure that agreement is maintained; if not, clinician-client agreement training is reintroduced. The client's transfer phase is not complete until six consecutive self-evaluation checks are passed, with the client's scores on the final six rating sessions meeting target behavior requirements.

When the residential portion of treatment is completed, the client returns to the clinic for a series of weekly sessions which form a further self-evaluation training phase. This phase precedes initiation of the maintenance schedule outlined in Table 8-1 and is used to verify that the client accurately evaluates the relevant speech behaviors and is ready to begin self-managed maintenance. The procedure is summarized in Table 8-2.

From Table 8-2 it can be seen that the client obtains two 1300-syllable recordings in three conditions: telephoning, at home, and at work or school. Each sample is scored by the client before being checked by the clinician. When two consecu-

Table 8-1. The Core Maintenance Procedure

Weeks between Stages	Stage Attempted	Failed Criterion Performance* Return to:	Passed with Criterion Performance* Proceed to:
1 wk	MP1 (1)	MP1 (1) R	MP1 (2)
1 wk	MP1 (2)	MP1 (1)	MP2 (1)
2 wk	MP2 (1)	MP1 (1)	MP2 (2)
2 wk	MP2 (2)	MP1 (1)	MP4 (1)
4 wk	MP4 (1)	MP1 (1)	MP4 (2)
4 wk	MP4 (2)	MP1 (1)	MP8 (1)
8 wk	MP8 (1)	MP1 (1)	MP8 (2)
8 wk	MP8 (2)	MP1 (1)	MP16 (1)
16 wk	MP16 (1)	MP1 (1)	MP16 (2)
16 wk	MP16 (2)	MP1 (1)	MP32 (1)
32 wk	MP32 (1)	MP1 (1)	MP32 (2)
32 wk	MP32 (2)	MP1 (1)	Finish

*Criterion Performance: Zero percent syllables stuttered and < 3 on the speech naturalness scale on three 1300-syllable conversations and three 1300-syllable telephone conversations. Four weeks on maintenance session week 1 results in cessation of maintenance stage schedule. At this point it is concluded that the client is not benefiting from the schedule, and it is necessary to introduce alternative procedures.

Table 8-2. Self-Evaluation Phase Schedule Preceding
Client-Managed Core Maintenance Procedure*

Weeks between Stages	Stage Attempted	Failed, Retreat to:	Success, Progress to:
	SEM1	SEM1R	SEM2
1 wk	SEM2	SEM1	SEN1
1 wk	SEN1	SEM1	SEN2
1 wk	SEN2	SEM1	SEN3
1 wk	SEN3	SEM1	SEN4
1 wk	SEN4	SEM1	MP1 (1)
1 wk			

*At each stage the client must provide two 1300-syllable recordings in each of three conditions: telephoning, home, and work or school. In SEM1 and SEM2, all six 1300-syllable assignment recordings must be scored by the subject and must match the scores of the clinicians.

tive weeks of recordings are matched (SEM1 and SEM2), intermittent checks are made by the clinician on some of them (two of six per week). After six successive checks confirm that the client's recordings are accurate, the client scores all samples without those checks. The self-evaluation training phase is completed when the subject scores two consecutive weeks of recordings (a total of twelve 1300-syllable recordings), while achieving target behavior.

At this point, the client initiates the performance-contingent schedule shown in Table 8-1 and performs the same speech tasks, but moves through the hierarchy on the basis of self-recorded data. When MP4(1) is reached, or MP(1) is failed on two consecutive occasions, the client must return to the clinic. At MP4(1) the client brings all recordings to the clinic and the clinician randomly selects six samples. If any sample fails to match the client's ratings, which usually means departures from the target behavior, the client begins self-evaluation training once more. These clinician verification checks are also carried out again at MP32(2). If the client fails two successive attempts at MP1(1) at any time after completing the self-evaluation phase, the clinician-controlled performance-contingent schedule is introduced.

This self-evaluation procedure has been effective with some adult clients,[8] but others have needed the clinician-controlled performance-contingent schedule.[2] Informal checks on clients using this system are conducted in exactly the same way as those used for the clinician-controlled program: If the client stutters during any contact, he or she returns to the beginning of the self-evaluation phase. The most immediate advantage of this procedure is that it reduces the frequency of the client's contact with the clinician and, not unimportantly, reduces the amount of management time. At present, I am reasonably confident that this method of managing maintenance procedures produces a faster rate of passage through this phase and, almost by definition, the client's speech shows better evidence of maintained fluency.

Alternatives to the Core Transfer-Maintenance Procedures

Several alternatives have been developed to supplement the clinician-controlled performance-contingent schedule if MP1(1) is failed on successive occasions. They are introduced after careful investigation of the perceived difficulties reported by the client and significant others. Such difficulties ordinarily are of two types: difficulties in producing stutter-free speech regardless of circumstances or continuing evidence of situation-specific stuttering.

In the former, the client's speech is assessed during a criterion period following an instructional session. Usually, this session determines whether the client can sustain the target behavior during 5 minutes each of oral reading, monologue, and conversation in clinic conditions. Then, increasingly complex speaking conditions, as rated by the client, are introduced over two 8-hour treatment days. In effect, another hierarchy control schedule is instituted. Thereafter, the clinician-controlled performance-contingent schedule is reintroduced. To date, however, that has not been very successful. Two clients with whom this procedure has been used have served to identify either the inadequacy of the initial fluency-inducing treatment method or situations that repeatedly produce stutterings.

In the case of situation-specific stuttering, alternative treatment procedures have been carefully constructed around the situation. The situation is analyzed until its critical features appear to be identified. The alternative procedures that are used are best described by example. One of the most useful procedural principles is to pair fluency-associated conditions with a problem situation, for example, arranging for a clinician to enter the problem situation with the client and then systematically withdrawing the clinician's presence. This has been most effective with clients at home or using the telephone. Another alternative has been to role-play an event shortly before it occurs, such as speaking before a particular audience. This has been effective with one client but has failed with another. We have also used paired stimuli in certain situations, particularly the microrecorder (stimulus) that is used to record the client's speech. In the course of treatment the recorder appears to achieve considerable stimulus control properties. Consequently, some clients have simply carried the recorder in some problematic speaking situations. The most useful techniques have relied on frequent telephone contact with the client or arranging for the clinician to accompany the client during the problem-causing task. Both of these techniques have then been systematically faded using variations of the core maintenance schedule.

For the most part, our treatment programs involve rather formalized data-recording procedures coupled with tight success criteria. These same procedures can be coupled with less formal data collection methods and more liberal criteria. However, my experience with less stringent variations has been essentially vicarious. I could catalogue examples of clinicians who have liberalized this procedure and reported poor outcome, but that would not be useful without cataloguing information from those who may have succeeded with this approach. For the most part, though, my experiences have vindicated the continued use of a schedule with stringent performance criteria.

Discarded Transfer-Maintenance Procedures

I have found the following types of procedures with adults to be relatively ineffective.

Noncontingent Sessions

This is the simplest variation on a performance-contingent schedule: The client is required to attend clinic sessions scheduled at either regular or decreasingly frequent intervals. There is reasonably convincing evidence[7] that noncontingent schedules are much less effective than contingent schedules in sustaining therapy benefits.

Monetary Control

This requires the client to deposit money before the maintenance schedule begins, and it is retrieved, either partly or completely, contingent on the client achieving performance criteria. This procedure generally requires frequent readjustment and is difficult to calibrate. I have found that it does not improve the performance of clients on a performance-contingent schedule.

Management by Significant Others

This occurs when a peer, teacher, or parent manages the recording schedule or delivers consequences whenever the client achieves performance criteria. My experience has ranged across the spectrum of possibilities: The significant other is frequently either undercommitted or overcommitted to the procedure. In the former instance, the person either is unreliable or liberalizes management criteria. In the latter, the procedure may be managed in such an officious way that the client avoids speaking or contact with that person. I have also found that similar problems occur when this procedure involves the use of other clinicians. Most problems seem to occur when the client's maintenance schedule is managed by a clinician in another city. There is variation in the clinical commitment of different clinicians, no matter how carefully the procedures are described.

Group Sessions or Group Control

This refers to procedures in which group discussion sessions with different clients are an essential component of maintenance. I have discarded this method as essential, with mixed feelings. The role model of a successful client may certainly encourage another to continue treatment. It may also solve problems that are not evident in individual treatment settings. But these advantages are often exaggerated. Furthermore, when clients are treated during the establishment phase in a group setting, they almost always continue to have contact with each other and exchange information, usually in a group setting. It is also worth noting that between-client contact may have some negative aspects. I have had two examples of successful clients whose interaction with clients experiencing less immediate success has seemingly led the latter to doubt their ability to benefit from treatment.

Organized groups of clients commonly meet to assist each other in maintaining fluency. And for some clients, it is evident that such groups assist with speech practice, role-playing practice, and other clinical procedures when formal therapy has ceased. Some of the concerns about benefits of these activities have been described recently.[12] A principal concern is that such meetings are often conducted by nonprofessionals who are not in a position to manage individual client problems carefully. This type of maintenance system may also tempt clinicians to abrogate their clinical responsibilities; if the clinician refers a client to this type of setting, it is not immediately obvious how the clinician can retain control over procedures that may be crucial to maintenance of that individual's performance. None of this is meant to diminish the virtues of such groups with respect to socialization, political representation for stutterers, or anything else. Indeed, controlled studies may yet show that their benefits exceed those achieved by clinician-directed maintenance procedures.

Booster-Therapy Sessions

I have already described what could be referred to as booster sessions when clients fail performance-contingent schedules. However, the latter procedures differ from regular brief clinical programs that may include abbreviated establishment and transfer procedures. My experience has been that such programs rarely produce the benefits achieved by returning the client to a complete therapy program.

Home Practice Schedules

Between-session practice, at home or elsewhere, is usually part of a performance-contingent schedule. Clients are told that they should schedule periods of speaking time to ensure that their stutter-free speech is not simply due to infrequent speaking. Most clients develop rigorous home-practice schedules in order to pass their maintenance schedule.

Some maintenance treatments depend solely upon the client adhering to formalized speech practice periods, usually at home. My experience has been that clients often vary their practice schedule whether or not it is working. The main problem with this method is that it is difficult to determine whether the practice effects carry over time or across speaking situations. That could easily be resolved if criterion tests were instituted. In that case, of course, this procedure would contain some of the necessary features of a performance-contingent schedule.

Counseling

This refers to group therapy or counseling designed to alleviate personal difficulties. My experience might be atypical, but almost all clients who have needed counseling during treatment did so because of difficulties independent of stuttering. That is not to say that those difficulties were unimportant to transfer or maintenance. In fact, the resolution of many problems may be essential to maintenance; counseling appears to have been as relevant as medical aid or financial assistance during the course of therapy. But I have never found that counseling alone produced maintained therapy benefits. I also include under this heading guidance about the benefits of sustained fluency or other cognitively oriented methods that may seem relevant to therapy success. Such instruction has been described elsewhere as a weak form of control, and that is my experience.

Additional Considerations

An overarching consideration in the conduct of this program is the continuing problem with stuttering event judgments. Like others, I am now increasingly concerned about the reliability of perceptual judgments of stuttering events, especially when such judgments form the basis for this type of program. It is obvious that different clients and clinicians may vary greatly in the consistency with which they are able to make perceptual judgments of stuttering events. Despite the use of training tapes to aid those judgments, this is an imperfect measure at best and subject to the vagaries of judgments made across the various circumstances. At worst, the measure may be completely misleading: It bypasses visual features when the data are obtained from audio recordings and does not address the problem of word avoidance. My own research has begun to confirm that groups of judges from different training institutions will make very different event counts on audio and on audiovisual samples of stutterers. Similar findings by other researchers raise serious questions about the utility of clinic programs that are structured around this measure. It is, of course, entirely possible that even with this imperfect measure, the program described here will still produce satisfactory clinical changes. At present, however, there are no obvious alternatives that are suitable for use in a context where frequency counts of stuttering events provide the basis for the treatment. Many clinical researchers are now devoting their energies to remedying this situation and searching for measurement procedures that are sufficiently reliable to provide a valid account of therapy effects. The use of intervals of speech that are judged to be stuttered or nonstuttered is one option that is being explored in my laboratory.

Assuming that stuttering event judgments still prove to be useful in a clinical context, some clinicians may rightly complain that the transfer and maintenance schedules depend on questionable sources of information: presence, or absence, of stuttering, speech rate, speech naturalness, and sometimes visual measures. These data do not measure how natural the client feels or experiences speech. Recently, several colleagues and I have been investigating the use of clinically viable methods of assessing and training the client to judge how natural speech feels. These investigations[13] have been based upon the finding that listeners, or clinicians, are able to use a 9-point scale to rate naturalness with exceptional reliability.[10] As a result, we have been working toward the development of procedures that will use this scale to measure how natural speech feels and the use of that measure in a performance-contingent schedule.

There are other ways of assessing normalcy, including ratings made by relatives or associates of the client. The difficulty with these measures is our uncertainty about their use in the clinical process, other than describing the extent to which a client's speech may resemble normal speech. Ideally, the critical dimensions of normalcy could be incorporated in the performance-contingent schedule. Some clinicians believe it is possible to use ratings of breathiness, phrasing, gentle contact, and so forth, within the clinical process, but neither the reliability nor the functional value of such measures has yet been adequately demonstrated.

Transfer-Maintenance Procedures for Young Children

The procedures used with young children differ only slightly from those described above for adults. The children are mainly under 8 years old, and almost all have been treated by procedures based on operant conditioning principles. Most of these treatment programs are based on gradually extending the length and complexity of utterances or time-out from speaking.[14] They have been either clinician- or parent-administered, under strictly prescribed schedules. A recent example of a parent-managed program by Onslow, Costa, and Rue[15] provides a useful outline of this type of therapy.

Generally, the lengthy maintenance procedures described in this chapter are rarely needed for young children. In a number of cases, comparisons of a performance-contingent schedule run up to MP8(2) with speech performance 12 months later have not found any relevant differences. The principal difference in the performance-contingent schedule used with young children is the composition of the speaking tasks, usually two 5-minute conversations with the clinician, two with their parent(s), and two with a friend. A speech rate criterion is usually ignored in favor of a speaking time measure since speech rate criteria for young children have not been developed (140 syllables per minute is a slow rate criterion used for children of 5 to 7 years). When necessary, speech rate modification has been used to achieve improved speech quality for some children. This is because the concept of speech naturalness is simply not meaningful for most children.

When parents manage maintenance procedures, the combination of regular telephone contact and recordings of their child's speech has been used to monitor progress on the performance-contingent schedule. The second successive failure at MP1(1) means that the program reverts to clinician control, and a schedule is designed around the reported source of difficulty. But, by either schedule, intermittent telephone contact is retained between the clinician and child. Other members of the clinic staff are also used to make informal checks.

Some clinicians may object that these stringent speech performance criteria, the rigorous schedule, and the emphasis on stutter-free speech could impose abnormal stress on a child. However, this emphasis on successful performance is probably offset by ensuring that clinicians and parents reinforce the child liberally throughout the maintenance program. At no time have I, or parents, detected that these procedures were causing distress to a child, although I am aware that this might occur in the absence of the customary sensitivities in dealing with children.

Some Final Comments

Finally, some mention should be made about follow-up assessments in the absence of a maintenance schedule. This still requires extensive research; however, it should be clear that by the time clients reach MP32(2) in a performance-contingent schedule, periodic checks of their fluency have been sustained over virtually 2 years. This evaluation process also includes informal and covert assessments that verify that the client's improved speech is reasonably durable. If follow-up data reveal otherwise, revisions are made on the performance-contingent schedule.

At present, I am unable to identify critical factors associated with sustained fluency in the performance-contingent schedule. I know only that clients usually succeed in opening a number of gates, which provide entry to decreasing amounts of assessment. It may be that this extended period of fluency depends on the client's exploitation of speech tactics, which, of course, may not be sustained during follow-up. All that can be claimed is that a start has been made on devising a generalization technology that offers some promise of improving the transfer and maintenance of therapy benefits.[16] I hope that it is a technology that will encourage other clinicians to investigate its efficacy. In the process, I hope to find many other viable maintenance-producing procedures.

Suggested Readings

Ingham RJ: The effects of self-evaluation training on maintenance and generalization during stuttering treatment. *J Speech Hear Disord* 1982; 47:271–280.
  This paper describes an experimental investigation of the use of self-evaluation training for maintenance and generalization. The procedures can be applied in a conventional clinic setting.

Ingham RJ: Generalization and Maintenance of Treatment, in Curlee R, Perkins W (eds): *Nature and Treatment of Stuttering: New Directions.* San Diego, College-Hill Press, 1984.

Ingham RJ, Onslow M: Generalization and maintenance of treatment benefits for children who stutter. *Semin Speech Lang* 1987; 8:303–326.

These two references review and critically evaluate generalization and maintenance procedures in the treatment of children and adults who stutter.

References

1. Ingham RJ: The experimental analysis and evolution of a stuttering therapy. *Semin Speech Lang* 1991; 12:336–348.
2. Ingham RJ: Evaluation and Maintenance in Stuttering Treatment: A Search for Ecstasy with Nothing but Agony, in Boberg E (ed): *Maintenance of Fluency.* New York, Elsevier, 1981.
3. Ingham RJ, Packman A: Treatment and generalization effects in an experimental treatment for a stutterer using contingency management and speech rate control. *J Speech Hear Disord* 1977; 42: 394–407.
4. Ingham RJ: *Residential Prolonged Speech Stuttering Therapy Manual.* Santa Barbara, Department of Speech and Hearing Sciences, University of California, Santa Barbara, 1987.
5. Ingham RJ: Stuttering, in Bellack AS, Hersen M, Kazdin AE (eds): *International Handbook of Behavior Modification and Therapy,* ed 2. New York, Plenum Press, 1990.
6. Ingham RJ, Andrews G: Details of a token economy stuttering therapy programme for adults. *Aust J Human Commun Disord* 1973; 1:13–20.
7. Ingham RJ: Modification of maintenance and generalization during stuttering treatment. *J Speech Hear Res* 1980; 23:732–745.
8. Ingham RJ: The effects of self-evaluation training on maintenance and generalization during stuttering treatment. *J Speech Hear Disord* 1982; 47:271–280.
9. Fowler SC, Ingham RJ: *Stuttering Treatment Rating Recorder.* Santa Barbara, Department of Speech and Hearing Sciences, University of California, Santa Barbara, 1986.
10. Martin RR, Haroldson SK, Triden KA: Stuttering and speech naturalness. *J Speech Hear Disord* 1984; 49:53–58.
11. Bandura A: Self-efficacy: Toward a unifying theory of behavioral change. *Psychol Rev* 1977; 84:191–215.
12. Onslow M, Ingham R: Whither prolonged speech: The disquieting evolution of a stuttering therapy procedure. *Aust J Human Commun Disord* 1989; 17:67–81.
13. Ingham RJ, Ingham JC, Onslow M, Finn P: Stutterers' self-ratings of speech naturalness: Assessing effects and reliability. *J Speech Hear Res* 1989; 32:419–431.
14. Costello JM: Current Behavioral Treatments for Children, in Prins D, Ingham RJ (eds): *Treatment of Stuttering in Early Childhood: Methods and Issues.* San Diego, College-Hill Press, 1984.
15. Onslow M, Costa L, Rue S: Direct early intervention with stuttering: Some preliminary data. *J Speech Hear Disord* 1990; 55:405–416.
16. Ingham RJ: Generalization and Maintenance of Treatment, in Curlee R, Perkins W (eds): *Nature and Treatment of Stuttering: New Directions.* San Diego, College-Hill Press, 1984.

9

Cluttering
Another Fluency Syndrome

DAVID A. DALY, ED.D.

Introduction

Cluttering is a congenital fluency syndrome disorder, frequently co-occurring with stuttering, which has interested medical and speech specialists for decades. Despite sincere interest in this combined speech-language syndrome by physicians such as Froeschels,[1] Weiss,[2] and Arnold and Luchsinger,[3] and by speech pathologists such as Tiger and colleagues,[4] Diedrich,[5] and myself,[6] the disorder of cluttering has been largely ignored by the speech-language pathology profession. Thirty-five years ago Weiss[2] called cluttering the "orphan" in the family of speech-language pathology, because he believed that this intriguing disorder was neglected and had been treated as an illegitimate relative of stuttering.

Weiss, perhaps more than any other single person, has familiarized speech-language pathologists and physicians with cluttering. He thought that Hippocrates's theory describing stuttering as the improper balance between thought and speech was more applicable to cluttering. In 1968, Weiss presented a comprehensive review of cluttering as a multidimensional problem at the International Convention of Logopedics and Phoniatrics in Paris. This report,[7] published in 1967, described the history, symptomatology, and therapy efforts up to that time. In this article, he reminded readers that "cluttering has always been with us" and identified landmark contributions written during the 1960s. Included were Luchsinger's 1963 book,[8] the first complete volume focusing on cluttering; Arnold and Luchsinger's[3] chapter on cluttering and tachyphemia; and of course, Weiss' text *Cluttering*,[2] which many clinicians, myself included, consider to be a classic. This 1964 text provided American speech-language pathologists with one source, written in English, devoted specifically to cluttering.

After thorough study of these works, and others sprinkled throughout the international literature, I am persuaded that interested readers can best inform themselves about cluttering problems by first reading Weiss' article in *Folia Phoniatrica*[7] and his follow-up article for pediatricians published in *Pediatrics Clinics of North America*.[9] In my view, Weiss has synthesized his many years of investigation into these two articles, and the information provided is practical as well as of theoretical interest.

Additional information can be gleaned from a series of descriptive and experimental articles on cluttering published in *Logos* in the 1960s and in a special 1970 issue of *Folia Phoniatrica* (vol. 22, no 4–5) that was dedicated to Deso Weiss. Also highly recommended is Arnold and Luchsinger's[3] description of cluttering, which remains, in my view, the most scholarly, comprehensive analysis in the literature and which many readers may want to examine in-depth.

More recent viewpoints on etiologies and treatments for cluttering have been presented by Tiger and colleagues,[4] Diedrich,[5] Burk,[9] and myself.[6] However, a new book devoted exclusively to the multifaceted aspects of cluttering by Myers and St. Louis[10] and their colleagues should rekindle both researchers' and clinicians' interests in individuals who present these challenging combinations of communication deficits.

Definition of Cluttering

A central problem, of course, is to define cluttering. Like stuttering, cluttering is difficult to define. To borrow a phrase coined by Winston Churchill in a 1939 speech describing how Russia might respond in a sensitive political situation, cluttering is "a riddle wrapped in a mystery inside an enigma." Its varied and inconsistent symptomatology has led to various definitions and diverse etiological perspectives.

If cluttering is related to stuttering, but is not stuttering, just what is it? I agree with Weiss[7] who asserted that ". . . cluttering is not a specific and isolated disturbance of speech." He maintained that "cluttering is the verbal manifestation of central language imbalance." Others, however, define cluttering primarily as a speech defect. For example, *Webster's Third New International Dictionary*[11] defines cluttering as "a speech defect in which phonetic units are dropped, condensed, or otherwise distorted as a result of overly rapid agitated speech utterance." The College of Speech Therapists in London[12] defines cluttering speech as being characterized by uncontrollable speed, which results in truncated, dysrhythmic, and incoherent utterances. St. Louis[13] sees cluttering as a speech-language disorder whose chief characteristics are: (1) abnormal fluency that is not stuttering and (2) a rapid and/or irregular speech rate. Diedrich,[5] writing in a text about articulation disorders, stated that "cluttering is a problem in maintaining sequential articulatory units with little self-consciousness about their difficulty." He added that cluttering should be regarded as a problem in self-monitoring speech output.

Many etiologies of cluttering have been proposed, but most authors favor a constitutional basis. For example, de Hirsch[14] proposed that cluttering results from disturbances in a child's basic developmental patterns that operate on all levels of central integration. Moreover, she believed that the perceptual, motor, and verbal problems attributed to cluttering were due to an immature or impaired central nervous system.

Arnold and Luchsinger,[3] in their seminal chapter, proposed that cluttering is a disability to formulate language that results in confused, hurried (tachyphemia), and slurred diction. They maintained that tachyphemia stemmed from a congenital, inheritable, and constitutional limitation of the total psychosomatic personality structure. They also noted that "this concept of an organic, familial, and dysphasia-like syndrome of disturbed language function is shared by all recent authors."

Froeschels[15] believed that cluttering was caused by an incongruity between thinking and speaking. In contrast, Freund[16,17] proposed that cluttering was a psychosyndrome, with concomitant constitutional speech and language inadequacies. He postulated that in some cases, cluttering was the underlying basis for stuttering. Op't Hof and Uys[18] hypothesized that cluttering was a complex disorder that was comprised of deficits in articulation, receptive and expressive language, and perceptual-motor problems in addition to a disorder of fluency.

Tiger, Irvine, and Reis[4] argued that cluttering should be conceptualized as a constellation of learning disabilities (LDs). They made a strong case by describing the striking similarities between symptoms of cluttering and LDs. Inasmuch as LD is widely viewed as a pervasive disability affecting the lives of millions of children and adults, and inasmuch as more and more stutterers and clutterers have been identified as also having LDs, such possible relationships and interlinking variables should be investigated more thoroughly.

I[19] contend that cluttering is a disorder of both speech and language processing which manifests itself as rapid, dysrhythmic, sporadic, unorganized, and frequently inarticulate speech by a person who is largely unaware or unconcerned with his difficulty.

Years ago, Perkins[20] asserted that cluttering was a microcosm of speech therapy. He suggested that clinicians could find nearly all of the prominent speech and language disorders in the cluttering population. Specifically, he considered cluttering as but one of many symptoms of a general language disability including grammatical deficiency, impaired reading, bizarre handwriting, poor musical ability, and poor coordination. But most important, Perkins identified rate and erratic rhythm problems as central features of cluttering.

Despite these and numerous other views that have been suggested, Weiss'[2] definition, continues to capture most of cluttering's clinical manifestations:

> Cluttering is a speech disorder characterized by the clutterer's unawareness of his disorder, by a short attention span, by disturbances in perception, articulation, and formulation of speech processes preparatory to speech and based on a hereditary disposition. Cluttering is the verbal manifestation of Central Language Imbalance, which affects all channels of communication (e.g., reading, writing, rhythm and musicality) and behavior in general.

This definition views cluttering as a constellation of symptoms, that is, a clinical syndrome that is often interrelated with stuttering but that can occur independent of stuttering. This chapter is intended to inform clinicians about the fluency disruptions and related characteristics associated with cluttering, as well as the diagnostic and treatment strategies that have been found to be useful in dealing with this fascinating constellation of symptoms. A final objective is to legitimize cluttering as a fluency syndrome that warrants study and management by speech-language clinicians.

Characteristics of Cluttering

Varied symptoms are typical of cluttering. Myers and St. Louis[10] report that as many as 62 separate characteristics of cluttering have been described in the literature. In his 1964 book, Weiss[2] listed but three obligatory symptoms that were pathognomonic and essential for diagnosis: (1) excessive repetitions of speech, (2) short attention span and poor concentration, and (3) lack of complete awareness of the problem. Weiss also listed over a dozen facultative symptoms that are often present but not mandatory. Interested clinicians and researchers may want to read Weiss' 1964 work in its entirety. In addition, my[6] review of the literature and integration of information that supports or clarifies Weiss' listing may also be helpful.

Later, Weiss[9] presented a revised list of 21 symptoms, which are listed below. The first five symptoms are obligatory and must be present in every case.

Obligatory symptoms:

1. Repetitions are excessive (8 to 10 repetitions).
2. Lack of awareness (does not believe his or her speech deviates).
3. Weakness of concentration and shortness of attention span.
4. Perceptual weakness.
5. Poorly organized thinking (speaks before clarifying thoughts).

Facultative symptoms:

1. Excessive speech rate (tachylalia most conspicuous symptom).
2. Interjections (long drawn-out vowels occur frequently).
3. Vowel stops (pauses before initial vowel).
4. Articulatory and motor disabilities (deletes phonemes/dyslalic).
5. Grammatical difficulties (inattentive to details and grammar).
6. Vocal monotony (lack of speech melody or intonation).
7. Respiration (jerky).
8. Delayed speech development (late talkers).

Associated symptoms:

1. Reading disorder (a frequent problem that Weiss suggests may be used for diagnostic confirmation).
2. Writing disorder (motor and imagination difficulties).
3. Lack of rhythmical and musical ability (poor singing).
4. Restlessness and hyperactivity (fidgeting is typical).
5. Electroencephalographic (EEG) findings (deviations on EEG common).
6. Lag in maturation (occurs often).
7. Heredity (familial factor/organic flavor).
8. Subgroups (e.g., receptive versus expressive; or a grouping of overhurried speech, hesitation and repetition, and talking in circles).

Clinical Evaluation

Assessment of fluency problems in children and adults who stutter has been described by other authors in this book. For clients suspected of cluttering, more comprehensive evaluations are usually necessary. I agree with colleagues like Hood,[21] Gregory and Hill,[22] and Riley and Riley[23,24] who recommend in-depth speech and language evaluations including attention, auditory processing, motor, and educational aspects. The challenge is to differentiate stutterers with concomitant problems (see publications by Bloodstein,[25] Blood and Seider,[26] myself,[27] Nippold,[28] and Preus,[29,30]) from those clients who more appropriately fit the cluttering classification. Such differentiation, in my experience, is best accomplished by assessing selected quantitative and qualitative features of cluttering.

Quantitative Features of Cluttering

There are eight quantitative features that should be investigated. First, marked acceleration of speech rate is a leading symptom of cluttering. Martin and associates[31] analyzed cluttered speech spectrographically and verified the occurrence of rapid and variable rate, rushes of compressed speech, and articulatory inadequacy. A discriminating sign of cluttering is an increase in rate between and within multisyllabic words. Seeman and Novak[32] and Seeman[33] referred to "interverbal acceleration," while Luchsinger[8] commented on clutterers' "intraverbal acceleration." Both types of acceleration are common. Wyatt[34] has also discussed clutterers' propulsive impulse to speak with increasing speed. Tachylalia is common in cluttering, and Wohl[35] labeled the tendency for clutterers' speech to become faster and faster as it proceeds as "festinating."

Second, short attention span and poor concentration should be verified. Pearson,[36] Weiss,[2] and others recommend objective testing for this obligatory symptom. A number of auditory and visual memory tests are commercially available. I[19] recently described a sentence imitation test developed with colleagues, for measuring immediate auditory memory skills. Normative data are available for children ages 4 through 18 years.[37] Formal testing is necessary to accurately assess poor concentration or attention span difficulties.

Third, vowel stops, or pauses, at the beginning of vowel-initial words without signs of frustration or fear or excessive muscle tonus or contractions are common. Sound prolongations are rare.

Fourth, clutterers repeat single syllables, short words, and phrases with disturbing frequency. Six, eight, or ten units of effortless repetitions, with no apparent concern, are typical. Such repetitions are obligatory.

Fifth, articulation errors, particularly on /r/ and /l/ phonemes, are common. Sheperd[38] and Arnold[39] observed that such misarticulations may persist into adulthood. Froeschels[1] reported that up to 50% of clutterers show dyslalias. It should be remembered, however, that the literature is also replete with evidence of significant articulation problems among youngsters who stutter.[40-46] Indeed, Bloodstein[47] concluded that functional difficulties in articulation and immature speech are confirmed throughout the stuttering literature. Thus, articulation errors, in and of themselves, are not diagnostically significant. Nevertheless, many clutterers tend to exhibit immature articulation abilities also. They often reduce consonant clusters into single-consonant productions[38] and show signs of oral apraxia.[48] Detailed testing is usually necessary.

Sixth, some clutterers show voice disturbances. Dalton and Hardcastle[49] and Weiss[7] commented on clutterers' vocal monotony. Some clutterers begin speaking loudly initially, then trail off to a murmur. A nasal quality may also be present.[3]

Seventh, Weiss[2] stated that clutterers are notoriously poor readers. He noted that clutterers often skip small words and round off phrases in apparent disregard of the fact that their version differs from the printed text. Some may start reading perfectly fine but begin making mistakes which suggest that they are skimming rather than reading. Concentration appears to be a problem for some of those clutterers who neglect details. Weiss[9] believed that a reading disability could be a decisive diagnostic sign of cluttering if classification was uncertain. Some stutterers are poor readers, too, although Conture and Van Naerssen[50] contend that most stutterers' reading skills are well within normal limits. Nippold and Schwartz[51] report inconsistent research findings, and further research into the reading abilities of both stutterers and clutterers is needed.

Eighth, a writing sample of at least one page should be obtained. Initially reported by Orton[52] and Spadino,[53] de Hirsch[54] described clutterers' poor written integration of ideas and space. Weiss[2] maintained that cluttering affected all channels of communication, and Roman-Goldzieher[55] presented evidence that clutterers' writing samples are uninhibited, sprawling, disorderly, and full of repetitions and deletions. I strongly recommend an assessment of writing abilities. One page usually indicates whether a client can follow a story line or train of thought. The lack of organization that characterizes the speech of many clutterers is often more evident in written samples. Recent preliminary research[56] indicates that reading and writing disorders are fruitful areas of investigation for differentiating clutterers from stutterers.

Qualitative Features of Cluttering

There are other features of cluttering that are more difficult to measure that should be considered in making a diagnosis of cluttering. Seven variables that may have diagnostic significance are described below. First, Froeschels[15] and others observed that clutterers do not think faster than they can speak, but speak quickly, before they have thought their ideas through. Their speech often appears disorganized and confusing as they go whizzing along, frequently getting ahead of themselves. Frequent changes in topics and incomplete sentences are suggestive not only of cluttering but of LD as well (see Lerner[57]). Gregory and Hill[22] reported word-retrieval difficulties in 55% of their stutterers who underwent comprehensive evaluations. Word-finding problems are quite common for clutterers, also.

Second, clutterers evidence frequent slips of the tongue. Bakwin and Bakwin[58] and Arnold[59] give examples of such transpositions as "The Lord is a shoving leopard." I[6] commented on the tendency for clutterers to make verbal faux pas. For example, an adult cluttering client asked me to attend an important business meeting with him. Although his presentation to supervisors was short, several transpositions were observed. For example, he said, "At this plant in time" thinking he had said, "At this point in time." He also substituted four other words during his 5-minute presentation, including "interrupted" for "interpreted" and "taking" for "talking." He left the audience confused, and his proposal was tabled for further discussion. More important, he did not receive the promotion he expected. Yet, this executive seemed oblivious to the mistakes he had made.

Third, many clutterers are physically immature, clumsy, and uncoordinated. De Hirsch[54] has documented clutterers' maturational delays in sitting, walking, and talking. And, it is not uncommon for clutterers to look and act much younger than their age. Orton[52] and Arnold and Luchsinger[3] have commented on the high percentage of cluttering clients with sinistrality (left-handedness) or mixed laterality. Other clutterers may appear inattentive, restless, and/or hyperactive. Such behaviors in clutterers may or may not be related to an attention deficit disorder (ADD). Cantwell and Baker[60] and Epstein[61] discussed the relationship of ADD to learning problems, and I[27] found several LD students among a group of language-disordered stutterers. An obvious question is whether these disorders have a common etiology or whether they present as independent impairments. Years ago, West, Kennedy, and Carr[62] speculated that stuttering and speech retardation could co-occur in some individuals, because they inherited a common predisposition to both conditions. The same could be true for cluttering and ADD.

Fourth, a weakness in musical ability and rhythm has been identified by many investigators (e.g., Arnold and Luchsinger,[3] Grewel[63]). I[6] found that many cluttering clients could not imitate a simple rhythmic pattern. Some clutterers report not liking music of any kind; others contend that they cannot sing.[59] Such symptoms may reflect deficits in auditory attention or perception that were noted earlier.

Fifth, a familial factor is clearly present in cluttering. Weiss[9] maintained that even though shifting symptomatology may make cluttering appear to be a functional disorder, it is hereditary. He wrote, "We are convinced that the hereditary nature of cluttering will be demonstrated in a definitive manner." Kidd[64] discussed several genetic models of stuttering, but the genetic findings he reported for stutterers may be skewed, in my opinion, because clutterers and stutterers were not differentiated. Poulos and Webster[65] recently reported that thorough interviews with stuttering clients and/or family members revealed that nearly two-thirds of other family members stuttered. They suggested that the origin of "developmental stuttering," in a significant proportion of clients, might be related to brain damage. There is reason to believe that cerebral dysfunction and/or heredity may play an even more prominent role in cluttering than in stuttering. It is common for relatives of clutterers to evidence the same or similar symptoms. During case history interviews I always ask the following series of questions: "Does anyone in the family stutter?" "Does anyone in the family stammer?" "Does anyone in the family clutter?" Frequently, positive responses are given to one or more questions. If so, I ask another related question: "Does the person's speech or behavior resemble anyone else's in the family?" More often than not, parents may respond: "He talks (or acts) like uncle Tim. That's why we brought him here in the first place. Can you do anything to help him?" Speech-language pathologists need to ask these kinds of questions and to diagram family trees whenever possible. Cluttering and stuttering often occur within the same families or simultaneously in the same individual.

Sixth, a number of personality traits of clutterers have been described. Terms used to characterize them include: impulsive, fidgety, hasty, hyperactive, careless, clumsy, untidy, slipshod, sloppy, impatient, and short-tempered. Most reports are based only on clinical observations, but the traits reported by different researchers are remarkably similar. Dalton and Hardcastle[66] object to such characterizations because they portray clutterers as a stereotyped personality; nevertheless, these same traits have also been used by psychologists and educators to describe children and adults with LD. It is my opinion that future research will verify that cluttering and LD are frequently interrelated.

Researchers' observations on clutterers' aptitudes, which may also be pertinent to these traits or characteristics, report that clutterers prefer scientific or exacting occupations. The majority of my clients classified as clutterers have been engineers, mathematicians, computer programmers, etc. School-age clutterers often report that their favorite subjects in school were math and/or science; they seldom favor English, social studies, or the like. Arnold and Luchsinger[3] summarized clutterers' aptitudes as follows: ". . . clutterers tend toward a one-sided concentration of talent in the exact disciplines of knowledge—that is, they often become good scientists, but usually remain rather poor speakers." These preferences and aptitudes are consistent with observations that clutterers are usually average or above average in intelligence. Many clutterers I have worked with were exceptionally bright. As Arnold[59] stated: "Low I.Q. does not belong to the tachyphemia syndrome."

The seventh and most important qualitative feature is lack of awareness. This subjective variable can be difficult to assess. Even the most insensitive clients occasionally acknowledge some awareness of their dysrhythmic, rapid, unintelligible speech. Most clutterers, however, seem unconvinced that their speech deviates from normal, and this lack of awareness is a critical and obligatory symptom.

When working with children less than 12 years old, I ask specific questions to assess awareness. Questions such as, "Do people ask you to repeat what you say?", "Do you ever repeat so much that people ask you to slow down?", "Are you ever afraid that people will make fun of your speech?" can yield significant clinical information. It is important to ask such questions directly and to probe deeply enough to gather relevant data. Reports of lack of frustration and/or fearlessness regarding speaking should be considered when making a diagnostic decision.

For adolescents and adults suspected of cluttering I employ another inventory. The Perceptions of Speech Communication (PSC) is a 60-item inventory that I adapted from Woolf's[67] Perception of Stuttering Inventory (PSI). The original PSI was altered by substituting "speaking difficulty" whenever "stuttering" was used. Thus, the altered inventory does not mention stuttering in its title or items, which permits its use with clutterers and other communicatively disordered clients. For example, the PSC has proved useful with adolescent and adult voice cases for determining how much they were aware or worried about their speaking ability. A low score indicates lack of awareness; a high score, the opposite. Several colleagues and I[68] compared high school students' scores on Woolf's PSI form with those on the PSC form and found that normal-speaking high school students checked an average of ten items on *either* inventory. Data[69] on Woolf's PSI adolescent stuttering clients showed an average of 27 items checked. Clinical experience with the modified perceptions inventory (PSC) with adolescent and adult clutterers has revealed that they usually check less than six items. This suggests that many clutterers are partially aware of their speaking difficulty, at least for fleeting periods of time.

Some individuals with a number of cluttering symptoms check many items on the PSC. This suggests that they are more aware, concerned, or perhaps apprehensive about their speech errors than most clutterers. Perhaps the correct diagnosis for these individuals is "clutterer-stutterer." The two disorders occur together with some regularity, and several authors[2,16,48,63] propose a more widespread use of this double diagnosis. Lack of awareness is an obligatory symptom of cluttering, and interested clinicians and researchers may find the adapted PSC inventory useful, a copy of which is included in Appendix A.

A New Cluttering Checklist for Clinicians and Researchers

Conducting a thorough evaluation of a client suspected of cluttering is not easy. In 1981, I described the use of an inventory for differential diagnosis of stutterers that assembled much of the information available about a client and his family on one form.[27] This early inventory was especially helpful for grouping stuttering clients into different developmental tracks. At present, however, whenever a fluency client is a suspected clutterer, or possibly a clutterer-stutterer, I use a new checklist for gathering pertinent information. This 33-item checklist (similar to Cooper's chronicity predictive checklist for stuttering[70]) presents features that numerous clinical researchers believe are indicative of cluttering. The interviewer questions the client or parent and then records the extent to which each statement is judged to be true for the client. Each item is rated 0 through 3, with a total of 99 points possible on the checklist.

Preliminary data suggest that a score of 60 or above is usually sufficient to support a diagnosis of cluttering. Scores between 30 and 60 may be indicative of a clutterer-stutterer. Several items on the checklist appear to be more critical for diagnosing cluttering than others:

- #2. Started talking late; onset of words and sentences delayed.
- #3. Fluency disruptions started early; no remissions; never very fluent.
- #7. Rapid rate (speaks too fast); tachylalia; speaks in spurts.
- #9. Jerky breathing pattern; respiratory dysrhythmia.
- #10. Slurred articulation (omits sounds or unstressed syllables).
- #12. Speech better under pressure; e.g., during short periods of heightened attention.
- #14. Distractible; attention span problems; poor concentration.
- #20. Reading disorder is a prominent disability.
- #25. Seems to think faster than he can talk or write.
- #33. Lack of self-awareness; unconcerned attitude over inappropriateness of many behaviors and responses.

I have found the checklist useful for structuring an interview, gathering information, and making decisions about cluttering and invite other researchers to use it. A copy can be found in Appendix B.

Prevalence of Cluttering

The number of clutterers in the United States is not known, but most authors agree that the syndrome is comparatively rare. In an in-depth study of 138 chronic stutterers,[27] only four could be rigorously classified as "pure clutterers." Thus, less than 3% of the total stuttering group were identified as "true" clutterers. Even if these four clutterers are considered a subgroup of the 33 track II stutterers (the category of speech-language delayed, articulation-impaired stutterers in Van Riper's tracking system[71]), prevalence rises only to 12%.

Freund[16] reported comparatively few "pure clutterers" among his fluency clients. He proposed using the label "stutterer-clutterer," as he worked with many clients who showed both stuttering and cluttering symptoms. Grewel[63] suggested that probably half of the children who presented as stutterers were motor clutterers or clutterer-stutterers. Langova and Moravek[72] reported that 16% of their patients were clutterers, 54% were stutterers, and the remaining 30% were stutterer-clutterers. Weiss[2] agreed that the symptoms frequently co-occur and proposed that cluttering was the primary disturbance and stuttering a secondary complication. This view is consistent with that of Seeman,[48] who reported that in about 50% of his clients, stuttering had its origin in cluttering.

In 1967, Weiss[7] indicated that one-sixth of his total fluency patients were "pure" clutterers and another one-sixth were "pure" stutterers. The remaining four-sixths of his fluency patients were designated as a combination of clutterer-stutterers who were further divided into four separate categories, depending upon the relative proportion of cluttering-stuttering symptoms judged to be present. Weiss believed that cluttering is usually observed before stuttering develops and that it persists to varying degrees during the early stages of stuttering until the efforts of the stutterer suppress it. He also hypothesized that ". . . it [cluttering] reappears towards the end of the treatment when stuttering diminishes."[7]

I[6] reported that about 5% of the fluency clients treated in a residential summer camp program were "pure" clutterers. The largest group were stutterers (55%); however, a sizable group (40%) were classified as clutterer-stutterers. These proportions agree with those reported by Dalton and Hardcastle[49] who, like many other clinicians, report seeing relatively few "pure" clutterers. Preus[73] reports that about 35% of the fluency clients he sees in Norway should be classified as cluttering stutterers. My clinical experience, and a review of reports from other clinical researchers, suggest that about every third stutterer seen for treatment is likely a clutterer-stutterer. One thing seems certain: many fluency clients present symptoms of both disorders, and a strong case can be made for their having concomitant LD,[4] apraxia of speech,[5] or attention deficits or language disorders.[22] Cluttering children and adults are most perplexing; they are challenging populations and require speech-language pathologists' best clinical efforts.

Comparative listings of characteristics that are believed to distinguish cluttering and stuttering have been catalogued by several authors.[16,72,74] Weiss' list,[7] however, may be best known and is included here (Table 9-1) for comparative purposes. This table is based on information that was compiled 25 years ago, and the number of clutterers and stutterers on which these characteristics are based is not known. Undoubtedly, many of these distinguishing characteristics need verification. Three specific examples are: (1) Langova and Moravek's[72] data on clutterers' abnormal EEG findings need replication, particularly since more sophisticated

Table 9-1. Weiss' (1967) Comparative Table Showing Various Differences between Stuttering and Cluttering*

	Stuttering	*Cluttering*
Interpretation	Functional; secondary	Hereditary; primary central language imbalance (lack of maturation of CNS mostly absent)
Underlying disturbance	Neurovegetative dysfunctional	
Awareness of disorder	Strong	Mostly absent
Speech characteristics		
Specific symptoms	Clonic and tonic inhibition	Hestitation, repetition (without inhibition)
Rate of delivery	Rather slow	Mostly quick
Sentence structure	Mostly correct	Often incorrect
Fear of specific sounds	Present	Absent
Heightened attention	Worse	Better
Relaxed attention	Better	Worse
Foreign language	Worse	Better
Gesturing	Stiff, inhibited	Broad, uninhibited
Reading aloud		
Well-known text	Better	Worse
Unknown text	Worse	Better
Writing characteristics	Compressed; high-pressure strokes	Loose, disorderly
School performance	Good to superior	Underachiever
Psychological attitudes	Embarrassed, inhibited	Carefree, sociable
	Painstaking, compulsive	Impatient, impulsive
	Grudge-bearer	Easily forgetting
	Penetrating	Superficial
Experimental responses:		
Alcohol	Better	Worse
Lee effect	Better	Worse
EEG	Borderline normal	Often deviant
Chlorpromazine	Worse	Better
Dexfenmetrazine	Better	Worse
Course	Fluctuating; spontaneous improvements and relapses	Persistent
Therapy	Attention should be diverted from details; psychotherapy	Concentration on details
Prognosis	Depends on emotional adjustment	Depends on acquiring concentration

*From Weiss.[7] Reprinted with permission.

tests and techniques are now available. (2) Weiss' conclusion that clutterers perform differently than stutterers under delayed auditory feedback (DAF) is at odds with my experience. Individuals from each group respond both positively and negatively (i.e., the Lee effect) to DAF. (3) Weiss believed that stutterers' treatment should focus on diverting their attention away from speech details or on psychotherapy, but many current clinical researchers[42,75-78] in fact focus fluency therapy on speech details successfully. Clearly, careful study of these and other variables is needed, on large numbers of clutterers and stutterers, before definitive conclusions can be drawn.

Clinical Management

Specific treatment goals vary, depending upon (1) the age of the client, (2) the length of time cluttering has been a problem, (3) whether cluttering and stuttering coexist, and (4) the nature and severity of the symptoms observed. A client's speech and language performance relative to his or her chronological age should be investigated. Children's use of "fillers" and possible word-finding difficulties should be explored, along with their articulation proficiency. Evidence of such obligatory signs as multiple word and phrase repetitions and lack of awareness of speech disfluencies and disruptions should be sought. Motor coordination skills, speech rate, and family history relative to fluency disorders are other factors worthy of scrutiny.

Conture[42] reminds us that the age of the disorder is as important as the age of the child. Some rules of thumb that I follow in planning treatment for cluttering are: The younger the child, the more I involve the parents in demonstrations and home practice. If oral-motor coordination deficits or weaknesses are identified, a variety of oral diadochokinetic activities should be incorporated in treatment. Riley and Riley's specific oral-motor training program[79] has proved effective with several such youngsters whom I have seen. The Rileys simplified the sequences of syllable combinations by beginning with all-voiced productions and report[80] that 78% of their disfluent clients improved their oral-motor coordination abilities following 14 hours of training, a finding that warrants replication. The cluttering youngsters I have seen have responded well to oral-motor training also, and I highly recommend such activities.

A cluttering child's attention span and ability to concentrate warrant clinical exploration. I agree with Gregory and Hill[22] who recommend training to increase attention span, if a youngster shows attentional problems, before formal work on fluency is initiated. Memory work is often necessary; however, I have found that working on several aspects of speech processing and production concurrently can be advantageous. Thus, in one therapy session with a cluttering child, I might include language therapy activities, articulation work, memory activities, and oral-motor coordination exercises. Such activities should build upon a primary therapeutic objective of producing a slower, more deliberate speech rate. For children 6 years and older, I often use DAF to shape an exaggerated, drone-type speech quality. With children under six years old I may simply play a "robot speech game" in which we both keep our voices on 100% of the time by dragging one syllable into the next. Most youngsters enjoy this "robot speech game," which also reduces their typically rapid speech rates and provides opportunities to reinforce their slower, more intelligible utterances. Parents are instructed to play the "robot speech game" for brief periods several times a day. Such home practice and modeling can be powerful in effecting change, and a potential side effect is that parents' rapid speech rates may be reduced, too.

This treatment program for young clutterers consists of an amalgamation of several different therapies that are intended to provide a concatenation of therapy activities that will keep the child interested and, as much as possible, focused on speech improvement. It is my opinion that fluency therapy alone is not sufficient for most clutterers or clutterer-stutterers because of the multidimensional nature of this syndrome. Moreover, treatment of such multifactored, speech-language disordered individuals usually takes much longer than for clients who stutter only. My study[27] of stutterers' response to intensive therapy indicated that those stutterers with concomitant speech/language/motor problems took longer than those who presented stuttering symptoms alone. The prognosis for clutterers may or may not be poorer than for pure stutterers, as Dostalova and Dosuzkov[81] and others contend, but clinicians should accept that their prognosis may be different.

Several authors,[3,6] have observed that story telling represents a significant problem for many young clutterers and stutterers. In such cases, I have found commercially available, sequenced picture stories to be most helpful. I begin with simple four-picture sequences and tell a story as the cards are arranged appropriately. Next the child retells the story while looking at the correct picture sequence. Then, the child is asked to arrange different cards and to tell a story their sequence suggests. Finally, the length and complexity of subsequent stories are increased by choosing longer card sequences.

Many elementary school-age cluttering youngsters appear to benefit from having the clinician write their story (e.g., on a large experience chart) as they dictate it. The clinician can help to organize or revise the story as it is written. Next, the client and clinician read the story aloud in unison. Finally, the client reads the story aloud. I have found that alternating the dictation and recording tasks is helpful in assisting some clients not only with organization and reading skills, but also with writing skills. I frequently audiotape or videotape a client's final effort and point out the clarity of his or her speech, improved fluency, and reading rate. In addition, all cluttering clients seem to benefit from instructions to briefly pause after every comma or period and to use those pauses in conversation or reading to take a breath. The simple reminder to inhale at punctuation marks often has significant therapeutic value.

Most adolescent and adult clients who clutter display similar problems. With confirmed cluttering clients I analyze their disfluency pattern, search for possible memory deficits, and assess awareness levels. Once these symptoms are addressed, I begin to focus on other facultative and associated symptoms. However, it is not uncommon for some older clutterers or clutterer-stutterers to announce that they do not want to be involved in treatment. Several authors[9,74,82] have commented on clutterer reluctance to cooperate in therapy. In fact, "aggressive," "impulsive," and "impatient" have been used to describe such clients. Indifference, belligerence, or hostility directed at a clinician trying to help a client presents quite a challenge, and clinicians should be forewarned that some clutterers direct verbal abuse at clinicians in a manner similar to that of head trauma patients.

A number of cluttering clients show little interest in their manner of speaking. Some appear unable to perceive their expressive mistakes. Still other cluttering clients seem unwilling or unable to utilize the clinician's suggestions and guidance. I recommend that speech-language pathologists be persistent and supportive. Experience has suggested that enthusiasm and motivation, along with persistence, seem to be factors that can motivate "difficult" clients. I am always reluctant to dismiss a client early in treatment, and if a client announces that he or she is withdrawing from therapy, I make it clear that my door remains open for future sessions. Perhaps my early personal experiences of repeated failure with my own stuttering therapy sharpened this perspective. After years of clinical experience with stutterers and clutterers, I believe that it is essential to foster a client's hope, which may kindle the desire to seek assistance later, with me or elsewhere.

Rapid speech rate, or tachylalia, occurs so frequently among clutterers that separate mention and treatment procedures are warranted. Instructions or verbal reprimands to slow down are usually worthless. Like many stutterers, clutterers have been admonished to reduce their speech rate for years. Reading or saying words one at a time, perhaps with accompanying finger tapping, helps some clients; however, a simple rate control program, described in detail by Burk[9], has also been highly effective. To normalize fast speech rates of clients, Burk has them read aloud a set of sample readings, first in unison with the clinician, then alone. The client then records the sample readings at several different rates. I have found it helpful to begin with the slowest rate, about 30 words per minute. The client then re-reads the material four more times, speeding up each time until the fifth reading is as fast as the client can produce it. In between each recording, the clinician comments on the client's rate. For example, before the second reading the clinician might say, "Now the passage will be read a little faster, but still slower than normal." After the client has read the same material five times (the last being the fastest speech), the clinician says, "Now the material will be read a final time. This time, _____ (client's name) will read it at a 'perfect rate,' that is, at a speed close to the third reading which was well within normal limits and easy to listen to and understand." At the conclusion of this reading the clinician adds something like, "That concludes this tape. The last reading is an ideal, perfect rate for _____ (client's name)." The audiocassette is copied and given to the client as the "anchor tape." I ask the client to listen to it many times during the first week after it is recorded and thereafter whenever he or she wonders if the rate is too fast. When the client begins speaking too fast in subsequent therapy sessions, I simply play a copy of the tape, or ask the client which of the five rates he or she is speaking. Burk's rate control program[9a] can be modified for individual clients, but the concept seems sound and has been exceedingly helpful with my tachylalic clients. I highly recommend its use in any treatment program for rapid-speaking fluency clients.

Most clinicians agree that increasing a clutterer's awareness of the particular speech pattern is essential to success. Cooper[83] recommends teaching clients what he terms the "language of fluency." He maintains that progress is unrealistic unless fluency clients can verbalize what they are doing and why. Clutterers, as well as stutterers, should be informed and educated on the rationale for practicing each skill. I believe that clients' ability to describe what they are doing in treatment increases their responsiveness to the procedure. With all but the very young cluttering client, heightened awareness is typically my first treatment goal.

Myers and Bradley[84] advocate close attention to such pragmatic features of clutterers' communication as turn taking. Clutterers may need assistance in alternating between speaker-listener roles, or compulsive talkers often need help in recognizing cues of frustrated listeners. Self-monitoring is difficult for many clutterers, and clinical simulations and video/audiotape review can be helpful. I begin by alternately reading aloud with a client such practice materials as sentences of various lengths. Next, we may read dialogues from a script. Finally, we practice taking turns during brief "staged" conversations. As turn-taking performance improves, I gradually increase our conversation time.

Because many cluttering clients appear to suffer from auditory inattentiveness and seemingly do not perceive speech errors, I often use repeated videotape playback viewings. During these viewings, it is not uncommon for a clutterer to ignore or deny inarticulate utterances or rapid, repetitive speech. A procedure I have found to be beneficial when this occurs is to temporarily shift the focus during video playback to the client's speech productions. This positive focus curtails arguments and counterproductive client comments about other speech errors. I work hard to catch the clutterer doing something right, then attend to that desirable behavior. I may play the video again and again, commenting on the appropriateness of the desirable behavior. Sometimes it is necessary to build up a clutterer's self-esteem before it is helpful to focus on interferring, undesirable behaviors. Experience indicates that attending to what a client can do is more productive than attending to what he or she does poorly. Since most clients have access to video playback machines at home, I often videotape short samples of their better speech and ask them to take the video home to view with parents or spouse. This technique has been described in more detail elsewhere[85] and illustrates my belief that anything that increases a client's awareness of successful speech efforts should be emphasized.

I favor the use of DAF with clutterers for a variety of reasons. First, DAF helps clients reduce their speech rate, and as rate is reduced, speech is more intelligible. Second, the continuous voicing pattern of speech elicited with DAF effects a more deliberate, exaggerated oral-motor response pattern. This monotone speech pattern, or "drone," can more easily be imitated by clients after they have first experienced it with DAF. The heavily phonated-type speech provides a solid foundation of slow rate upon which to build other speech parameters.

Although an occasional clutterer (or stutterer) may complain about the disruption that DAF causes, I have not observed the "expressive speech aggravation" that Langova and Moravek[72] reported for 89% of their cluttering clients. While some clients do not like DAF, none has refused to wear it "for a few necessary sessions." I agree with Perkins[86] and his coworkers that the slower, more deliberate speech rate promoted by the DAF facilitates the acquisition of other elements of fluent speech.

An alternate feedback source can be provided through a vibrotactile device described by Shames.[87] The clutterer places a transducer over the laryngeal area and feels the vocal folds vibrate as he or she speaks into the microphone of this vibrotactile device. Most of our cluttering clients prefer to receive either tactile feedback or auditory feedback separately. Some clients clearly favor one type of feedback over the other. A few clients elect to wear both the auditory and the tactile feedback devices simultaneously. I do not insist on a specific sequence. Each clutterer experiences both feedback devices in order to promote a heightened awareness of the speech production process in the laryngeal and oral areas. As Van Riper[71] suggested over 20 years ago, a client needs to attend to the control he or she does have over the execution of air, voice, and movements.

Recently, I[75] described the use of cognitive training for both stutterers and clutterers. Breathing exercises and relaxation techniques have been effective with some cluttering clients. One objective is to help them mentally rehearse, as well as orally rehearse, speaking successes. With relaxation and mental imagery practice, many clients report picturing themselves as being more intelligible and fluent in the future. Lazarus[88] provides many excellent visualization or mental imagery exercises that can be adapted to the needs of specific stuttering and cluttering clients. The use of imagery, positive self-talk, and affirmation-training procedures with a number of other significant health and behavior problems has been described in the literature.[89–91] Respected researchers[89,92–95] reported dramatic successes when using these cognitive procedures with such problems as phobias, fears, and several medical diseases. I have studied and used these procedures with fluency clients for the last decade[75,96] and believe that they show great promise for individuals who clutter and/or stutter. It is my opinion that these procedures increase clients' mental rehearsal and visualization skills and can result in more durable success with chronic clutterers and stutterers.

Case Studies

Three case studies briefly illustrate the types of cluttering clients I have seen.

Case 1

Chet, a 10-year, 4-month-old fifth grader was referred for a possible stuttering problem. His mother, who seemed to be a high-strung, impatient individual who spoke rapidly, reported that teachers had complained of her son's rapid and unintelligible speech. Testing revealed that Chet misarticulated the /r/, /l/, and /s/ sounds. Repetitive disfluencies occurred on only 3% of his speech. Although his speech misarticulations and repetitions were long-standing and both parents were professional people, he had never received therapy. Chet read well, but too rapidly. Subsequent analyses indicated that his reading and speaking rates were not faster than his peers, but apparently too rapid for his oral-motor coordination system. Chet spoke in spurts, with the ends of many sentences trailing off into unintelligible murmurs. Testing also revealed deficits in auditory memory abilities. Chet used the DAF reluctantly but responded well during the first few sessions. His slightly slower speech rate off the machine was reinforced and recorded on videotape, which he was asked to view with his parents at home. An audiotape rate control program, as described by Burk,[9] was made for self-comparisons. Chet was making progress and responding well to treatment, and I was surprised when his parents announced following the sixth session that they had observed little progress and were discontinuing him in therapy. While early self-dismissal from treatment is not uncommon for adults who clutter, such parental termination of therapy for younger clients is unusual. As always, the door was left open should services be requested in the future.

Case 2

Gaylord was an 11-year, 2-month-old sixth grader whom we treated for 18 months. His father was a chemical salesman; mother, a music teacher. Two older sisters were talented musically. Gaylord showed little interest or talent in music, even after taking weekly piano and violin lessons for over 2 years. Case history reports indicated slow motor development and left-right hand confusion. Gaylord was left-handed and seemed quite clumsy when first evaluated, apparently trying to accomplish every task as rapidly as possible. He was small for his age, acted immature, and was reported to play with children much younger than himself. Testing indicated frequent misarticulations and tachylalia. His conversational speech contained many interjections, or filler words. Word and phrase repetitions were common. His writing was sloppy, almost unreadable. He evidenced difficulty sequencing ideas and organizing stories.

Therapy was provided twice a week for 3 months, weekly for 4 months, then biweekly for 3 months. Monthly booster sessions were provided thereafter. Basically, treatment consisted of rate reduction and deliberate phonation activities described in my fluency program.[75] Oral-motor coordination exercises, patterned after Riley and Riley's syllable training program,[79] were helpful, and telling and retelling stories with picture-sequencing cards benefited his memory and organizational abilities.

Gaylord worked hard in therapy, and his parents provided supportive home practice. Stars, stickers, and pennies were used in the clinic to reinforce longer, slower, fluent utterances. Gaylord's parents kept a practice chart at home, on which points for practice time were accumulated for a highly desired reward—a new bicycle. Specific school activities were practiced in therapy, and teachers reported successful performance in the classroom. Slow, definite progress was observed. Parents reported improved speech at home and church, and Gaylord's teachers indicated better performance at school. Therapy was discontinued when Gaylord started the eighth grade.

I had not treated Gaylord for several years but recently saw his mother at a shopping mall. She reported that he was a freshman in a computer-engineering program at a prestigious university. He had scored exceedingly high on the mathematics and science portions of the Scholastic Aptitude Test, but quite poorly on the verbal portion. Gaylord's mother reported that although he continued to speak too rapidly at times, he was doing quite well over all.

Case 3

Burt was a 43-year-old engineer, who came at his company's recommendation. He reported that colleagues complained that he spoke too fast and mumbled and said that he frequently was asked to repeat. Burt stated that his brother and a cousin stuttered and that his 18-year-old son spoke even faster than he. Testing revealed a conversational speech rate of 174 words per minute. Sporadic deletions of smaller words like "the," "this," and "could," and transpositions and substitutions such as "taking" for "talking" and "at this part in time" for "at this point in time" left listeners confused. Burt was aware of his speech difficulty, checking 28 of 60 items on Woolf's PSI.[67] Adult stuttering clients check an average of 30 items on this inventory. In view of his occasional repetitions, rapid speech rate, language confusion, and growing awareness of his difficulty, my diagnosis was clutterer-stutterer. Burt's company requested that I design an initial ten-session speech plan, which would be evaluated and continued if progress was evident. Burt attended the ten sessions and made good progress. He responded especially well to the audiotape rate control program and videotape comparison procedures. He discontinued therapy after making a company presentation in which he transposed several words. He said that he was satisfied with his progress and would continue to practice on his own. I shared my hope that he would reconsider and continue treatment as his company had recommended. A year has passed and there has been no word from Burt. Client withdrawal, or failure to enroll in therapy, is a common problem with this fluency syndrome.

Conclusion

This chapter has described cluttering as a fluency syndrome that is related to, but independent of stuttering. A number of definitions and specific symptoms that distinguish cluttering from stuttering have been provided. The point was made that "pure" cluttering is relatively rare and that more commonly the two disorders (cluttering and stuttering) occur simultaneously. The international literature suggests that cluttering and stuttering co-occur in about 40% to 50% of the cases. Treatment approaches that address the varied dimensions of this syndrome were recommended. It is my contention that attention should be directed to clutterers' possible deficits in oral-motor coordination, memory, language, and speech articulation. Therapy might also need to include specific organizational and sequencing activities. My experience is consistent with the clinical observations of Weiss,[2] who contended that cluttering could affect all channels of communication. Because related reading and writing disorders are common in both children and adults who clutter, a team approach that utilizes the talents of other professionals may be necessary.

Speech rate and fluency modification techniques appear to be critically important for the successful remediation of clutterers' difficulties but frequently are not the central focus of therapy. I have found it profitable to work on several dimensions of a clutterer's problem, within each session. Procedures and activities that help cluttering clients heighten their awareness to the multifaceted aspects of their problem and to the specific purposes of therapy seem to be particularly powerful. Finally, the need for persistence and repetition with these clients cannot be overemphasized.

Suggested Readings

Daly DA: *The Clutterer*, in St. Louis KO (ed): *The Atypical Stutterer: Principles and Practice of Rehabilitation*. New York, Academic Press, 1986.
   A comprehensive review of the various definitions and characteristics of cluttering by numerous investigators. Differentiations of stuttering and cluttering, as well as assessment and treatment procedures, are presented.
de Hirsch K: Stuttering and cluttering. *Folia Phoniatr (Basel)* 1970; 22:311–324.
   De Hirsch presents a developmental orientation suggesting that cluttering children may show disturbances in their rhythmic flow of speech that are related to a genetic predisposition or vulnerability in the language area. Clues for differential diagnosis and treatment are presented.
Arnold, GE, Luchsinger R: *Voice-Speech-Language, Clinical Communicology: Its Physiology and Pathology*. Belmont, CA, Wadsworth, 1965.
   This Herculean contribution by two physicians presents the most scholarly, in-depth analysis of

cluttering (tachyphemia) up to that time. These authors discuss the possible relationship between disordered rhythm and disorders of music and motor ability. Mandatory background reading for serious investigators and clinicians.

Weiss DA: Cluttering. *Folia Phoniatr (Basel)* 1967; 19:233–263.

Weiss' most comprehensive description of cluttering as a central language imbalance. This article is a published report to the International Association of Logopedics and Phoniatrics in Paris. His theoretical framework is described and illustrated with figures and tables. Weiss elaborates on the numerous features of cluttering and highlights faulty integration of language as the main criterion of cluttering, with or without acceleration of speech delivery. This article represents a culmination of his most serious writings.

Weiss DA: Cluttering: Central language imbalance. *Pediatr Clin North Am* 1968; 15:705–720.

Pediatricians are told that the problem of cluttering is an undefinable relative of stuttering. He urged physicians to take the rapid-fire repetitive speech and confused way of speaking shown by most cluttering children most seriously. Weiss explained that clutterers do not necessarily think faster than they can speak, but rather speak before they think through their ideas. Weiss emphasizes his clinical observation that most clutterers are in fact clutterer-stutterers. He stresses the point that young clutterers are more amenable to treatment than older clutterers. Students and clinicians will find this article most informative.

References

1. Froeschels E: Contribution to the relationship between stuttering and cluttering. *Logopaedic Phoniatr* 1955; 4:1–6.
2. Weiss DA: *Cluttering*. Englewood Cliffs, NJ, Prentice-Hall, 1964.
3. Arnold GE, Luchsinger R: *Voice-Speech-Language, Clinical Communicology: Its Physiology and Pathology*. Belmont, CA, Wadsworth, 1965.
4. Tiger RJ, Irvine TL, Reis RP: Cluttering as a complex of learning disabilities. *Lang Speech, Hear Serv Schools* 1981; 11:3–14.
5. Diedrich WM: Cluttering: Its Diagnosis, in Winitz H (ed): *Treating Articulation Disorders: For Clinicians by Clinicians*. Baltimore, University Park Press, 1984.
6. Daly DA: The Clutterer, in St. Louis KO (ed): *The Atypical Stutterer: Principles and Practice of Rehabilitation*. New York, Academic Press, 1986.
7. Weiss DA: Similarities and differences between stuttering and cluttering. *Folia Phoniatr (Basel)* 1967; 19:98–104.
8. Luchsinger R: *Poltern*. Berlin-Charlottenberg, Manhold Verlag, 1963.
9. Weiss DA: Cluttering: Central language imbalance. *Pediat Clin North Am* 1968; 15:705–720.
9a. Burk K: Cluttering: A Rate Control Program. Presented at the annual convention of the American Speech-Language-Hearing Association, Detroit, November, 1986.
10. Myers FM, St. Louis KO: *Cluttering: A Clinical Perspective*. Leicester, England, FAR Communications, in press.
11. Gove PB (ed): *Webster's Third New International Dictionary*, Boston, Merriam, 1981.
12. *Terminology for Speech Disorders*. London, College of Speech Therapists, 1959.
13. St. Louis KO: On Defining Cluttering, in Myers F, St. Louis KO (eds): *Cluttering: A Clinical Perspective*. Leicester, England, FAR Publications, in press.
14. de Hirsch K: Stuttering and cluttering: Developmental aspects of dysrhythmic speech. *Folia Phoniatr (Basel)* 1970; 22:311–324.
15. Froeschels E: Cluttering. *J Speech Disord* 1946; 11:31–36.
16. Freund H: Studies in the interrelationship between stuttering and cluttering. *Folia Phoniatr (Basel)* 1952; 4:146–168.
17. Freund H: Observations on tachylalia. *Folia Phoniatr (Basel)* 1970; 22:280–288.
18. Op't Hof J, Uys IC: A clinical delineation of tachyphemia (cluttering). *S Afr Med J* 1974; 10:1624–1628.
19. Daly DA: Helping the Clutterer: Therapy Considerations, in Myers F, St. Louis KO: *Cluttering: A Clinical Perspective*. Leicester, England, FAR Communications, in press.
20. Perkins WH: *Human Perspectives in Speech and Language Disorders*. St. Louis, Mosby, 1978.
21. Hood SB: The Assessment of Fluency Disorders, in Singh S, Lynch J (eds): *Diagnostic Procedures in Hearing, Language, and Speech*. Baltimore, University Park Press, 1978.
22. Gregory HH, Hill D: Stuttering Therapy for Children. *Semin Speech Lang Hear* 1980; 1:351–363.
23. Riley G, Riley J: Motoric and linguistic variables among children who stutter: A factor analysis. *J Speech Hear Disord* 1980; 45:504–514.

24. Riley G, Riley J: Evaluation as a Basis for Intervention, in Prins D, Ingram RJ: *Treatment of Stuttering in Early Childhood*. San Diego, College-Hill Press, 1983.
25. Bloodstein O: The development of stuttering: I. Changes in nine basic features. *J Speech Hear Disord* 1960; 25:219–237.
26. Blood GW, Seider R: The concomitant problems of young stutterers. *J Speech Hear Disord* 1981; 46:31–33.
27. Daly A: Differentiation of stuttering subgroups with Van Riper's developmental tracks: A preliminary study. *J Nat Student Speech-Language-Hear Assoc* 1981; 9:89–101.
28. Nippold MA: Concomitant speech and language disorders in stuttering children: A critique of the literature. *J Speech Hear Disord* 1990; 55:51–60.
29. Preus A: *Identifying Subgroups of Stutterers*. Oslo, Norway, Universitietsforlaget, 1981.
30. Preus A: The cluttering type of stutterer. *Scand J Logoped Phoniatr* 1987; 12:3–19.
31. Martin R, Kroll R, O'Keefe B, Painter C: Cluttered Speech: Spectrographic Data. Presented at the annual convention of the American Speech-Language-Hearing Association, Cincinnati, November 1983.
32. Seeman M, Novak A: Ueber die Motorik bei Polteren. *Folia Phoniatr (Basel)* 1963; 15:170–176.
33. Seeman M: Relations between motorics of speech and general motor ability in clutterers. *Folia Phoniatr (Basel)* 1970; 22:376–378.
34. Wyatt GL: *Language Learning and Communication Disorders in Children*. New York, The Free Press, 1969.
35. Wohl MT: The treatment of the non-fluent utterance—A behavioral approach. *Br J Disord Commun* 1970; 5:66–76.
36. Pearson L: Studies in tachyphemia: V. Rhythm and dysrhythmia in cluttering associated with congenital language disability. *Logos* 1962; 5:51–59.
37. Daly DA, Ostreicher HJ, Jonassen SA, Darnton SW: Memory for Unrelated Sentences: A Normative Study of 480 Children. Presented at the annual convention of the International Neuropsychological Society, Atlanta, 1981.
38. Sheperd G: Studies in tachyphemia: II. Phonetic description of cluttered speech. *Logos* 1960; 3:73–81.
39. Arnold GE: Studies in tachyphemia: I. Present concepts of etiologic factors. *Logos* 1960; 3:24–45.
40. Andrews G, Harris M: *The Syndrome of Stuttering*. London, Heinemann Medical Books, 1964.
41. Berry M: The developmental history of stuttering children. *J Pediatr* 1938; 12:209–217.
42. Conture EG: *Stuttering*. Englewood Cliffs, NJ, Prentice-Hall, 1982.
43. Daly A: Considerations for Treating Stutterers with and without Concomitant Articulation Disorders. Presented at the annual convention of the American Speech-Language-Hearing Association, Toronto, November 1982.
44. Morley ME: *The Development and Disorders of Speech in Childhood*. Edinburgh, Scotland, Livingstone, 1957.
45. Riley G, Riley J: A component model for diagnosing and treating children who stutter. *J Fluency Disord* 1979; 4:279–293.
46. Williams DE, Silverman FH: Note concerning articulation of school-age stutterers. *Percept Mot Skills* 1968; 27:713–714.
47. Bloodstein O: Stuttering as Tension and Fragmentation, in Eisenson J (ed): *Stuttering: A Second Symposium*. New York, Harper & Row, 1975.
48. Seeman M: Speech Pathology in Czechoslovakia, in Rieber RW, Brubaker RS: *Speech Pathology: An International Study of the Science*. Philadelphia, JB Lippincott, 1966.
49. Dalton P, Hardcastle WJ: *Disorders of Fluency and Their Effects on Communication*. London, Elsevier North-Holland, 1977.
50. Conture EG, Van Naerssen E: Reading abilities of school-age stutterers. *J Fluency Disord* 1977; 2:295–300.
51. Nippold MA, Schwartz IE: Reading disorders in stuttering children: Fact or fiction? *J Fluency Disord* 1990; 15:175–189.
52. Orton ST: *Reading, Writing, and Speech Problems in Children*. New York, Norton, 1937.
53. Spadino EJ: *Writing and Laterality Characteristics of Stuttering Children*. New York, Teachers College, 1941.
54. de Hirsch K: Studies in tachyphemia: IV. Diagnosis of developmental language disorders. *Logos* 1961; 4:3–9.
55. Roman-Goldzieher K: Studies in tachyphemia. VI. The interrelationship of graphologic and oral aspects of language behavior. *Logos* 1963; 6:41–58.
56. Daly DA, McPhail JC: Differentiation of Clutterers and Stutterers through Written Expression. Presented at the annual convention of the Michigan Speech-Language-Hearing Association, Kalamazoo, MI, 1992.

57. Lerner J: *Learning Disabilities: Theories, Diagnosis, and Teaching Strategies*. Boston, Houghton Mifflin, 1989.
58. Bakwin RM, Bakwin H: Cluttering. *J Pediatr* 1952; 40:393–396.
59. Arnold GE: Studies in tachyphemia: III. Signs and symptoms. *Logos* 1960; 3:82–95.
60. Cantwell DP, Baker L: Association between attention deficit-hyperactivity disorder and learning disorders. *J Learning Disabilities* 1991; 24:88–95.
61. Epstein MA: The boundaries of attention deficit disorder. *J Learning Disabilities* 1991; 24:78–86.
62. West R, Kennedy L, Carr A: *The Rehabilitation of Speech*. New York, Harper & Bros, 1947.
63. Grewel F: Cluttering and its problems. *Folia Phoniatr (Basel)* 1970; 22:301–310.
64. Kidd KK: Genetic models of stuttering. *J Fluency Disord* 1980; 5:187–202.
65. Poulos MG, Webster WG: Family history as a basis for subgrouping people who stutter. *J Speech Hear Res* 1991; 34:5–10.
66. Dalton P, Hardcastle WJ: *Disorders of Fluency*. London, Whurr Publishers, 1989.
67. Woolf G: The assessment of stuttering as struggle, avoidance, and expectance. *Br J Disord Commun* 1967; 2:158–171.
68. Daly DA, Oakes D, Breen K, Mishler C: Perception of Stuttering Inventory: Norms for Adolescent Stutterers and Nonstutterers. Presented at the annual convention of the American Speech-Language-Hearing Association, Los Angeles, November 1981.
69. Daly DA, Darnton SW: Intensive Fluency Shaping and Attitudinal Therapy with Stutterers: A Follow-up Study. Presented at the annual convention of the American Speech-Language-Hearing Association, Houston, November 1976.
70. Cooper EB: The development of a stuttering chronicity predictive checklist for school-age stutterers: A research inventory for clinicians. *J Speech Hear Res* 1973; 38:215–223.
71. Van Riper C: *The Nature of Stuttering*. Englewood Cliffs, NJ, Prentice-Hall, 1971.
72. Langova J, Moravek M: Some results of experimental examinations among stutterers and clutterers. *Folia Phoniatr (Basel)* 1964; 16:290–296.
73. Preus A: Cluttering and Stuttering: Related, Different, or Antagonistic Disorders, in Myers F, St. Louis KO (eds): *Cluttering: A Clinical Perspective*. Leicester, England, FAR Communications, in press.
74. Van Riper C: Stuttering and cluttering: The differential diagnosis. *Folia Phoniatr (Basel)* 1970; 22: 347–353.
75. Daly DA: *The Freedom of Fluency: A Therapy Program for the Chronic Stutterer*. Moline, IL, Lingui-Systems, 1988.
76. Peters H, Starkweather CW: The interaction between speech motor coordination and language processes in the development of stuttering: Hypotheses and suggestions for research. *J Fluency Disord* 1990; 15:115–125.
77. Shames G, Florance C: *Stutter-Free Speech: A Goal for Therapy*. San Antonio, Harcourt Brace Jovanovich, 1980.
78. Webster RL: Empirical Considerations Regarding Stuttering Therapy, in Gregory HH (ed): *Controversies about Stuttering Therapy*. Baltimore, University Park Press, 1979.
79. Riley G, Riley J: *Oral Motor Assessment and Treatment: Improving Syllable Production*. Austin, TX, Pro-Ed, 1985.
80. Riley G, Riley J: Oral motor discoordination among children who stutter. *J Fluency Disord* 1986; 11:335–344.
81. Dostalova N, Dosuzkov T: Uber die drei Hauptforem des Neurotische Stotterns. *Ther Vocis Loquellae* 1965; I:273–276.
82. Langova J, Moravek M: Some problems of cluttering. *Folia Phoniatr (Basel)* 1970; 22:325–336.
83. Cooper EB: Mentally Retarded Stutterer, in St. Louis KO (ed): *The Atypical Stutterer: Principles and Practice of Rehabilitation*. New York, Academic Press, 1986.
84. Myers FM, Bradley C: Clinical Management of Cluttering from a Synergistic Framework, in Myers FL, St. Louis KO: *Cluttering: A Clinical Perspective*. Leicester, England, FAR Communications, in press.
85. Daly DA: Use of the home VCR to facilitate transfer of fluency. *J Fluency Disord* 1987; 12:103–106.
86. Perkins WH: Replacement of stuttering with normal speech: II. Clinical procedures. *J Speech Hear Disord* 1973; 38:295–303.
87. Shames G: New therapy for stuttering utilizes vibrotactile feedback. *Psychiatr Times Med Behav* 1989; June.
88. Lazarus AA: *In the Mind's Eye*. New York, Guilford Press, 1984.
89. Cousins N: *Head First: The Biology of Hope*. New York, EP Dutton, 1989.
90. Helmstetter S: *What To Say When You Talk To Yourself*. New York, Pocket Books, 1986.
91. Meichenbaum D, Cameron R: The clinical potential of modifying what clients say to themselves. *Psychother Theory Res Prac* 1974; 11:103–117.

92. Bandler R: *Using Your Brain for a Change: Neuro-Linguistic Programming,* Moab, UT, Real People Press, 1985.

93. Robbins A: *Unlimited Power.* New York, Simon & Schuster, 1986.

94. Siegel B: *Love, Medicine, and Miracles,* New York, Harper & Row, 1986.

95. Simonton OC, Simonton S: *Getting Well Again,* New York, Bantam Books, 1978.

96. Daly DA, Thompson J, Simon C: Treatment of Cluttering with Stutter-Free Speech and Mental Imagery. Presented at the annual convention of the American Speech-Language-Hearing Association, Washington, DC, November 1985.

APPENDIX A: PERCEPTIONS OF SPEECH COMMUNICATION

S _____   PSC Total

A _____   _____

Name _____   E _____

Address _____   Date _____

Directions

Here are sixty statements about speech behavior. Some of these may be characteristic of **your** speech. Read each item carefully and respond as in the example below.

Characteristic
of me
□ Repeating sounds.

Put a check mark (✔) under **characteristic of me** if "repeating sounds" is part of your speech; if it is **not characteristic,** leave the box blank.

Characteristic of me refers only to what you do **now,** not to what was true of your speech in the past and which you no longer do; and not what you think you should or should not be doing. Even if the behavior described occurs only occasionally or only in some speaking situations, if you regard it as characteristic of your speech, check the box under **characteristic of me.** Be accurate in your judgments.

Characteristic
of me

□ 1. Avoiding talking to people in authority (e.g., a teacher, employer, or clergyman).

□ 2. Feeling that interruptions in your speech (e.g., pauses, hesitations, or repetitions) will lead to speaking difficulty.

□ 3. Making the pitch of your voice higher or lower when you expect to get "stuck" on words.

□ 4. Having extra and unnecessary facial movements (e.g., flaring your nostrils during speech attempts).

□ 5. Using gestures as a substitute for speaking (e.g., nodding your head instead of saying "yes" or smiling to acknowlege a greeting).

□ 6. Avoiding asking for information (e.g., asking for directions or inquiring about a train schedule).

□ 7. Whispering words to yourself before saying them or practicing what you are planning to say long before you speak.

□ 8. Choosing a job or hobby because little speaking would be required.

□ 9. Adding an extra and unnecessary sound, word, or phrase to your speech (e.g., "uh," "well," or "let me see") to help yourself get started.

Characteristic
of me

☐ 10.   Replying briefly using the fewest words possible.
☐ 11.   Making sudden jerky or forceful movements with your head, arms, or body during speech attempts (e.g., clenching your fist, jerking your head to one side).
☐ 12.   Repeating a sound or word with effort.
☐ 13.   Acting in a manner intended to keep you out of a conversation or discussion (e.g., being a good listener, pretending not to hear what was said, acting bored, or pretending to be in deep thought).
☐ 14.   Avoiding making a purchase (e.g., going into a store or buying stamps in the post office).
☐ 15.   Breathing noisily or with great effort while trying to speak.
☐ 16.   Making your voice louder or softer when speaking difficulty is expected.
☐ 17.   Prolonging a sound or word (e.g., m-m-m-m-my) while trying to push it out.
☐ 18.   Helping yourself to get started talking by laughing, coughing, clearing your throat, gesturing, or some other body activity or movement.
☐ 19.   Having general body tension during speech attempts (e.g., shaking, trembling, or feeling "knotted up" inside).
☐ 20.   Paying particular attention to what you are going to say (e.g., the length of a word, or the position of a word in a sentence).
☐ 21.   Feeling your face getting warm and red (as if you are blushing), as you are struggling to speak.
☐ 22.   Saying words or phrases with force or effort.
☐ 23.   Repeating a word or phase preceding the word on which speaking difficulty is expected.
☐ 24.   Speaking so that no word or sound stands out (e.g., speaking in a singsong voice or in a monotone).
☐ 25.   Avoiding making new acquaintances (e.g., not visiting with friends, not dating, or not joining social, civic, or church groups).
☐ 26.   Making unusual noises with your teeth during speech attempts (e.g., grinding or clicking you teeth).
☐ 27.   Avoiding introducing yourself, giving your name, or making introductions.
☐ 28.   Expecting that certain sounds, letters, or words are going to be particularly "hard" to say (e.g., words beginning with the letter "s").
☐ 29.   Giving excuses to avoid talking (e.g., pretending to be tired or pretending lack of interest in a topic).
☐ 30.   "Running out of breath" while speaking.
☐ 31.   Forcing out sounds.
☐ 32.   Feeling that your periods of smooth speech are unusual, that they cannot last, and that sooner or later you will have speaking difficulty.
☐ 33.   Concentrating on relaxing or not being tense before speaking.
☐ 34.   Substituting a different word or phrase for the one you had intended to say.
☐ 35.   Prolonging or emphasizing the sound preceding the one on which speaking difficulty is expected.
☐ 36.   Avoiding speaking before an audience.
☐ 37.   Straining to talk without being able to make a sound.
☐ 38.   Coordinating or timing your speech with a rhythmic movement (e.g., tapping your foot or swinging your arm).
☐ 39.   Rearranging what you had planned to say to avoid a "hard" sound or word.

(Continued on next page)

Characteristic
of me

☐ 40. "Putting on an act" when speaking (e.g., adopting an attitude of confidence or pretending to be angry).

☐ 41. Avoiding the use of the telephone.

☐ 42. Making forceful and strained movements with your lips, tongue, jaw, or throat (e.g., moving your jaw in an uncoordinated manner).

☐ 43. Omitting a word, part of a word, or a phrase which you had planned to say (e.g., words with certain sounds or letters).

☐ 44. Making "uncontrollable" sounds while struggling to say a word.

☐ 45. Adopting a foreign accent, assuming a regional dialect, or imitating another person's speech.

☐ 46. Perspiring much more than usual while speaking (e.g., feeling the palms of you hands getting clammy).

☐ 47. Postponing speaking for a short time until certain you can use smooth speech (e.g., pausing before "hard words").

☐ 48. Having extra and unnecessary eye movements while speaking (e.g., blinking your eyes or shutting your eyes tightly).

☐ 49. Breathing forcefully while struggling to speak.

☐ 50. Avoiding talking to others of your own age group (your own or the opposite sex).

☐ 51. Giving up the speech attempt completely after getting "stuck" or if difficulty is anticipated.

☐ 52. Straining the muscles of your chest or abdomen during speech attempts.

☐ 53. Wondering whether you will have difficulty speaking and how it will sound if you do.

☐ 54. Holding your lips, tongue, or jaw in a rigid position before speaking or when getting "stuck" on a word.

☐ 55. Avoiding talking to one or both of your parents.

☐ 56. Having another person speak for you in a difficult situation (e.g., having someone make a telephone call for you or order for you in a restaurant).

☐ 57. Holding your breath before speaking.

☐ 58. Saying words slowly or rapidly preceding the word on which speaking difficulty is expected.

☐ 59. Concentrating on how you are going to speak (e.g., thinking about where to put your tongue or how to breathe).

☐ 60. Using your speech difficulty as a reason to avoid a speaking activity.

> The Perceptions of Stuttering Inventory (PSI) from which this inventory (PSC*) was adopted was developed by Dr. Gerald Woolf, currently at Montclair State College, Upper Montclair, New Jersey, and originally published in the *British Journal of Disorders of Communication*, 1967, 2, 158–177.

Do you now or have you ever had a speech problem?   Yes ☐   No ☐
If Yes, please specify.

Foreign dialect   Yes ☐   No ☐

---

*PSC adapted by David A. Daly, University of Michigan, 1978.

APPENDIX B: DALY'S CHECKLIST FOR POSSIBLE CLUTTERING—EXPERIMENTAL EDITION

Client's Name _____   Date _____

Instructions: Please respond to each descriptive statement below. Your answers should reflect how well you believe the statement describes the child/adult:

STATEMENT TRUE FOR CLIENT	Not at all 0	Just a little 1	Pretty much 2	Very much 3
1. Repeats syllables, words, phrases	0	1	2	3
2. Started talking late; onset of words and sentences delayed	0	1	2	3
3. Fluency disruptions started early; no remissions; never very fluent	0	1	2	3
4. Speech very disorganized; confused wording	0	1	2	3
5. Silent gaps or hesitations common; interjections; many "filler" words	0	1	2	3
6. Stops before saying initial vowel; no tension; drawn-out vowels	0	1	2	3
7. Rapid rate (speaks too fast); tachylalia; speaks in spurts	0	1	2	3
8. Extrovert; high verbal output; compulsive talker	0	1	2	3
9. Jerky breathing pattern, respiratory dysrhythmia	0	1	2	3
10. Slurred articulation (omits sounds or unstressed syllables)	0	1	2	3
11. Mispronounciation of /r/, /l/, and sibilants	0	1	2	3
12. Speech better under pressure; e.g., during short periods of heightened attention	0	1	2	3
13. Difficulty following directions; impatient/ uninterested listener	0	1	2	3
14. Distractible; attention span problems; poor concentration	0	1	2	3
15. Story-telling difficulty; (trouble sequencing events)	0	1	2	3
16. Demonstrates word-finding difficulties resembling anomia	0	1	2	3
17. Inappropriate reference by pronouns is common	0	1	2	3
18. Improper language structure; poor grammar and syntax	0	1	2	3
19. Clumsy and uncoordinated; motor activities accelerated (or hasty)	0	1	2	3
20. Reading disorder is a prominent disability	0	1	2	3
21. Disintegrated and fractionated writing; poor motor control	0	1	2	3
22. Writing shows transposition of letters and words (omits letters and syllables)	0	1	2	3
23. Left-right confusion; delayed hand preference	0	1	2	3
24. Initial loud voice; trails off to a murmer; mumbles	0	1	2	3

(Continued on next page)

STATEMENT TRUE FOR CLIENT	Not at all 0	Just a little 1	Pretty much 2	Very much 3
25. Seems to think faster than he can talk or write	0	1	2	3
26. Above average in mathematical and abstract reasoning abilities	0	1	2	3
27. Poor rhythm, timing or musical ability (may dislike singing)	0	1	2	3
28. Improper stress patterns of speech; poor melodic accenting of syllables	0	1	2	3
29. Appears younger than age; small and/or immature	0	1	2	3
30. Other family member with same/similar problem; heredity	0	1	2	3
31. Untidy, careless, hasty, impulsive or forgetful	0	1	2	3
32. Impatient, superficial, and/or short-tempered	0	1	2	3
33. Lack of self-awareness; unconcerned attitude over inappropriateness of many behaviors and responses	0	1	2	3

TOTAL SCORE _____

DIAGNOSIS _____

Other Relevant Information Determined by Interviewer:

(Circle correct answer)

*Identified in school as learning disabled.   Yes   No   Recommended   Don't know
for testing

*Current receiving speech/language therapy   Yes   No   Recommended   Don't know

*Comments: _____

_____

_____

Clinician _____

Experimental Edition by
David A. Daly, 1991

10

Stuttering Associated with Acquired Neurological Disorders

Nancy Helm-Estabrooks, Sc.D.

Introduction

Acquired Neurological Stuttering

In 1978, two papers described groups of adults in whom onset of stuttering was associated with neurological events. In one paper Rosenbek and colleagues[1] described seven brain-damaged patients who developed "cortical stuttering" after cerebral vascular accidents (CVAs). The damage involved the left cerebral hemisphere in five of the seven cases, although the sites of lesions did not conform to any particular pattern. Of the remaining two patients, one had bilateral disease and one had a right parietal lobe lesion. In the second paper my colleagues and I described acquired stuttering in ten adults, six of whom had experienced strokes (CVAs) and four of whom had incurred traumatic brain injury.[2] We observed that persistent stuttering was associated with bilateral pathology, and transient stuttering was associated with unilateral, but multifocal, pathology.

Although adult onset of stuttering associated with neurological disorders had been described prior to these 1978 studies, references to it before this time were somewhat rare. Since 1978, however, this phenomenon received sufficient attention that by 1991 approximately 50 papers had been published describing single cases or groups of patients with so-called "neurogenic" stuttering. Included among these publications is a national survey in which 81% of more than 100 speech-language pathologists reported that they had seen patients with acquired stuttering.[3]

The crucial question to be asked about all studies of neurogenic or acquired stuttering is: What behaviors have investigators defined or described as "stuttering"? The term "stuttering" has classically been used to indicate a constellation of signs and symptoms displayed by individuals who begin to show signs of notable speech dysfluency as children. Many clinicians, therefore, are not comfortable with the application of this label to the speech of adults with no childhood history of stuttering. The World Health Organization (WHO) definition of stuttering, however, does not refer to the period of life in which this phenomenon appears. Instead, it chooses to focus on speech behavior alone, defining stuttering as

> disorders in the rhythm of speech in which the individual knows precisely what he wishes to say but at the time is unable to say it because of an involuntary repetition, prolongation, or cessation of a sound.[4]

Two concepts proposed in the WHO definition deserve special comment here. The first is that of "disorders," which implies that stuttering is not a unitary disorder. This seems to be true of developmental stuttering. For example, it is known[5] that some forms of developmental stuttering persist into adulthood while most others disappear prior to puberty. Some forms of developmental stuttering appear to be idiopathic while others may be genetically determined. Some forms of developmental stuttering are associated with language and learning problems while others appear to be isolated motor speech phenomena.

So too, acquired stuttering appears not to be a unitary disorder.[6] Some forms of acquired stuttering are transient while others are persistent. Some forms are associated with speech, language, and cognitive disorders while others are not. Perhaps most importantly, various types of acquired stuttering have been described in association with temporary, progressive, and nonprogressive neurological conditions affecting various brain areas, including the cerebral cortex, basal ganglia, cerebellum, and brain stem. This suggests that acquired stuttering can result from damage to or involvement of the pyramidal, extrapyramidal, corticobulbar, and cerebellar motor systems. One study in which computed tomography (CT) scans were used to confirm lesion sites in acquired stuttering is that of Ludlow and her colleagues.[7] They comprehensively examined ten men who exhibited this speech disorder for up to 15 years after sustaining penetrating missile wounds. Acquired stuttering in these cases was associated with lesions of the subcortical pyramidal and extrapyramidal systems, and not with lesions directly involving the cortex.

The second concept in the WHO definition that deserves special comment is that "the individual knows precisely what he wishes to say." This implies that the individual is not stuttering because of an aphasia or a word-finding problem. But, *acquired* stuttering has often been linked to aphasia. Arnold and Luchsinger,[8] for example, discussed three varieties of acquired stuttering: *aphasic stuttering*, in which the speech dysfluencies are a part of the language disorder; *stuttering with aphasia*, thought to represent a psychological reaction to the aphasia; and *dysarthric stuttering*, which may occur during the recovery phase of any type of aphasia, especially expressive aphasia.

Subsequent reports have shown that while acquired stuttering and aphasia may co-occur, they are probably independent phenomena. Supporting this contention is the evidence that aphasic patients are rarely said to "stutter," and that the majority of patients with acquired stuttering appear not to be aphasic.[3] In the diagnosis of acquired stuttering, therefore, it is crucially important to rule out language problems as a basis for the dysfluency and to establish that the individual has retrieved the words and the sounds that comprise the words.

If the term "acquired stuttering" is to be used then the definition as put forth by the WHO probably should be expanded to include the following statement: To be labeled as "acquired stuttering," onset of the dysfluent speech must occur in adulthood in the absence of a childhood history of developmental stuttering.

Worsening and Reappearance of Stuttering with Neurological Disease

In addition to those cases in which stuttering appears for the first time in adulthood, several cases have been reported in which *childhood stuttering reappeared or worsened with the onset of neurological disorders*. For example, in their report of 16 cases of neurogenic stuttering, Mazzucchi and colleagues[9] described three patients in whom mild forms of developmental stuttering were exacerbated either by CVAs or head trauma. A fourth patient had recurrence of childhood stuttering with onset of a left temporal lobe stroke. Similarly, several colleagues and I reported on a 61-year-old, ambidextrous man who outgrew his childhood stuttering only to have it reappear after a stroke.[10]

Recurrence of childhood stuttering was the first symptom of an Alzheimer's-like dementia in a 62-year-old man described by Quinn and Andrews.[11] This successful businessman had onset of stuttering 7 months before the appearance of other neurological signs. More recently, I saw a 64-year-old man who experienced recurrence of stuttering with onset of a progressive, parkinsonian-like form of dementia.

Thus, stuttering may worsen or recur in the presence of neurological dysfunction. In keeping with these observations, a definition of "acquired stuttering" must allow for those cases in which the reappearance or worsening of stuttering in adulthood is part of the neurological condition. Perhaps it is time for a new term that can serve as an umbrella to cover all of these cases. Consider for example, *stuttering associated with acquired neurological disorders* (SAAND) and the following working definition:

> Stuttering refers to disorders in the rhythm of speech in which the individual knows precisely what he or she wishes to say but at the time is unable to say it because of an involuntary repetition, prolongation, or cessation of a sound. When this behavior first occurs, notably worsens, or recurs in the presence of acquired neurological problems, it is diagnosed as *stuttering associated with acquired neurological disorders (SAAND)*.

Disappearance of Stuttering with Neurological Changes

Before proceeding to a discussion of the clinical evaluation of SAAND, I should note that there is some published evidence that developmental stuttering may cease in adults with changes in neurological status. The cases described by Jones[12] are examples of this phenomenon. Four male stutterers, all with personal and family histories of left-handedness, underwent neurosurgical procedures (three for aneurysm, one for tumor). Presurgical carotid amobarbital (Amytal) tests showed bilateral representation for speech in all cases. Following surgery, all four ceased to stutter, and amobarbital testing now showed unilateral representation for speech.

Miller[13] described two male patients whose severe childhood stuttering continued into adulthood until they developed multiple sclerosis (MS) and the stuttering began to remit. As MS progressed, the stuttering lessened until they no longer stuttered, although other speech problems appeared. Both patients had clinical evidence of bilateral cerebellar disease.

Finally, I had an opportunity to work with an ambidextrous man with severe developmental stuttering that remitted with head injury.[10] This young man sustained a right subdural hematoma and loss of consciousness for 10 days' duration. Upon awakening, he spoke at a slower rate than before with signs of mild dysarthria but no stuttering. To quote Miller: "These cases serve to emphasize the complexity with which neurologic lesions can alter human speech, even result in a paradoxical improvement in oral communication."[13]

Clinical Evaluation of Stuttering Associated with Acquired Neurolgical Disorders

The Case History

A detailed case history is of the utmost importance in the differential diagnosis of SAAND. To underscore this point, consider the following two cases in which the primary diagnosis was that of *psychogenic* stuttering. In the first case, Deal[14] described a 28-year-old male who began to stutter after attempting suicide. The means of this suicide attempt were not stated, but the patient was in a methadone program at the time (indicating that he was a drug abuser). At age 16 he had attempted suicide by cutting his throat and stuttered for "approximately seven or eight days afterward." There is no mention of whether he had experienced loss of consciousness with this or the later attempt. Furthermore, this man had a history of arrests for car theft and other behaviors that placed him in the group at high risk for head trauma. Lastly, he was "well-known" to the psychiatry service, which raises the possibility that he had received antidepressive or antipsychotic drugs.

A second case thought to be "psychogenic in onset" was described by Attanasio.[15] This investigator, however, stated that there was a "possible neurologic base" for the stuttering that began in an adult male who was experiencing marital difficulties. This behavior worsened until it became "full-blown" at the time of divorce a few years later. But Attanasio goes on to say that "what cannot be ignored is the fact that he had epilepsy." Furthermore, the man had experienced his first seizure at age 11, and was taking primidone (Mysoline) and phenobarbital at time of speech evaluation at age 36. He had experienced his last "grand mal" seizure at age 33.

These so-called "psychogenic" cases are of interest here because they suggest some of the many *neurological* factors that might lead to SAAND. Among other conditions, stuttering has been described in relation to *drug use*,[16,17] *head trauma*,[18] *anoxia*,[6] and *epilepsy*.[19]

Sometimes, however, there appears to be no neurological basis for the development of "stuttering" in adulthood, but there is a history of psychological problems. In other cases, the individual may stand to gain from the speech disorder. Some years ago, two colleagues and I[20] described three such cases, two of whom were veterans of the armed services. Both had long histories of psychological problems and had repeatedly sought government compensation for stress they experienced while in the service. Their "stuttering" appeared suddenly, was not observed in all situations, and disappeared after a few months without treatment. The third person experienced transient stuttering that began during a severe anxiety attack and disappeared within a week. As a rule of thumb, when adult-onset stuttering occurs in persons with no neurological indicators, but in whom there is psychological dysfunction and/or secondary gain (either monetary or emotional), the question of a psychogenic etiology should be raised. In all such cases, however, it is important first to rule out any neurological factors that might lead to a diagnosis of SAAND.

As a final consideration, I should mention that onset of SAAND may be associated with psychologically traumatic events occurring in persons with known neurological disease. For example, I once saw a man with Parkinson's disease who experienced a sudden worsening of his speech problems and onset of stuttering-like behaviors after being side-swiped by a trailer truck on the highway. Although he experienced no apparent physical injuries, it was thought that the release of various neurochemicals associated with great fright was responsible for the onset of stuttering-like speech behaviors in this man with an already compromised nervous system. Interestingly, he had a lifelong history of ambidexterity. His ambidexterity also raised the long-standing issue of anomalous dominance for language in persons with either developmental or acquired stuttering.[10] Unfortunately, both Deal[14] and Attanasio[15] failed to report the handedness of their patients with "psychogenic" stuttering. They are not alone, however, in omitting this important information. Market and colleagues,[3] for example, did not ask respondents to list handedness in their survey of persons with acquired stuttering. Without more thorough investigations of the handedness history of patients and their families, the extent to which left-handed and ambidextrous people are more at risk for SAAND remains uncertain. If anomalous dominance does play a role in this disorder, then such patients might be expected to report a higher incidence of learning disabilities and other behaviors associated with left-handedness.[21]

In this section, evidence has been offered suggesting that careful case histories are crucial in the diagnosis of SAAND. Sometimes the results of the personal interviews and speech and language examinations will lead to referrals to a neurologist and a neuropsychologist for further evaluation. Probably more commonly, the patient will have been referred to speech-language pathologists by a physician or a psychologist. In either instance, an interdisciplinary approach to the diagnoses and management of individuals with SAAND is usually necessary for optimal results. A case history format for interviewing individuals with adult onset of stuttering-like behaviors is presented in Appendix A. It is expected that the experienced clinician will expand the scope of inquiry as suggested by the answers provided by the patient.

Observations and Tests

SPEECH AND LANGUAGE TASKS

As noted above, a complete case history is the first and, perhaps, most important step in the diagnosis of SAAND. The second step is to determine the presence or absence of aphasia or word-finding problems. According to the definition of

SAAND, the person "knows precisely what he or she wishes to say but at the time is unable to say it because of an involuntary repetition, prolongation, or cessation of a sound." There are many standardized tests that can be used to examine for aphasia. Two tests that together can be given to a nonaphasic person in under 1 hour are the Aphasia Diagnostic Profiles (ADP),[22] and the Boston Naming Test (BNT).[23] Both tests have norms for both aphasic and nonaphasic individuals. By comparing the performance of a person with adult-onset stuttering with the norms tables provided for these two standardized tests, the clinician may begin to determine whether the speech dysfluencies displayed are likely the result of word-finding problems or of a motor speech dysfunction.

The third step in diagnosing SAAND involves determination of whether dysfluencies occur regardless of word class. Typically, patients with SAAND display speech dysfluencies on both small, grammatical words (functors) and high-information words (substantives). In contrast, adults with developmental stuttering are more likely to stutter only on substantive words. Samples of narrative and expository speech and oral repetition can be obtained by using the ADP or subtests from other clinical exams such as the Boston Diagnostic Aphasia Examination (BDAE).[24] Of course, all speech samples obtained in the SAAND examination should be *tape-recorded* for careful analyses. Ideally, videotapes should be made to record any accessory behaviors, such as facial grimacing, eye blinking, and fist clenching, that may accompany the instances of stuttering. But even in the absence of videotaping, clinicians should watch for these symptoms, note their presence, and describe their nature. The presence or absence of accessory behaviors is important in the diagnosis of SAAND because typically these symptoms are absent or less striking in patients whose stuttering is known to be associated with neurological disorders.

The fourth step in the diagnosis of SAAND is to establish whether the patient displays an *adaptation effect* as indicated by fewer and fewer dysfluencies on repeated readings of a passage. It has been estimated that about 70% of developmental stutterers evidence adaptation.[25] Persons with SAAND are less likely to show this effect. To determine the presence of adaptation, two standard passages containing all the sounds in the English language are recommended: "The Rainbow Passage"[26] and "The Grandfather Passage."[27]

Fifth, the clinician needs to determine whether the person suspected of having SAAND produces dysfluencies on highly automatized speech tasks such as counting to 30; reciting the months of the year, "The Lord's Prayer," or "The Pledge of Allegiance"; and singing popular songs. Persons with SAAND are more likely to produce dysfluencies when performing such tasks than are those with developmental stuttering. That is, persons with SAAND will show less variability in dysfluency across tasks than will those with developmental stuttering. All the speech tasks used to diagnose SAAND are outlined in Table 10-1.

After recording these samples, the clinician must then analyze them for moments and types of dysfluencies, noting on which tasks dysfluencies occurred and whether they occurred on initial or medial phonemes, grammatical or substantive words. It is important also to note whether these dysfluencies took the form of repetitions, prolongations, or blocks and whether certain phonemes were more likely than others to elicit dysfluencies. The speech behaviors associated with SAAND are summarized in Table 10-2.

Table 10-1. Speech and Language Tasks Recommended for Diagnosing SAAND

Standardized tests
    Aphasia Diagnostic Profiles[22]
    Boston Naming Test[23]
Standard speech passages (repeated readings)
    "The Rainbow Passage"[26]
    "The Grandfather Passage"[27]
Automatized recitations
    Counting to 30
    Months of the year
    "The Pledge of Allegiance" or "The Lord's Prayer"
Singing familiar songs

As a final note, SAAND should be distinguished from the neurological speech disorder called *palilalia*. In this disorder, whole words and phrases, rather than individual sounds, are repeated often with increasing speed and decreasing distinctness. Palilalia is most often associated with diseases affecting the basal ganglia, particularly postencephalitic Parkinson's disease. For example, I reported on such a patient who, when asked his name, repeated, "My name, my name, my name. . ." over 30 times.[28]

OTHER TESTS

Individuals who have been diagnosed as having SAAND, by definition also suffer from some neurological disorder. Depending on the nature, site, and extent of brain involvement, this neurological disorder may give rise to problems other than stuttering that are important to treatment decisions. I noted above the possibility that stroke patients with acquired stuttering may also have some degree of aphasia that will affect word finding. Consider also that some patients with dementia develop SAAND but they also commonly experience memory problems from the earliest stages of the disease. Similarly, head trauma, which probably is the most common cause of SAAND,[3] also may be associated with memory loss. Closed head injury, in particular, often results in shearing of neuronal axons and swelling of brain tissue, causing complex behavioral sequelae and cognitive deficits affecting memory and initiation skills. Obviously, memory problems will interfere with the learning of new strategies for speaking, and initiation problems may result in the failure to implement the use of communication aids such as a pacing

Table 10-2. Speech Behaviors Associated with SAAND

1. There is no adaptation effect.
2. Repetition, prolongations, and blocks are not restricted to initial syllables.
3. Dysfluencies occur on grammatical as well as substantive words.
4. Stuttering may occur across speech tasks.
5. The speaker may be annoyed but does not appear anxious.
6. There are rarely secondary symptoms such as facial grimacing, eye blinking, or fist clenching associated with the moments of dysfluency.

board.[28] Depending on the etiology of SAAND, therefore, the speech-language pathologist may need to probe other skill areas with such tests as the Arizona Battery for Communication Disorders in Dementia,[29] the Brief Test of Head Injury,[30] or the Scales of Cognitive Ability for Traumatic Brain Injury.[31] In addition, reports of neuropsychological and neurological examinations may be crucial for selecting patients for treatment of SAAND and for choosing appropriate management techniques.

Case Selection Criteria

In the foregoing section I stressed the importance of obtaining thorough case histories and formal test results in diagnosing SAAND and any coexisting cognitive deficits. Based on the information gleaned from these inquiries, decisions can be made as to whether a particular patient is a candidate for therapeutic intervention and, if so, what specific approach is likely to produce positive results.

Probably the first question to be asked in selecting SAAND patients for therapeutic intervention is: *Does the stuttering represent a communication handicap?* In some cases the dysfluencies are so mild that although noticeable, they do not appreciably interfere with communication. In other cases, the stuttering is part of a larger communication problem (such as aphasia) that must take precedence in the rehabilitation program. If stuttering is judged to represent a significant speech handicap, then the next question to be asked is: *Is the individual motivated to work on the problem?* One of the behavioral features of SAAND (see Table 10-2) is that patients may be somewhat annoyed, but not highly anxious about the stuttering. Probably depending on the neuropathology of their disorders, other patients may show total indifference to their dysfluencies. Such individuals may be poor candidates for any therapeutic program that involves behavior modification. Similarly, patients with initiation problems may fail to implement newly learned strategies and techniques when left to their own devices. For example, I saw a highly dysfluent patient who could speak without repetition of sounds and words when using a pacing board[32] but who never initiated use of this aid. This did not deter us from giving him the board and training him to pace his speech, but at the same time his caretakers were trained to place it in his hands and encourage him to use it when talking.

Another question to be asked regarding SAAND treatment candidacy is: *Does the patient have a rapidly progressing neurological disorder?* If so, then even severe stuttering may represent a minor problem in the overall scheme of life. For example, two studies[33,34] described adult-onset stuttering in patients with dialysis dementia. These patients had been given extensive dialysis therapy for kidney disease when stuttering appeared along with early signs of confusion and dementia. As their conditions worsened, the patients became mute and finally died. Because of the severe and progressive nature of their disease, these patients probably were not candidates for speech therapy. Similarly, I examined a patient who developed severe stuttering 3 weeks after the first neurological signs of an inoperable brain tumor.[20] Although there was time to perform a speech and language examination, it was mutually agreed that the remaining time was too short to spend in speech therapy.

Sometimes patients will be candidates for drug therapy, which requires interdisciplinary cooperation between a speech-language pathologist and a neurologist. For example, Baratz and Mesulam[19] described a 42-year-old woman who developed seizures and began to stutter following a closed head injury. When her seizures were brought under control with phenytoin (Dilantin), her speech dysfluencies diminished.

Thus, the selection of SAAND patients for various therapeutic interventions will depend on the overall health status of each individual as well as the etiology of the stuttering, its neuropathological correlates, and any concomitant behavioral disorders.

Clinical Management

Treatment Goals

Because SAAND is a speech problem of adults, ideally each patient will take an active part in setting treatment goals. These goals will be determined in part according to each individual's life-style, work status, age, general health, etc. For example, a salesperson with a relatively mild degree of nonfluency may consider stuttering to be a significant handicap. In contrast, a bedridden person who can communicate basic needs may not consider himself or herself significantly handicapped by the stuttering. In some cases, however, memory and other cognitive deficits may prevent the patient from participating in the goal-setting process. In such cases, clinicians, family members, and/or caretakers will determine the extent to which stuttering interferes with the communicative needs of the individual patient. The next step after the clinical evaluation, therefore, is to establish the level of the handicap and document the situations in which communication suffers as a result of stuttering. This information, which may be obtained using a formal questionnaire, then can be used to establish treatment goals. Readministration of such a questionnaire also can serve as one measurement of treatment effectiveness.

Treatment Procedures

A review of the literature indicates that SAAND has been treated with surgery, various pharmacological agents, thalamic stimulation, transcutaneous nerve stimulation (TNS), delayed auditory feedback (DAF) and auditory masking, biofeedback and relaxation, and speech-pacing techniques. In the following sections, each of the treatments that have been described will be considered, beginning with surgery.

SURGICAL INTERVENTION

In 1979 Donnan[35] described a 65-year-old woman who developed stuttering concurrently with an episode of cerebral ischemia. Donnan described her stuttering as "rapid, easy repetition of the initial sound syllable of every other word." He reported that the woman displayed no sound blocks or facial grimacing, agnosia, or apraxia. Slight word-finding problems were present. A carotid angiogram showed left carotid stenosis with elevated plaques due to hemorrhaging beneath the plaques. An endarterectomy was performed, and upon recovering from the anesthesia, the woman "was found to be completely free from stutter." The postsurgical angiogram showed uninterrupted left carotid blood flow. In such cases the role of the speech clinician is limited to documenting the nature and severity of stuttering associated with carotid artery disease and its treatment. The therapeutic intervention is carried out by the surgeon. Another treatment for SAAND that is implemented by a physician, with the speech clinician only documenting the effectiveness of the intervention, involves the use of pharmacological agents.

PHARMACOLOGICAL AGENTS

There is evidence to suggest that drugs may have either a negative or positive effect on speech fluency. Above, I cited Baratz and Mesulam's case[19] in which stuttering associated with head injury and seizures diminished when the seizures were brought under control with phenytoin. McClean and McClean[36] reported that their patient with post–head injury seizures stuttered when treated with phenytoin but reduced his dysfluency levels when switched to carbamazepine. These cases suggest that when stuttering occurs in patients with documented or suspected seizures, the choice of antiepileptic agents should be carefully explored.

Stuttering also has been associated with dopamine receptor–blocking drugs like phenothiazine. Nurnberg and Greenwald[17] described two patients with chronic schizophrenia who developed severe stuttering when phenothiazine levels were high enough to eliminate psychosis. These investigators then had to find a dosage that would manage both the psychosis and stuttering at acceptable levels for daily living.

Quader[16] described two patients in whom stuttering was associated with the administration of amitriptyline, a tricyclic antidepressant. In both cases speech returned to normal when the drug was discontinued. Similarly, Elliott and Thomas[37] reported onset of stuttering in a 22-year-old woman who was treated with alprazolam for anxiety and depression. A double-blind, placebo-controlled study verified the negative effect of alprazolam on speech fluency. This drug is thought to have some pharmacological effects that are similar to those of tricyclics.

Together these reports indicate that SAAND may result from or be eliminated by the administration of various pharmacological agents. In such cases the speech clinician will work in consultation with the physician to achieve optimal management of the stuttering in relation to other medical or psychological disorders.

THALAMIC STIMULATION

In a unique report, Bhantnagar and Andy[38] described a 61-year-old man with stuttering associated with a long history of trigeminal pain. Over an 18-year period he was treated with various medications and bilateral trigeminal ganglion blocks. Methysergide maleate (Sansert) was the only drug that reduced speech dysfluencies but it had adverse affects on kidney function. There were no co-occurring aphasia or memory problems, and the patient showed no adaptation effect, anxiety, or secondary characteristics. A surgical procedure was used to implant a chorionic stimulation electrode in the left centromedian thalamic nucleus for relief of chronic pain. Through a battery-operated stimulator, the patient could self-stimulate three or four times a day for 20-minute periods. This resulted in remarkable improvement in speech fluency as well as considerable pain reduction.

TRANSCUTANEOUS NERVE STIMULATION

In 1977 Butler and I reported the case of a 68-year-old woman who experienced a series of minor strokes to both cerebral hemispheres.[39] Severe stuttering occurred after the fifth stroke, which also produced a transient left hemiparesis. The woman was left-handed but had been converted to use her right hand for writing. Her language skills remained essentially intact, but she had mild dysarthria and markedly dysfluent speech with severe blocking or prolongations of initial and medial syllables, especially consonant blends. Trials with a speech-pacing board increased her dysfluency as she tried to speak in a deliberate, syllable-by-syllable manner. But when an electrolarynx was vibrated against her left hand, moments of stuttering during an oral reading task decreased from 38 to 8. We wondered whether the noise produced by the electrolarynx was acting as a masking device. To test this, we applied a TNS unit to the bicipital groove of her left arm. This unit, originally developed for pain control, was also successful in reducing this patient's speech dysfluencies.

DELAYED AUDITORY FEEDBACK AND AUDITORY MASKING

There is some evidence to suggest that patients with SAAND may show a positive response to auditory masking. In 1984 Rentschler and colleagues[40] described a 41-year-old man who developed stuttering following drug overdose with chlorazepate dipotassium (Tranxene) (and possibly chlordiazepoxide hydrochloride [Librium]). Binaural white noise masking at 95 dB resulted in fluent speech. With reduced levels of noise intensity, stuttering returned. In our VA clinic, the Edinburgh Masker[41] has been used to reduce dysfluency in some patients with SAAND.

Marshall and Starch[42] used DAF to successfully treat a 32-year-old man who developed SAAND after a closed head injury. The DAF procedures were introduced 4 years after the injury occurred, and were in keeping with the protocol used by Curlee and Perkins[43] with developmental stutterers. Earlier, Downie and associates[44] reported that DAF was effective with two Parkinson's patients with speech disorders. One of the two had stuttering-like hesitations.

BIOFEEDBACK AND RELAXATION

Biofeedback techniques similar to those employed with developmental stuttering have been used for the treatment of SAAND. One such patient experienced onset of moderately severe stuttering after a series of small strokes.[6] His articulation and grammar were normal and he showed no evidence of oral apraxia. Using an electromyographic (EMG) biofeedback unit, an integrated baseline of masseter tension level was obtained for 5 minutes of conversation, followed by 5 minutes of relaxation techniques. He then was asked to maintain a lower tension level, by observing and responding to biofeedback for 5 more minutes of conversation.

After a 4-month, twice-weekly course of this biofeedback/relaxation therapy and home relaxation exercises, he was discharged with only mild stuttering. Similarly, Rubow and colleagues[45] used EMG biofeedback and relaxation training to successfully treat a man with SAAND following a stroke.

SPEECH PACING

Some patients with SAAND may respond to pacing techniques that involve slowing the speech rate and speaking one syllable at a time.[1] Often, however, patients do not respond to instructions for producing slower, paced speech because of an underlying neurological drive to speak at faster rates. This appears especially true of individuals with Parkinson's disease. For such patients a *pacing board* may be required. The pacing device I first described in 1979[28] had six multicolored squares with raised dividers. The patient was encouraged to tap his or her forefinger from square to square while speaking in a syllable-by-syllable manner. Both a large board and a more portable, pocket-size board for those patients who can manage finer finger movements are now available,[32] but other even smaller pacing devices may prove as effective as a pacing board. For example, one of my Parkinson's patients with SAAND was able to control his speech rate and stuttering by pacing himself with a toggle switch mounted on a piece of wood. A 1983 article[46] described another small device that fits over the patient's forefinger. Holes are punched in Kay-splint material and then the material is molded over the finger. The patient paces his or her speech by moving the thumb from hole to hole. I have found that some patients progress from using a pacing instrument to tapping the table, to tapping their thigh, eliminating the need for an overt device.

According to the survey conducted by Market et al,[3] clinicians most commonly use slow speech rate techniques, easy voice onset approaches, or a combination of the two for treatment of SAAND. Although 82.2% reported positive results, no specific descriptions of the therapy protocols were provided.

Expected Outcome

Given the many approaches to the treatment of SAAND, one might expect that there is an effective form of therapy for each individual with stuttering associated with acquired neurological disorders. But as I have stressed elsewhere in this chapter, SAAND is not a unitary disorder, nor is it typically unidimensional. It is, therefore, difficult to predict how well a specific patient will respond to therapeutic intervention. Sometimes, clinicians and patients must make compromises, as in cases where a certain drug is best for alleviating a neurological or psychiatric symptom but also results in some speech dysfluency. Parkinson's patients with SAAND seem to respond well to a variety of techniques whereas stroke patients with SAAND seem harder to treat. Fortunately, in many of these latter cases, stuttering may be a transient phenomenon. SAAND is not uncommon following closed head injury and may be associated with seizure activity. Control of the epilepsy also may result in control of the stuttering. Patients with rapidly progressing disorders such as tumors will probably not be candidates for formal treatment, although supportive counseling may be required. Thus, one cannot make a blanket statement about the expected outcomes of SAAND patients and their response to treatment. Instead, one should consider each patient individually, beginning with the case history, progressing through the clinical evaluation, and finally choosing what appears to be the best approach to management and treatment.

Conclusion

SAAND is one of the most interesting, puzzling, and challenging speech problems of adults confronting speech-language pathologists. There is mounting evidence that a variety of transient, static, and progressive neurological disorders may result in dysfluent speech patterns labeled "stuttering" by clinicians, family members, and patients themselves. In fact, the evidence is so compelling, clinicians should consider adult onset of stuttering as a symptom of possible neurological dysfunction. Fluent speaking is, perhaps, the most refined motor act performed by humans, requiring the complex coordination of many different muscle groups. It is, therefore, sensitive to even small changes in neurological status. It may be for this reason that stuttering occurs in a wide range of neurological disorders, from Parkinson's disease to closed head injury. If this fact is ignored, clinicians may be overlooking an important indicator of neurological disease. For example, a man was referred to our clinic with sudden onset of mildly dysfluent speech. He had been sent to the psychiatry unit of the hospital when the admitting physician found "no postive neurological signs." Psychiatry, however, found no psychiatric basis for the speech problem in this man, who had a long history of good mental health. When he was evaluated in the speech department, about a week later, a slight right facial weakness was detectable. A few months later he died of a brain tumor. The lesson to be learned is that adult onset of stuttering should first be considered a potentially positive neurological sign. The early diagnosis of SAAND may lead to successful treatment of a neurological disorder causing the stuttering, or to successful treatment of the communication disorder itself.

Acknowledgements.   I would like to thank Martin Albert, Marjorie Nicholas, and Richard Curlee for their helpful comments on this chapter.

Suggested Readings

Helm NA, Butler RB, Benson DF: Acquiring stuttering. *Neurology* 1978; 28:1159–1165.
   This report of ten patients with acquired stuttering was the first to describe specific neuropathological, neuropsychological, and language correlates of transient and persistent forms of this disorder. As such, it is widely cited and its findings have been used as reference points for comparing cases examined in subsequent reports.
Jones RK: Observations on stammering after localized cerebral injury. *J Neurol Neurosurg Psychiatry* 1966; 29:192–195.
   This is a highly controversial report of four patients who ceased to stutter after neurosurgery for various brain abnormalities. Jones' findings have not been replicated and, therefore, have been repudiated. Over the past 10 years, however, several cases of cessation of stuttering with the onset of neurological disease or brain injury have been described. These more recent cases lend some support to Jones' over 25-year-old findings.
Ludlow C, Rosenberg M, Salazar A, Grafman J, Smutok A: Site of penetrating brain lesions causing chronic acquired stuttering. *Ann Neurol* 1987; 21:60–66.
   In this well-controlled and scientific study of acquired stuttering, Ludlow and her colleagues compared test performance and CT scans of ten men who developed stuttering after penetrating missile wounds with those of other head-injured and normal subjects. The findings indicate that acquired

stuttering is a motor control disorder most commonly associated with unilateral subcortical and extrapyramidal system lesions in this form of brain damage.

Mazzucchi A, Moretti G, Carpeggiani P, Parma MA, Paini P: Clinical observations in acquired stuttering. *Br J Disord Commun* 1981; 16:19–30.

Mazzuchi and her colleagues compiled information on 16 cases of acquired stuttering associated with traumatic or vascular cerebral lesions. This information is presented in tables that make it easy to compare patients on such parameters as etiology, speech abnormalities, aphasia, and neurological and neuropsychological findings.

References

1. Rosenbek JC, Messert B, Collins M, Wertz RT: Stuttering following brain damage. *Brain Lang* 1978; 5–6:82–96.
2. Helm NA, Butler RB, Benson DF: Acquired stuttering. *Neurology* 1978; 28:1159–1165.
3. Market KE, Montague JC, Buffalo MD, Drummond SA: Acquired stuttering: Descriptive data and treatment outcomes. *J Fluency Disord* 1990; 15:21–33.
4. *Manual of the International Statistical Classification of Diseases, Injuries and Causes of Death*, vol 1. Geneva, World Health Organization, 1977.
5. Andrews G, Craig A, Feyer A, Hoddinott S, Howie R, Neilson M: Stuttering: A review of research findings and theories circa 1982. *J Speech Hear Disord* 1982; 47:226–246.
6. Helm-Estabrooks N: Diagnosis and Management of Neurogenic Stuttering in Adults, in St. Louis KO (ed): *The Atypical Stutterer: Principles and Practices of Rehabilitation*. New York, Academic Press, 1986, pp 198–217.
7. Ludlow C, Rosenberg M, Salazar A, Grafman J, Smutok A: Site of penetrating brain lesions causing chronic acquired stuttering. *Ann Neurol* 1987; 21:60–66.
8. Arnold GE, Luchsinger R: *Voice-Speech-Language, Clinical Communicology: Its Physiology and Pathology*. Belmont, CA, Wadsworth, 1965.
9. Mazzucchi A, Moretti G, Carpeggiani P, Parma MA, Paini P: Clinical observations in acquired stuttering. *Br J Disord Commun* 1981; 16:19–30.
10. Helm-Estabrooks N, Yeo R, Geschwind N, Freedman M, Weinstein C: Stuttering: Disappearance and reappearance with acquired brain lesions. *Neurology* 1986; 36:1109–1112.
11. Quinn PT, Andrews G: Neurologic stuttering: A clinical entity? *J Neurol Neurosurg Psychiatry* 1977; 40:699–701.
12. Jones RK: Observations on stammering after localized cerebral injury. *J Neurol Neuorsurg Psychiatry* 1966; 29:192–195.
13. Miller AE: Cessation of stuttering with progressive multiple sclerosis. *Neurology* 1986; 35:1341–1343.
14. Deal J: Sudden onset of stuttering: A case report. *J Speech Hear Disord* 1982; 47:301–304.
15. Attanasio JS: A case of late-onset or acquired stuttering in adult life. *J Fluency Disord* 1987; 12: 287–290.
16. Quader SE: Dysarthria: An unusual side effect of trycyclic antidepressants. *Br Med J* 1977; 9:97.
17. Nurnberg HG, Greenwald B: Stuttering: An unusual side effect of phenothiazines. *Am J Psychiatry* 1981; 138:386–387.
18. Marshall RC, Neuburger SI: Effects of delayed auditory feedback on acquired stuttering following head injury. *J Fluency Disord* 1987; 12:355–365.
19. Baratz R, Mesulam M: Adult-onset stuttering treated with anticonvulsants. *Arch Neurol* 1981; 38:132–133.
20. Helm NA, Butler RB, Canter GJ: Neurogenic acquired stuttering. *J Fluency Disord* 1980; 5:55–68.
21. Geschwind N, Behan P: Left-handedness: Association with immune disease, migraine and developmental learning disorder. *Proc Natl Acad Sci USA* 1982; 79:5097–5100.
22. Helm-Estabrooks N: *Aphasia Diagnostic Profiles*. Chicago, Riverside Publishing, 1992.
23. Kaplan E, Goodglass H, Weintraub S: *Boston Naming Test*. Philadelphia, Lea & Febiger, 1983.
24. Goodglass H, Kaplan E: *Boston Diagnostic Aphasia Examination*. Philadelphia, Lea & Febiger, 1983.
25. Newman PW: Adaptation performance of individual stutterers: Implications for research. *J Speech Hear Res* 1963; 6:293–294.
26. Fairbanks G: *Voice and Articulation Drill Book*. New York, Harper, 1960.
27. Darley FL, Aronson AE, Brown JR: *Motor Speech Disorder*. Philadelphia, WB Saunders, 1975.
28. Helm NA: Management of palilalia with a pacing board. *J Speech Hear Disord* 1979; 44:350–353.
29. Bayles K, Tomoeda C: *Arizona Battery for Communication Disorders in Dementia*. Tuscon, AZ, Canyonlands Press, 1991.
30. Helm-Estabrooks N, Hotz G: *Brief Test of Head Injury*. Chicago, Riverside Publishing, 1991.
31. Adamovich B, Henderson J: *Scales of Cognitive Ability for Traumatic Brain Injury*. Chicago, Riverside Publishing, 1991.

32. Helm-Estabrooks N, Kaplan E: *Boston Stimulus Boards*. Chicago, Riverside Publishing, 1989.
33. Rosenbek JC, McNeil MR, Lemme ML, Prescott JE, Alfy AC: Speech and language findings in a chronic hemodialysis patient: A case report. *J Speech Hear Disord* 1975; 40:2.
34. Madison D, Baeher E, Bazell M, Hartman K, Mahurkar S, Dunea G: Communicative and cognitive deterioration in dialysis dementia: Two case studies. *J Speech Hear Disord* 1977; 42:238–246.
35. Donnan GA: Stuttering as a manifestation of stroke. *Med J Aust* 1979; 1:44–45.
36. McClean MD, McClean A: Case report of stuttering acquired in association with phenytoin use for post-head-injury seizures. *J Fluency Disord* 1985; 10:241–255.
37. Elliott RL, Thomas BJ: A case report of alprazolam-induced stuttering. *J Clin Psychopharmacol* 1985; 5:159–160.
38. Bhatnagar SC, Andy OJ: Alleviation of acquired stuttering with human centremedian thalamic stimulation. *J Neurol Neurosurg Psychiatry* 1989; 52:1182–1184.
39. Helm NA, Butler RB: Transcutaneous nerve stimulation in acquired speech disorder. *Lancet.* 1977; 2:1177–1178.
40. Rentschler GJ, Driver LE, Callaway EA: The onset of stuttering following drug overdose. *J Fluency Disord* 1984; 9:265–284.
41. Dewar A, Dewar AD, Austin WTS, Brash HM: The long term use of an automatically triggered auditory feedback masking device in the treatment of stammering. *Br J Disord Commun* 1976; 14:219–229.
42. Marshall RC, Starch SA: Behavioral treatment of acquired stuttering. *Aust J Commun Disord* 1984; 12:87–92.
43. Curlee RF, Perkins WH: Conversational rate control therapy for stuttering. *J Speech Hear Disord* 1969; 34:245–250.
44. Downie AW, Low JM, Linsay DD: Speech disorders in parkinsonism: Use of delayed auditory feedback in selected cases. *J Neurol Neurosurg Psychiatry* 1981; 44:852–853.
45. Rubow RT, Rosenbek JC, Schumaker JG: Stress management in the treatment of neurogenic stuttering. *Biofeedback Self Regul* 1986; 11:77–78.
46. Pacing devices developed. *ASHA* 1983; 25(4):16.

APPENDIX A: SAAND CASE HISTORY

Date: Examiner:

Name:

Address:

Telephone: Date of Birth:

Years of Education: Age Completed:

Strongest Academic Areas:

Weakest Academic Areas:

Remedial Instruction:

Employment History:

Previous History of Speech or Language Problems:

Family History of Speech or Language Problems:

Personal and Family Handedness:

Health history (with dates) including head trauma; periods of unconsciousness, high fever, seizures, or convulsions; alcohol or drug abuse; use of any prescription drugs affecting the central nervous system; and hospitalizations.

Individual's Description of His or Her Problems at This Time:

Index

Achievement landmarks, 126, 128, 132
Acquired neurological disorders, 142, 205–217
  clinical evaluation, 208–213
  clinical management, 213–217
  and school-age stuttering, 207
  and speech rate, 216
  treatment procedures, 213–216
  treatment results, 216–217
Across-settings generalization, 86–88
Adaptation effect, 210
ADD *see* Attention deficit disorder
Adolescent and adult stuttering, 115–135
  acquired neurological disorders, 205–217
  audio recordings, 133
  clinical management, 122–132
  cluttering, 191–192
  expected outcomes, 132–134
  fluency training, 139–164
  pretreatment evaluation, 118–122
ADP *see* Aphasia Dignostic Profiles
Adult stuttering *see* Adolescent and adult stuttering
Animal tracks therapy, 104
Aphasia, 206, 210, 211
Aphasia Dignostic Profiles (ADP), 210
Arm squeezing therapy, 108
Articulation errors, 183–184
Articulatory rate, 72
Assignments, fluency training, 157–158, 161–162
Attention deficit disorder (ADD), 185
Attention span, 183, 185, 190
Attention therapy, 123
Attitude change, 41, 120
Atypical disfluency, 26, 28, 32–36
Audio recordings

adolescent and adult stuttering, 133
  behavior treatment, 70
  cluttering, 191
  fluency training, 147, 148
  school-age stuttering, 55
Auditory awareness, 194
Auditory masking, 215
Automatization therapy, 131
Awareness therapy, 107, 186
  see also Auditory awareness;
    Kinesthetic awareness; Tactile
    awareness

Beginning stuttering, 1–20
  books and articles about, 17
  clinical evaluation, 2–15
  clinical management, 15–20
  differential evaluation-differential
    therapy, 23–37
  indicators, 4–5, 8–9
  school-age, 55–61
Behavior treatment, 68–88
  adolescent and adult stuttering, 117–118, 126, 133
  beginning stuttering, 18–20
  clinical evaluation, 68–74
  clinical management, 74–88
  differential evaluation-differential
    therapy, 30–31
  school-age stuttering, 62–63
Beyond-treatment measurement, 78
Biofeedback, 215–216
BNT *see* Boston Naming Test
Booster-therapy sessions, 174–175
Borderline atypical disfluency, 28
Boston Naming Test (BNT), 210
Breath curve, 105–106
Breath holding, 106

Breathing therapy, 149–150, 194
Brochure for Parents of Children Who Stutter (Ramig), 52

CAFET *see* Computer-Assisted Fluency Establishment Trainer
Carryover and transfer fluency, 110–112
Case history interview
  acquired neurological disorders, 208–209, 219
  adolescent and adult stuttering, 118–119
  beginning stuttering, 3–6
  behavior treatment, 68–69
  cluttering, 194–196
  differential evaluation-differential therapy, 29
  fluency training, 141–142
  school-age stuttering, 47–48
Case selection criteria
  acquired neurological disorders, 212
  adolescent and adult stuttering, 120–122
  beginning stuttering, 11–15
  behavior treatment, 74
  fluency training, 143–146
  school-age stuttering, 49–50
Cassettes *see* Audio recordings
Cerebral disorders, 144, 185
Cerebral vascular accidents (CVA), 205
Children *see* Parent-child interactions; Preschool-age stuttering; School-age stuttering
Chronic stuttering
  case selection criteria, 12
  fluency training, 139–164
  indicators, 5–6, 9–10
  treatment transfer-maintenance, 166–177
  see also Confirmed stuttering
Client/clinician sessions, 124, 126–130
Clinical evaluation
  acquired neurological disorders, 208–213
  adolescent and adult stuttering, 118–122
  beginning stuttering, 2–15
  behavior treatment, 68–74
  cluttering, 183–190
  differential evaluation-differential therapy, 23–31, 37

fluency training, 141–146
  school-age stuttering, 46–50
Clinical laboratory, 125, 128, 131
Clinical management
  acquired neurological disorders, 213–217
  adolescent and adult stuttering, 122–132
  beginning stuttering, 15–20
  behavior treatment, 74–88
  cluttering, 190–196
  differential evaluation-differential therapy, 31–36, 37–42
  fluency training, 146–163
  indirect, 15, 17, 19–20
  school-age stuttering, 50–55, 101–112
  see also Treatment goals; Treatment procedures; Treatment results
Cluttering, 145, 179–196
  books and articles about, 179–180
  characteristics, 182, 187–190
  clinical evaluation, 183–190
  clinical management, 190–196
  definition, 180–181
  evaluation forms, 200–204
  qualitative features, 184–187
  quantitative features, 183–184
Cognitive therapy, 122, 133, 194
Communication attitude test, 10
Communication disorders, 69
Communication styles, 33
Communicative stress, 31–32
Computer-Assisted Fluency Establishment Trainer (CAFET), 105, 106
Computers, 72
Confirmed stuttering, 61–66
  see also Chronic stuttering
Consonant-vowel combinations, 39
Contrasting therapy, 107
Coping technique, 156–157
Cortical stuttering, 205
Counseling *see* Group therapy; Parent-teacher counseling
"Crystal goblet phenomenon", 116–118
CVA *see* Cerebral vascular accidents

DAF *see* Delayed auditory feedback
Defense Style Questionnaire, 148
Delayed auditory feedback (DAF), 190, 193, 215

Delayed maturation, 52, 185
Dementia, 207, 211
Desensitization, 58, 126
Detection therapy, 128
Developmental stuttering, 206
Different feet therapy, 105
Differential evaluation-differential
    therapy, 23–42
  books and articles about, 32
  differential evaluation, 23–25, 37
  differential therapy, 31–36, 37–42
    attitude change, 41
    parent-teacher counseling, 41–42
    speech modification, 38–41
  prevention and management, 23–37
  school-age stuttering, 37–42
  treatment results, 42
Direct clinical management, 20
Disability characteristics, 115, 116–117,
    118, 121
Disfluency episodes, 32–33
Disfluency types, 26, 27, 28
Do You Stutter: A Guide for Teens
    (booklet), 47
Drug therapy, 213, 214
Dysarthric stuttering, 206

Easy phrase initiation, 150
Elephant symbolism, 111
ELU *see* Extended length of utterance
Emotional reactions
  adolescent and adult stuttering, 120
  beginning stuttering, 5–6, 10
  differential evaluation-differential
    therapy, 41
  school-age stuttering, 51–52
Evaluation *see* Clinical evaluation;
    Differential evaluation-differential
    therapy; Speech evaluation
Exploration phase, 123–124
Extended length of utterance (ELU), 76,
    77, 78, 82–86, 90–98

Fail criterion, 78
Families *see* Friends and relatives
    evening; Hereditary factors;
    Parent-child interactions; Siblings
Feedback procedures, 79–82
  schedules, 81–82
  selection of positive and negative
    stimuli, 79–81

Feelings *see* Emotional reactions
Fluency analysis, 25–29, 142–143
Fluency development, 34–36, 59–60, 115
Fluency instatement, 149–151
Fluency rules program (FRP), 101–113
  carryover and transfer, 110–112
  revised rules, 102, 109–110
  secondary rules, 107–109
  therapy outcome, 112–113
  universal rules, 102–105
Fluency shaping, 151–154
Fluency threshold, 60
Fluency training, 139–164
  clinical evaluation, 141–146
  clinical management, 146–163
  expected outcomes, 163–164
Friends and relatives evening, 160–161
FRP *see* Fluency rules program

Generalization and transfer therapy, 36
"Gentle not soft" therapy, 107
Gentle voice onset/offset, 150
GILCU *see* Gradual increase in length
    and complexity of utterance
Goals *see* Treatment goals
Gradual increase in length and
    complexity of utterance (GILCU), 76
Group sessions, 174
Group therapy, 175

Handicap characteristics, 115, 117, 118, 121
Hard contact therapy, 108
Head trauma, 211–212
Hereditary factors, 185–186
Hierarchy control, 167
Holmes Social Readjustment Scale for
    Children, 29
Home practice schedules, 175

Identification issues, 63–64
If Your Child Stutters: A Guide for Parents
    (booklet), 32, 47
Impairment characteristics, 115, 118
In block corrections, 65–66
Independence nurturing *see* Self-
    management
In-depth speech and language
    evaluation, 25
Indicators
  beginning stuttering, 4–5, 8–9
  chronic stuttering, 5–6, 9–10

Indirect clinical mangement, 15, 17, 19–20
Instatement procedures, 151
Intensive fluency training *see* Fluency
    training
Interaction *see* Parent-child interactions
Interruption therapy, 128
Introductions assignment, 161
Iowa Scale of Stuttering Severity, 48–49

Johnson, Wendell, 117

Kinesthetic awareness, 64

Language evaluation, 25, 30–31
Language tasks, 209–211
Learning disabilities, 184, 185, 186
Lily pads therapy, 108
Linkage therapy, 131–132

Maintenance
    fluency training, 163
    see also Treatment transfer-maintenance
Management *see* Clinical management
Maturation *see* Delayed maturation;
        Physical immaturity
Measurement procedures, 77–79
Memory disorders, 211, 212
Mergerization therapy, 131
Metronome, 103
Mirror therapy, 109, 127
Modeling therapy, 104, 123, 127, 130
Modification techniques
    beginning stuttering, 18
    differential evaluation-differential
        therapy, 38–41
    school-age children, 62, 64–65
Monetary control, 173
Monologue, 16, 54, 143
Motivation therapy, 123
Motor reproduction therapy, 123
Motor targets, 132
"Mr. Voice Box" therapy, 106–107
Multiple sclerosis (MS), 207–208
Musical ability, 185

National Stuttering Project, 47–48, 52
Nerve stimulation, 215
Neurological disorders *see* Cerebral
        disorders; Acquired neurological
        disorders
Nintendo, 111

Noncontingent sessions, 173

Observational learning, 123
Observations and tests
    acquired neurological disorders, 209–
        212
    adolescent and adult stuttering, 119–
        120
    beginning stuttering, 6–10
    behavior treatment, 69–74
    differential evaluation-differential
        therapy, 24–25
    fluency training, 142–143
    school-age stuttering, 48–49
Old ears therapy, 104, 105
Outcomes *see* Treatment results

Palilalia, 211
Parent-child interactions
    beginning stuttering, 9, 13–14, 19
    differential evaluation-differential
        therapy, 23–24, 25, 27, 29–30
    school-age stuttering, 104–105
Parent-teacher counseling
    beginning stuttering, 15–16
    behavior treatment, 87
    differential evaluation-differential
        therapy, 31–37, 41–42
    school-age stuttering, 50–55
    treatment transfer-maintenance, 174
Parkinson's disease, 209, 211
Pass criterion, 78
Peers, 87, 174
Perceptions of Speech Communication
        (PSC), 186–187
Perception of Stuttering Inventory (PSI),
        186–187
Performance mastery, 122, 126, 131
Personal efficacy, 120
Personality traits, 186
Pharmacological agents *see* Drug therapy
Phrase continuity, 150
Phrasing and pausing, 150
Physical immaturity, 185
Piano fingers therapy, 108–109
Placebo-controlled research, 139
Play therapy, 15, 26–27
Preinstatement session, 149
Preschool-age stuttering
    beginning stuttering, 1, 5, 12, 15, 17,
        20

behavior treatment, 76
cluttering, 190–191
differential evaluation-differential
    therapy, 23, 34
treatment transfer-maintenance, 176–
    177
Presentation, 150–151
Pressure play, 27, 29
Primary fluency rules, 105–107
Prince Henry program (Australia), 140
Prince Henry Yardstick, 142–143
Progress reports, 154, 158–160, 162
Prolongations *see* Sound prolongations;
    Within-word repetitions
Prosody, 150
PSC *see* Perceptions of Speech
    Communication
Pseudostuttering, 56–58
PSI *see* Perception of Stuttering Inventory
Psychogenic stuttering, 208
Pullouts, 65–66

Questionnaires, 120, 142, 148

"Radical behaviorism", 118
Radio assignment, 161–162
Railroad train therapy, 104
Rate control, 149
Rating sessions, 151–153, 157
Reading skills, 184
Recordings *see* Audio recordings; Video
    recordings
Reinforcement systems, 99–100
Relatives *see* Friends and relatives
    evening; Hereditary factors;
    Parent-child interactions; Siblings
Relaxation techniques, 194, 215–216
Replacement therapy, 128, 130
Response hierarchies, 35
Results *see* Treatment results
Retention therapy, 123
Riley Stuttering Severity Instrument, 48–
    49, 113, 119

SAAND *see* Stuttering associated with
    acquired neurological disorders
St. Vincent's Hospital (Sydney, Australia),
    140
"Say a word once" therapy, 104–105
School-age stuttering, 45–67
    acquired neurological disorders, 207

books and articles about, 47–48, 52
clinical evaluation, 46–50
clinical management, 50–55
cluttering, 191
differential evaluation-differential
    therapy, 37–42
fluency rules program, 101–113
treatment goals, 55–66
treatment transfer-maintenance, 176–
    177
Screening tests, 6–7, 24–25, 69
SDA *see* Systematic Disfluency Analysis
Secondary characteristics, 62–63
Secondary fluency rules, 107–109
Self-efficacy theory, 116, 117
Self-judgment, 125
Self-management
    adolescent and adult stuttering, 124–
        125, 127–128, 130–132, 137–138
    behavior treatment, 86–87
    school-age stuttering, 61–62
    treatment transfer-maintenance, 170–
        172
Self-observation, 124–125, 131
Self-reactions, 125
Severity rating scales, 49–50
Siblings, 87
Situation modification, 18
Smooth speech technique, 141, 145, 149–
    151
Social learning theory, 116, 133
Social validity, 73
Soft articulatory contact, 150
Sound prolongations, 4, 5, 9, 17, 25
Speech breathing, 105
Speech disruptions, 4, 8, 9, 10, 18
Speech evaluation
    beginning stuttering, 17–18
    behavior treatment, 70–74
    cluttering, 200–204
    differential evaluation-differential
        therapy, 25, 30–31
Speech helpers therapy, 107–109
Speech holding, 106
Speech modification, 38–41
Speech naturalness, 72
Speech rate
    acquired neurological disorders, 216
    beginning stuttering, 17
    behavior treatment, 71–72
    cluttering, 183, 192

fluency training, 143
school-age stuttering, 102–104
Speech samples, 119–120
see also Standard talking samples
Speech tasks, 75–77, 161, 209–211
"Speech vacation", 55
SPM *see* Syllables per minute
Standard talking samples (STSs), 70–74,
    78, 86
Story telling, 27, 191
Stroke, 207, 211, 215–216
Stuttering
    acquired neurological disorders, 205–
        217
    adolescent and adult treatment, 115–135
    beginning identification and
        management, 1–20
    behavior treatment, 68–88
    books and articles about, 17, 32, 47–
        48, 52, 179–80
    cluttering and, 179–196
    differential evaluation-differential
        therapy, 23–42
    fluency training, 139–164
    school-age treatment, 45–67, 101–113
    treatment transfer-maintenance, 166–
        177
Stuttering associated with acquired
        neurological disorders (SAAND),
        207, 208–217, 219
Stuttering Prediction Instrument, 112
*Stuttering and Your Child: Questions and
        Answers* (booklet), 17, 32, 47
Suggestion therapy, 107
Surgical intervention, 213–214
Syllable repetitions *see* Within-word
        repetitions
Syllables per minute (SPM), 142
Symbolic therapy, 103
Systematic Disfluency Analysis (SDA),
        27, 28, 31

Tachylalia, 192
Tachyphemia, 179, 180–181, 186
Tactile awareness, 60, 64, 106, 194–195
Teacher counseling *see* Parent–teacher
        counseling
Teenagers *see* Adolescent and adult
        stuttering
Telephone therapy, 111–112, 119, 132, 133,
        148

Tense pauses, 5
Tension, 63–64, 116
Testing *see* Observations and tests;
        Screening tests
Thalamic stimulation, 214–215
"Time-out" period, 54
Tongue slips, 184–185
Transcutaneous nerve stimulation, 215
Transfer, fluency training, 154–163
Transfer-maintenance *see* Treatment
        transfer-maintenance
Treatment goals
    acquired neurological disorders, 213
    adolescent and adult stuttering, 122
    beginning stuttering, 16–17
    behavior treatment, 75
    fluency training, 146
    school-age stuttering, 55–66
    transfer-maintenance, 168
Treatment procedures
    acquired neurological disorders, 213–
        216
    adolescent and adult stuttering, 123–
        132
    beginning stuttering, 17–19
    behavior treatment, 75–86
    differential evaluation-differential
        therapy, 31–36, 37–42
    fluency training, 146–163
    school-age stuttering, 50–55, 101–112
    transfer-maintenance, 168–170
Treatment results
    acquired neurological disorders, 216–
        217
    adolescent and adult stuttering, 132–
        134
    beginning stuttering, 19–20
    behavior treatment, 86–88
    differential evaluation-differential
        therapy, 42
    fluency training, 163–164
    school-age stuttering, 66
Treatment transfer-maintenance, 166–177
    alternative procedures, 172–173
    core procedure, 167–172
    discarded procedures, 173–175
    miscellaneous considerations, 175–176
    objectives, 167
    for young children, 176–177
    see also Maintenance; Transfer
Turtle speech, 102–103

Turtle tracks therapy, 104, 105, 108
Typical disfluency, 26, 28, 31–32

Universal fluency rules, 102–105

Variation therapy, 128
Video games, 111, 112
Video recordings
  acquired neurological disorders, 210
  adolescent and adult stuttering, 119,
      125, 127, 128, 129, 130, 131, 132, 133
  beginning stuttering, 6, 7, 11, 18–19
  behavior treatment, 70
  cluttering, 191, 193
  differential evaluation-differential
      therapy, 27, 41
  fluency training, 148, 153–154
Voice disorders, 145, 184

Voluntary stuttering, 66
Vowel-consonant combinations, 39, 183

Weekend briefing, 155–156
WHO *see* World Health Organization
Williams, Dean, 117
Within-treatment measurement, 77–78
Within-word repetitions
  beginning stuttering, 4, 5, 8, 9, 11, 17
  behavior treatment, 72
  cluttering, 183
  differential evaluation-differential
      therapy, 25
Word-finding difficulty, 36
Work assignment, 161
World Health Organization (WHO), 205–
  206
Writing skills, 184